Atlas of Pediatric Laparoscopy and Thoracoscopy

Atlas of Pediatric Laparoscopy and Thoracoscopy

George W. Holcomb III, MD, MBA
Katharine B. Richardson Professor of Surgery
Department of Surgery
University of Missouri–Kansas City School of Medicine
Surgeon-in-Chief and Director, Pediatric Surgery Training Program
Department of Surgery
Children's Mercy Hospitals and Clinics
Kansas City, Missouri

Keith E. Georgeson, MD
Professor and Vice-Chairman
Department of Surgery
Director, Pediatric Surgical Sciences
Director, Division of Pediatric Surgery
Program Director, Pediatric Surgery Fellowship Program
Department of Surgery
The University of Alabama School of Medicine
Birmingham, Alabama

Steven S. Rothenberg, MD
Clinical Professor of Surgery
Department of Surgery
Columbia University College of Physicians and Surgeons
Attending Surgeon
Department of Pediatric Surgery
Morgan Stanley Children's Hospital of NewYork–Presbyterian
New York, New York
Chief of Pediatric Surgery
Chairman, Department of Pediatrics
Rocky Mountain Hospital for Children
Denver, Colorado

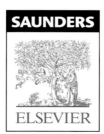

SAUNDERS

ELSEVIER

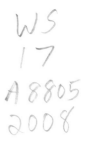

ATLAS OF PEDIATRIC LAPAROSCOPY AND THORACOSCOPY   ISBN: 978-1-4160-3373-8
Copyright © 2008 by Saunders, an imprint of Elsevier Inc.

Notice

Library of Congress Cataloging-in-Publication Data
Atlas of pediatric laparoscopy and thoracoscopy / [edited by] George W. Holcomb III, Keith E. Georgeson, Steven S. Rothenberg. – 1st ed.
      p.   ;   cm.
   Includes bibliographical references.
   ISBN 978-1-4160-3373-8
   1. Children–Surgery–Atlases.   2. Laparoscopic surgery–Atlases.   3. Thoracoscopy–Atlases.   I. Holcomb, George W.   II. Georgeson, Keith.   III. Rothenberg, Steven.
   [DNLM: 1. Child.   2. Laparoscopy–methods–Atlases.   3. Infant.   4. Thoracoscopy–methods–Atlases. WS 17 A8805 2008]
   RD137.3.A85 2008
   617.5'5059083–dc22   2007042121

Acquisitions Editor: Judith Fletcher
Developmental Editor: Martha Limbach
Publishing Services Manager: Tina Rebane
Senior Project Manager: Linda Lewis Grigg
Design Direction: Gene Harris

Printed in China

Last digit is the print number: 9   8   7   6   5   4   3   2   1

This book would not have been possible without the help of our personal surgical assistants. We dedicate this book to Meredith Kopp, RN, CPN, CNOR; Lee Hamby, SA; Aletta Harres, RN; and Mercy Varghese, ADN, CNOR.

For all pediatric surgeons around the world, the success of an operation depends on a team approach, and this book is also dedicated to the surgical teams who help us each and every day.

Contributors

Craig T. Albanese, MD
Professor of Surgery, Pediatrics, and Obstetrics and Gynecology, Department of Surgery, Stanford University School of Medicine; John A. and Cynthia Fry Gunn Director of Surgical Services, Lucile Packard Children's Hospital, Stanford, California
Robotic Kasai Procedure; Thoracoscopic Excision of Foregut Duplications

Maria H. Alonso, MD
Associate Professor of Clinical Surgery, Divisions of Pediatric Surgery and Transplantation, Department of Surgery, University of Cincinnati College of Medicine; Assistant Surgical Director, Renal Transplantation, Cincinnati Children's Hospital Medical Center, Cincinnati, Ohio
Laparoscopic-Assisted Donor Nephrectomy

Marjorie J. Arca, MD
Assistant Professor of Surgery, Department of Surgery, Medical College of Wisconsin; Pediatric Surgeon, Children's Hospital of Wisconsin, Milwaukee, Wisconsin
Thoracoscopic Decortication and Debridement for Empyema

Klaas (N) M.A. Bax, MD, PhD
Professor of Surgery, Erasmus University Faculty of Medicine; Pediatric Surgeon, Sophia Children's Hospital, Erasmus Medical Center Rotterdam, Rotterdam, The Netherlands
Laparoscopic Thal Fundoplication; Laparoscopic Repair of Duodenal Atresia and Stenosis; Thoracoscopic Aortopexy

Mary L. Brandt, MD
Professor and Vice Chair, Michael E. DeBakey Department of Surgery, Baylor College of Medicine; Pediatric Surgeon, Texas Children's Hospital, Houston, Texas
Laparoscopic Ovarian Surgery

Allen F. Browne, MD
Associate Professor of Surgery, Division of Pediatric Surgery, University of Illinois College of Medicine at Chicago; Attending Pediatric Surgeon, University of Illinois Medical Center and Rush Medical Center, Chicago, Illinois
Laparoscopic Adjustable Gastric Band Placement

Robert A. Cina, MD
Chief Resident, Department of Surgery, Division of Pediatric Surgery, The University of Alabama at Birmingham School of Medicine; Pediatric Surgeon, The Children's Hospital of Alabama, Birmingham, Alabama
Laparoscopic Total Colectomy with Pouch Reconstruction

Raul A. Cortes, MD
Surgical House Officer, Department of Surgery, University of Michigan Medical Center, Ann Arbor, Michigan
Laparoscopic Resection of Choledochal Cyst

Sanjeev Dutta, MD, MA, FRCSC, FACS
Assistant Professor of Surgery and Pediatrics, Stanford University School of Medicine; Associate Director, Goodman Simulation Center, Department of Pediatric Surgery, Stanford University Medical Center; Attending Surgeon Department of Pediatric Surgery, Lucile Packard Children's Hospital, Stanford, California
Robotic Kasai Procedure; Thoracoscopic Excision of Foregut Duplications

James D. Geiger, MD
Associate Professor of Surgery, Division of Pediatric Surgery, Department of Surgery, University of Michigan Medical School, Ann Arbor, Michigan
Robotic Excision of Choledochal Cyst

Keith E. Georgeson, MD
Professor and Vice-Chairman, Department of Surgery;
Director, Pediatric Surgical Sciences, and Director,
Division of Pediatric Surgery; Program Director,
Pediatric Surgery Fellowship Program, Department of
Surgery; University of Alabama School of Medicine,
Birmingham, Alabama

Laparoscopic Gastrostomy; Laparoscopic Antroplasty;
Laparoscopic Jejunostomy; Laparoscopic Management of
Ileocolic Intussusception; Laparoscopic Total Colectomy
with Pouch Reconstruction; Laparoscopic-Assisted Pull-
Through for Hirschsprung's Disease; Laparoscopic-Assisted
Anorectal Pull-Through

George W. Holcomb III, MD, MBA
Katharine B. Richardson Professor of Surgery,
Department of Surgery, University of Missouri–Kansas
City School of Medicine; Surgeon-in-Chief and
Director, Pediatric Surgery Training Program,
Department of Surgery, Children's Mercy Hospitals
and Clinics, Kansas City, Missouri

History of Minimally Invasive Surgery; Principles of
Laparoscopic Surgery; Laparoscopic Nissen Fundoplication;
Laparoscopic Cholecystectomy; Laparoscopic Adrenalectomy;
Laparoscopic Orchiopexy; Thoracoscopic Decortication and
Debridement for Empyema; Thoracoscopic Biopsy of a
Mediastinal Mass

Mark J. Holterman, MD, PhD
Associate Professor, Department of Surgery, University
of Illinois College of Medicine at Chicago; Chief,
Division of Pediatric Surgery, Department of Surgery,
University of Illinois Medical Center; Chief of
Pediatric Surgery, Department of Surgery and
Pediatrics, Rush University Medical Center, Chicago,
Illinois

Laparoscopic Adjustable Gastric Band Placement

Thomas H. Inge, MD, PhD
Associate Professor of Surgery and Pediatrics,
Department of Surgery, University of Cincinnati
College of Medicine; Attending Surgeon, Pediatric
General and Thoracic Surgery, Cincinnati Children's
Hospital, Cincinnati, Ohio

Laparoscopic Roux-en-Y Gastric Bypass

Michael S. Irish, MD
Assistant Adjunct Professor of Surgery, Department of
Surgery, University of Iowa Carver College of
Medicine, Iowa City; Attending Pediatric Surgeon,
Department of Pediatric Surgery, Raymond Blank
Children's Hospital, Des Moines, Iowa

Robotic Fundoplication in Infants and Children

Vincenzo Jasonni, MD
Professor of Pediatric Surgery, Department of Pediatric
Surgery and Obstetrics, University of Genoa Faculty of
Medicine; Chief, Pediatric Surgery and Other Surgical
Activities, Gaslini Children's Hospital, Genoa, Italy

Laparoscopic Esophagomyotomy

Robert E. Kelly, Jr., MD
Professor of Clinical Surgery, Department of Surgery,
Eastern Virginia Medical School; Chief, Department of
Surgery, Children's Hospital of the King's Daughters,
Norfolk, Virginia

The Minimally Invasive Pectus Excavatum Repair (Nuss
Procedure)

Michael P. La Quaglia, MD
Professor of Surgery, Department of Surgery, Weill
Medical College of Cornell University; Chief, Pediatric
Surgery, Department of Surgery, Memorial Sloan-
Kettering Cancer Center; Attending Surgeon,
Department of Pediatric Surgery, NewYork–
Presbyterian Hospital; Consulting Surgeon, Hospital
for Special Surgery, New York, New York

Thoracoscopic Lung Biopsy

Hanmin Lee, MD
Associate Professor, Department of Surgery, University
of California, San Francisco, School of Medicine;
Director, Fetal Treatment Center, UCSF Medical
Center, San Francisco, California

Laparoscopic Resection of Choledochal Cyst

Marc A. Levitt, MD
Associate Professor, Department of Surgery, University
of Cincinnati College of Medicine; Associate Director,
Colorectal Center, Cincinnati Children's Hospital
Medical Center, Cincinnati, Ohio

Laparoscopy in the Management of Fecal Incontinence and
Constipation

Danny C. Little, MD
Assistant Professor of Surgery, University of Arkansas
for Medical Sciences, Little Rock, Arkansas

Thoracoscopic Biopsy of a Mediastinal Mass

Thom E. Lobe, MD
Professor of Pediatrics, University of Tennessee
College of Medicine, Memphis, Tennessee; Pediatric
Surgeon, Raymond Blank Children's Hospital, Des
Moines; Clinical Professor of Surgery, Iowa University
Carver College of Medicine, Iowa City, Iowa

Thoracoscopic Thymectomy

Marcelo Martinez-Ferro, MD
Professor of Surgery and Pediatrics, Division of
Pediatric Surgery, CEMIC University; Chief, Division
of Surgery, Private Children's Hospital, Buenos Aires,
Argentina
Laparoscopic Portoenterostomy (Kasai Operation);
Thoracoscopic Repair of Esophageal Atresia without
Tracheosophageal Fistula

Girolamo Mattioli
Associate Professor of Pediatric Surgery, Giannina
Gaslini Research Institute and Children's Hospital,
University of Genoa Faculty of Medicine, Genoa, Italy
Laparoscopic Esophagomyotomy

Eugene D. McGahren, MD
Professor of Pediatric Surgery, Department of Surgery,
University of Virginia School of Medicine,
Charlottesville, Virginia
Laparoscopic Appendectomy

John J. Meehan, MD
Associate Professor of Surgery, Department of Surgery,
University of Washington School of Medicine;
Pediatric Surgeon, Department of General and
Thoracic Surgery, Seattle Children's Hospital and
Regional Medical Center, Seattle, Washington
Principles of Pediatric Robotic Surgery

Christopher R. Moir, MD
Associate Professor, Department of Surgery, Mayo
Clinic College of Medicine; Consultant, Department
of Surgery, Division of Pediatric Surgery, Mayo Clinic,
Rochester, Minnesota
Laparoscopic Ladd Procedure

Michael J. Morowitz, MD
Assistant Professor of Surgery and Pediatrics,
Department of Surgery, University of Chicago Pritzker
School of Medicine, Chicago, Illinois
Laparoscopic-Assisted Pull-Through for Hirschsprung's
Disease

Donald Nuss, MB, ChB, FRCSC, FACS
Professor, Departments of Surgery and Pediatrics,
Eastern Virginia Medical School; Pediatric Surgeon,
Children's Hospital of King's Daughters, Norfolk,
Virginia
The Minimally Invasive Pectus Excavatum Repair (Nuss
Procedure)

Daniel J. Ostlie, MD
Associate Professor of Surgery, Department of Surgery,
University of Missouri–Kansas City School of
Medicine; Pediatric Surgeon, Children's Mercy
Hospital and Clinics, Kansas City, Missouri
Laparoscopic Cholecystectomy

Alberto Peña, MD
Professor of Surgery, Department of Surgery,
University of Cincinnati College of Medicine; Director,
Colorectal Center, Department of Surgery, Cincinnati
Children's Hospital Medical Center, Cincinnati, Ohio
Laparoscopy in the Management of Fecal Incontinence and
Constipation

Craig A. Peters, MD
John E. Cole Professor of Urology, Department of
Urology, University of Virginia School of Medicine;
Chief, Division of Pediatric Urology, University of
Virginia Health System, Charlottesville, Virginia
Robotic Pyeloplasty

Alessio Pini Prato, MD
Research Fellow, Department of Gynecology and
Obstetrics, Division of Pediatric Surgery, University of
Genoa Faculty of Medicine; Registrar Pediatric
Surgeon, Giannina Gaslini Research Institute, Genoa,
Italy
Laparoscopic Esophagomyotomy

Igor V. Poddoubnyi, MD
Professor and Chairman, Department of Paediatric
Surgery, Moscow State University of Medicine and
Dentistry; Chief, Department of Pediatric Surgery,
Izmailovo Children's Hospital, Moscow, Russia
Laparoscopic Varicocelectomy

Frederick J. Rescorla, MD
Professor of Surgery and Director of Pediatric Surgery,
Indiana University School of Medicine; Surgeon-
in-Chief, Riley Hospital for Children, Indianapolis,
Indiana
Laparoscopic Splenectomy

Bradley M. Rodgers, MD
Chief of Pediatric Surgery, Department of Surgery,
University of Virginia School of Medicine;
Surgeon-in-Chief, University of Virginia Children's
Hospital, Charlottesville, Virginia
Thoracoscopy for Treatment of Spontaneous Pneumothorax

Steven S. Rothenberg, MD
Clinical Professor of Surgery, Department of Surgery, Columbia University College of Physicians and Surgeons; Attending Surgeon, Department of Pediatric Surgery, Morgan Stanley Children's Hospital of NewYork–Presbyterian, New York, New York; Chief of Pediatric Surgery and Chairman, Department of Pediatrics, Rocky Mountain Hospital for Children, Denver, Colorado

Laparoscopic Ileocolectomy for Crohn's Disease; Laparoscopic Segmental Colectomy; Minimally Invasive Diaphragmatic Plication; Principles of Thoracoscopy; Thoracoscopic Lung Biopsy; Thoracoscopic Lobectomy; Thoracoscopic Repair of Esophageal Atresia and Tracheoesophageal Fistula

Frederick C. Ryckman, MD
Professor of Surgery, Department of Pediatric Surgery, University of Cincinnati College of Medicine; Pediatric Surgeon, Cincinnati Children's Hospital Medical Center, Cincinnati, Ohio

Laparoscopic-Assisted Donor Nephrectomy

Shawn D. St. Peter, MD
Assistant Professor of Pediatric Surgery, Department of Pediatrics, University of Missouri–Kansas City School of Medicine; Director, Center for Prospective Clinical Trials, Department of Surgery, Children's Mercy Hospital, Kansas City, Missouri

History of Minimally Invasive Surgery

Felix Schier, MD
Professor and Chairman, Department of Pediatric Surgery, University of Mainz Faculty of Medicine, Mainz, Germany

Laparoscopic Repair of Inguinal Hernias

Greg M. Tiao, MD
Assistant Professor of Surgery, University of Cincinnati College of Medicine; Pediatric Surgeon, Cincinnati Children's Hospital Medical Center, Cincinnati, Ohio

Laparoscopic-Assisted Donor Nephrectomy

Michael V. Tirabassi, MD
Pediatric Endosurgery Fellow, Department of Surgery, Division of Pediatric Surgery, The University of Alabama of Birmingham School of Medicine; Pediatric Endoscopy Fellow, The Children's Hospital of Alabama, Birmingham, Alabama

Laparoscopic Gastrostomy

Jean-Stephane Valla, MD
Professor of Pediatric Surgery, University of Nice Medical School; Chief, Department of General Surgery and Urology, Lenval Hospital, Nice, France

Retroperitoneoscopic Nephrectomy

David C. van der Zee, MD, PhD
Pediatric Surgeon, University Medical Center Utrecht, Wilhelmina Children's Hospital, Utrecht, The Netherlands

Laparoscopic Duhamel Procedure

Mark L. Wulkan, MD
Associate Professor of Surgery and Pediatrics, Department of Surgery, Emory University School of Medicine; Director of Minimally Invasive Surgery, Children's Healthcare of Atlanta, Atlanta, Georgia

Laparoscopic Pyloromyotomy; Thoracoscopic Congenital Diaphragmatic Hernia Repair

Preface

Before 1988, very few general surgeons had heard of the term *laparoscopy*, much less performed a laparoscopic operation. Yet, over the next 5 years, an explosion in the use of this technology developed. By and large, pediatric surgeons were slower to adopt this approach compared with our adult general surgery colleagues. However, to varying degrees, it has now become a routine part of most pediatric surgeons' practices.

As the use of laparoscopy and thoracoscopy has matured among pediatric surgeons, many of the operations have become standardized. For the past few years, we have felt that an atlas of laparoscopy and thoracoscopy in infants and children would be a very useful reference book, not only for pediatric surgeons in practice but also for those in training.

The authors of each chapter have been carefully selected according to their interests and expertise with either the laparoscopic or thoracoscopic approach. Almost all pediatric surgical conditions are discussed. In addition, we have tried to ensure a broad representation of authors from many different continents and countries.

As most pediatric surgeons know, we have been involved with promoting the appropriate use of laparoscopy and thoracoscopy and with teaching this approach at numerous venues. This atlas represents our collective thoughts about the minimally invasive approach to a variety of pediatric surgical problems and hope that the readers will find it helpful in the care of their patients.

George W. Holcomb III
Keith E. Georgeson
Steven S. Rothenberg

Contents

VIDEO CLIPS

1
History of Minimally Invasive Surgery

Shawn D. St. Peter and George W. Holcomb III

Hippocrates, the father of Western medicine, detailed the use of a primitive anoscope to examine hemorrhoids in 400 BC. In the ruins of Pompeii (AD 70), a three-bladed speculum was identified that is similar to one used today. An Arabian named Abulkasim improved on Hippocrates' method around AD 1000 by reflecting light to examine the cervix. The dominant limitation to these fledgling attempts at endoscopy was an adequate light source to illuminate the area exposed by the other end of the instrument. Therefore, 15 centuries passed without a major advance in the field, until 1585, when Tgulio Caesare Aranzi began focusing sunlight through a flask of water and projecting the light into the nasal cavity.

THE 19TH CENTURY

More than 200 years later, in 1806, Philip Bozzini produced the first endoscope with a light source. His revolutionary development involved a series of mirrors to reflect light from a burning wax candle inside an aluminum device to the point of focus. His tool, which he termed the *Lichtleiter* (light conductor) and used as a cystoscope and vaginoscope, is considered the first true endoscope (Fig. 1-1). Unfortunately, the medical community's reception of the *Lichtleiter* was tragically unfavorable, which was perhaps predictable for such a giant leap. The instrument's potential was not understood, and it was condemned as "merely a magic lantern." After a review by the medical faculty of the University in Vienna, Bozzini was punished. However, his contributions fashioned the groundwork for others to make steady progress in the field of endoscopy. Nearly 200 years after his death, the concept of image projection on a screen would unlock the vast potential of minimally invasive surgery.

The *Lichtleiter* and its modified variants would be used by others and would account for the endoscopic evolution over the next century. Pierre Salomon Segalas introduced the *urethro-cystique* (a cystoscope), a variation of Bozzini's instrument, to the Académie de Sciences in Paris in 1826. Simultaneously, the American John Fisher was using a similar instrument clinically for vaginoscopy in Boston. His development was driven by the necessity to evaluate the cervix of shy young women for whom standard exposure would be traumatic.

A French surgeon named Antoine Jean Desormeaux began using a technological modification of the *Lichtleiter* for urologic procedures in the mid 1800s. He is considered by some to be the father of endoscopy, and he is certainly the father of cystoscopy. He modified Bozzini's scope by changing the light source from a candle to the flame from a solution of alcohol and turpentine. This solution produced a brighter and more condensable beam of light. Near the same time, in Dublin, Francis Cruise improved Desormeaux's work by enhancing illumination with a paraffin lamp. Cruise's instrument was more readily usable and was designed with attachments for examining the rectum, uterus, auditory canal, pharynx, and larynx. In his writings,

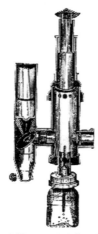

Figure 1-1. In 1806, Philip Bozzini developed the first endoscope with a light source. His instrument utilized a series of mirrors to reflect light from a burning candle inside an aluminum device to the point of focus. He termed this tool the *Lichtleiter*, which means "light conductor." This was considered the first true endoscope and was used initially as a cystoscope and vaginoscope.

Cruise mentioned that scopes might be modified for examination of the esophagus and stomach. In 1869, Commander Pantaleoni used a modified cystoscope to cauterize a hemorrhagic uterine growth. This procedure became the first therapeutic hysteroscopy.

Continuing along the same conceptual line with further modification, in 1877, a German physician, Maximilian Nitze, introduced the first modern-style endoscope with a distal light source. His *kystoskop* was designed by Viennese instrument maker Joseph Leiter, who used an incandescent platinum wire loop to illuminate the body cavity from inside, which allowed an image to be directed through lenses to the outside with magnification. Leiter used this instrument to inspect the urethra, bladder, and larynx.

In 1868, Adolf Kussmaul viewed the esophagus and stomach of a professional sword swallower. Although performed merely for demonstration and not clinically useful, it was very likely the first esophagoscopy. Therefore, he is considered by some to be the father of the current field. However, this arena was advanced more substantially by Johann Mikulicz, a surgeon in Vienna with a keen interest in the treatment of gastric cancer. He began performing clinically useful esophagoscopy in 1881 in an attempt to discover gastric tumors at an earlier stage. A prolific surgeon, Mikulicz documented 183 gastrectomies for gastric cancer during his relatively short career and became quite cognizant of its fatal nature. In fact, he died of gastric cancer at age 55.

THE EARLY 20TH CENTURY

In 1901, the first experimental laparoscopy was performed in an animal model. A German surgeon, George

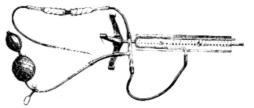

Figure 1-2. In 1901, the first experimental laparoscopy was performed in an animal model by George Kelling. After insufflation of the peritoneal cavity with sterile air, he peered into the abdomen with a cystoscope, which he called a *coelioskope*. The insufflator he used is shown.

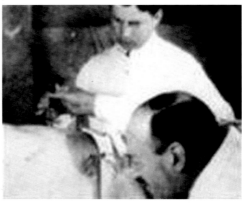

Figure 1-3. The first clinical description of laparoscopy and thoracoscopy is attributed to Hans Christian Jacobaeus. He used pneumoperitoneum and a light source on the distal end of his endoscope. He is seen peering through the lens of his laparoscope in this photograph.

Kelling, made a small incision in the abdomen of dogs, insufflated the peritoneal cavity with sterile air, and investigated the abdomen with a cystoscope. He created the term *coelioskope* for his visionary procedure. His clinical goal was to stop intra-abdominal hemorrhage from diseases such as ruptured ectopic pregnancy and pancreatitis. Although his work found little support, his research established the importance of a sterile pneumoperitoneum to allow visualization, an anchoring principle for future laparoscopy (Fig. 1-2).

Near the time of Kelling's animal experiments, the seeds of minimally invasive techniques in humans were being planted. Hans Christian Jacobaeus, an internist in Stockholm, introduced the term *laparothorakoskopie* in his unprecedented report on laparoscopy and thoracoscopy in humans. This sentinel paper was published in *Münchener Medizinische Wochenschrift* in 1911. He utilized a pneumoperitoneum and light source on the distal end of his endoscope (Fig. 1-3). Kelling took exception to the article and issued a letter to the editor that appeared 2 months later disputing the assertion that Jacobaeus introduced the technique in humans. Kelling contended he had successfully performed two laparoscopic cases in humans between 1901 and 1910. Regardless of the merit in Kelling's letter, his failure to publish his work in a timely manner will leave the record attributing the first clinical description of laparoscopy and thoracoscopy to Jacobaeus. Interestingly, in this paper, Jacobaeus reported thoracoscopy as a more promising procedure than laparoscopy.

In 1911 as well, Bertram M. Berheim at Johns Hopkins performed the first laparoscopy in the United States, which he asserts was prior to any knowledge of Jacobaeus's or Kelling's work. He used a $1/2$-inch-diameter proctoscope with a directed external light and coined the term *organoscopy*, a misnomer because he was inspecting the inside of a cavity, not an organ.

The enthusiasm Jacobaeus held for thoracoscopy over laparoscopy resulted from the pressing medical needs of his patients. He advocated an opposite working port to perform pneumolysis in those patients with tuberculosis, another founding principle in therapeutic thoracoscopy. This technique became widely practiced and therefore represents the first minimally invasive procedure to gain a reasonable level of acceptance. This initial period of minimally invasive surgery ended in 1945 with the discovery of streptomycin. Now that this disease could be managed medically, the use of thoracoscopy fell into a quiescent period.

The first large case series on the clinical use of laparoscopy appeared in 1920. An internist from Chicago, B. H. Orndoff, described 42 cases of diagnostic peritoneoscopy. He described the use of a sharp pyramidal trocar for an access port. The next substantial step occurred in 1929 when Heinz Kalk, a German gastroenterologist, developed a 135-degree lens system and described the addition of a working port. He used laparoscopy effectively in the diagnosis of hepatobiliary disease. Ten years after his invention, demonstrating remarkable confidence in his instrumentation, Kalk published a series of 2000 liver biopsies under local anesthesia without any mortality. During this time, in 1934, John C. Ruddock, an American internist, claimed laparoscopy to be a diagnostic technique superior to laparotomy. His work produced an important instrument in modern minimally invasive surgery: forceps with electrocoagulation capacity.

Another modern tool of laparoscopy was introduced in 1938 when Hungarian Janos Veress developed a spring-loaded blunt-tipped needle for draining ascites and evacuating fluid and air from the chest. His innovation was used to create a therapeutic pneumothorax for tuberculosis. Although he did not foresee application of this tool in minimally invasive surgery, the Veress needle has become an indispensable instrument for many laparoscopic surgeons. Although the device was, and still is, considered unsafe by some surgeons, an alternative approach, using the cut-down technique, would later be published in 1971 by H. M. Hasson, a gynecologist in Chicago.

In 1944, Raoul Palmer began examining the intra-abdominal reproductive organs of women in Paris. He used an umbilical port with insufflation and a rigid optic lighting system. Notably, his patients were placed in the Trendelenburg position to facilitate a view of the pelvis by passively allowing air into this space. Palmer monitored the intra-abdominal pressure during the procedure. Both of these concepts are now known to be important to modern laparoscopy.

THE DEVELOPMENT OF FIBEROPTIC TECHNOLOGY

The greatest advance during the middle of the 20th century was not a surgical application but the technological discovery of fiberoptics. In 1954, two separate articles describing imaging bundles appeared in *Nature*, one by Abraham van Heel of the Technical University in Delft, Holland, and the other by Harold H. Hopkins and Narinder Kapany of Imperial College in London. Hopkins, an English physicist, produced the first functional fiberoptic prototype in 1954. Van Heel, stimulated by a conversation with the American optical physicist Brian O'Brien, subsequently covered the fiber with a transparent layer having a lower refractive index. This protected the total-reflection surface from contamination and greatly reduced interfiber contamination.

The next step was made by Lawrence Curtiss, an undergraduate at the University of Michigan working under physician Basil Hirschowitz and physicist C. Wilbur Peters. Curtiss covered the optical fibers in glass. This glass-encased fiberscope, built as a gastroscope, made its clinical debut in 1957 in Ann Arbor. For the first time, the image was sufficient for photographs. Bergein F. Overholt, also working in Ann Arbor as a trainee at the time, helped develop the first flexible fiberoptic sigmoidoscope-colonoscope in 1963. After he presented his experience to the American Society of Gastrointestinal Endoscopy in 1967, the idea of colonoscopy was officially embraced.

THE LATE 20TH CENTURY

Now that technology had progressed enough to enable clear visualization of body cavities, the next opportunity for advancement rested in the hands of the surgeons. Few surgeons have had a more influential role in the development of minimally invasive surgery than Kurt Semm of Kiel, Germany. His story reflects the plight assumed by original thinkers when they begin to transform ideas into action. He began publicizing his work with presentations at German, Austrian, and Swiss gynecologic meetings in the early 1960s. A trained toolmaker as well as a physician, he developed an electronic carbon dioxide insufflator, producing a clear shift in the previous concept of air pneumoperitoneum. He also began to develop specific endoscopic tools with a designated function such as a uterine manipulator, a high-volume irrigation and aspiration device, knot-tying instruments, and a tubal patency testing device. Understanding the overwhelming potential of laparoscopy, he urged the general surgeons at Kiel University to perform a laparoscopic cholecystectomy in the late 1970s, more than a decade before general surgeons considered this a viable approach. Of course, his suggestion was ridiculed. Despite this skepticism, he performed the first laparoscopic appendectomy in 1981. After presentation of the technique at a surgical meeting in Germany, the President of the German Surgical Society wrote a letter to the Board of Directors of the German Gynecological Society requesting suspension of Semm's privileges. Apprehension, fear, and unfounded resistance should be anticipated by pioneers. Overcoming these prejudices is a necessary step for advancement.

The development of medical therapy for tuberculosis lessened physicians' interest in thoracoscopy. In the 1960s, there were occasional case reports describing its use, but there were no real accepted applications. Mediastinoscopy for evaluating resectability of pulmonary carcinomas became useful in the 1960s, as this procedure did not depend on advanced visualization or lighting systems and the instrumentation needed was rudimentary. In the early 1970s, thoracoscopy reemerged as a useful diagnostic technique. Brad Rodgers and Jim Talbert at the University of Virginia used thoracoscopy in children to visualize lung pathology and obtain biopsies. Around the same time, several small series of adult patients undergoing thoracoscopy in a similar manner began to appear in the world literature. The use of fiberoptics for these procedures allowed expansion of this technology beyond gynecology and set the stage for the coming era of minimally invasive surgery.

In the late 1970s, an inspired obstetrician and scientist in Bristol, England, Patrick C. Steptoe, used a laparoscopic technique to harvest oocytes to perform in vitro fertilization for infertile couples. With the help of Robert Edwards, a physiologist at Cambridge University, the first "test tube" baby, Louise Joy Brown, was born on July 25, 1978. A landmark in minimally invasive surgery, the birth of this 5-pound, 12-ounce baby girl with blue eyes and blond hair was also the birth of a new field in medicine.

The political climate in medicine began a gradual shift in the late 1970s that would strengthen the push toward modern minimally invasive surgery. In Hamburg, Germany, the Surgical Study Group on Endoscopy and Ultrasound (CAES) was created in 1976. In 1981, the Society of American Gastrointestinal Endoscopic Surgeons (SAGES) was conceived. The same year, the American Board of Obstetrics and Gynecology made laparoscopy a requirement for residency training. The first issue of the journal *Surgical Endoscopy* was published in 1987, and in 1988, the annual World Congress on Surgical Endoscopy made its debut in Berlin.

THE MODERN ERA

Meanwhile, the technical key to Pandora's box was found in 1982 when a real-time, high-resolution video camera was developed that could be attached to the endoscope. This miniature electronic camera (4 × 4 mm) had a charge-coupling device (CCD) that could convert the incoming optical image into electrical impulses that could be sent to a monitor, a recording device, or elsewhere. This development allowed a clear magnified image of the entire operating field to be shown on a monitor. Up to this point, the surgeon was hunched over, peering into the scope, with limited vision. Once a high-resolution, magnified intracorporeal image could be viewed on a monitor, the surgeon could stand upright and work with two operating hands without handling the camera. Moreover, additional assistants could then join the procedure with an equal view. Surgeons would no longer need to scrub to teach an operation, trainees could watch without being close to the field, and operations could easily be recorded and transmitted to separate sites. The limitation to minimally invasive surgery was instantly shifted to the imagination and willingness of the surgeons.

Five years after this critical innovation, the revolution in minimally invasive surgery began. The first laparoscopic cholecystectomy was reported in 1987 by Philippe Mouret in Lyon, France. The news of this surgical triumph spread, and the next calendar year witnessed laparoscopic cholecystectomies performed by several surgeons including Dubois (Paris), Perissat (Bordeaux), Nathanson and Cuschieri (Scotland), McKernan and Saye (Georgia), Reddick and Olsen (Tennessee), Groitl and Troidl (Germany), Katkhouda (France), Klaiber (Switzerland), and others. On the surface, it appears that few advances in the history of surgery have become so widely accepted so quickly. However, given the long struggle against resistance that minimally invasive surgery incurred initially, these early laparoscopic cholecystectomies represent the breaking points that led to the modern era of minimally invasive surgery. The evolution toward laparoscopy and thoracoscopy was a monumental shift in surgical capacity akin to the advent of general anesthesia and antiseptic agents. In the 5 years that followed, surgeons from every subspecialty began applying the surgical principles found in those original cholecystectomies. Shortly thereafter, laparoscopy became routinely used for colectomy, splenectomy, nephrectomy, adrenalectomy, appendectomy, small bowel resections, explorations, and more. Thoracoscopy became standard for decortication and wedge resections. This explosion of surgical advancement pressed commercial producers of surgical equipment to an inflection point of technological improvement. Staplers, clip devices, endoloops, ultrasonic shears, Ligasure technology (Covidien, Mansfield, MA), endoscopic ultrasound probes, and many innovative devices provided surgeons with fertile ground for advancing the field of minimally invasive surgery.

In the late 1990s, minimally invasive surgery experienced dueling processes of advancement. One was the use of a robot to push the technical limits of human laparoscopy. However, laparoscopy itself was advancing as experience and skills grew, allowing surgeons to overcome previous contraindications and limitations. The once unthinkable minimally invasive operations being mastered at some centers included gastric bypass, hepatoportoenterostomy (Kasai procedure), total abdominal colectomy with ileal pouch–anal anastomosis, and esophageal atresia repair. The notion of using tools to lessen injury to the patient was having effects in multiple fields. During this time, technological advances of expandable stents and percutaneous endovascular tools revamped the fields of vascular and cardiothoracic surgery. As the century turned, hospitals began building operating suites specifically designed for minimally invasive operations.

Today, we bear witness to an emerging phenomenon of proven efficacy. We stand beyond the point of no return as the surgical fields have irreversibly moved into the minimally invasive era. The scientist John Tyndall said, "We are truly heirs of all the ages; But, as honest men, it behooves us to learn the extent of our inheritance; And as brave ones not to whimper if it should prove less than we had supposed." Mindful of the well-founded surgical principles handed down from our predecessors, our role now is to continue to challenge dogmatic assumptions with the goal of easing the burden and stress that operations have on our patients and their families.

SELECTED REFERENCES

1. Gans SL: Historical development of pediatric endoscopic surgery. In Holcomb GW III (ed): Pediatric Endoscopic Surgery. Norwalk, CT, Appleton and Lange, pp 1-7, 1994
2. Spaner SJ, Warnock GL: A brief history of endoscopy, laparoscopy, and laparoscopic surgery. J Laparoendosc Adv Surg Tech 7:369-373, 1997
3. Litynski GS: Kurt Semm and the fight against skepticism: Endoscopic hemostasis, laparoscopic appendectomy, and Semm's impact on the "laparoscopic revolution." JSLS 2:309-313, 1998
4. Georgeson KE, Owings E: Advances in minimally invasive surgery in children. Am J Surg 180:362-364, 2000
5. Himal HS: Minimally invasive (laparoscopic) surgery. Surg Endosc 16:1647-1652, 2002
6. Modlin IM, Kidd M, Lye KD: From the lumen to the laparoscope. Arch Surg 139:1110-1126, 2004
7. Harrell AG, Heniford BT: Minimally invasive abdominal surgery: Lux et veritas past, present, and future. Am J Surg 190:239-243, 2005

PART ONE

LAPAROSCOPY

2

Principles of Laparoscopic Surgery

George W. Holcomb III

The general principles for performing a laparoscopic operation have not changed significantly since the laparoscopic revolution began in the late 1980s. Prior to the laparoscopic procedure, a preoperative conference should be held with the parents and the patient (if the age is appropriate) to discuss the nature of the laparoscopic operation and the risks and benefits of this approach. The benefits include reduced discomfort, reduced hospitalization, and faster return to routine activities (such as school or sporting activities). In addition, the cosmetic advantage of this approach is becoming increasingly appreciated. Finally, there appears to be a definite reduction in the risk of adhesive postoperative small bowel obstruction with this approach. Risks include a small (generally 1%) chance of conversion to an open operation, usually because of unclear anatomy and sometimes because of adhesions from previous open operations. In addition, as with the open approach, there is a small but definite incidence of injury to other structures, or of bleeding requiring transfusion.

The contraindications for the laparoscopic approach are few. The laparoscopic technique has been used for every general and thoracic surgical procedure in children. Its primary contraindication is a situation in which an adequate pneumoperitoneum cannot be created or a lung cannot be collapsed for a thoracic operation. Fortunately, this rarely occurs. Adhesions from previous procedures precluding adequate visualization are occasionally found. Bleeding that cannot be readily con-trolled may develop, but this is rare. Finally, because of chronic lung disease or uncorrected congenital cardiac disease, the patient may not be able to tolerate creation of a pneumoperitoneum for an abdominal operation or lung collapse for a thoracic procedure.

The preoperative evaluation and preparation of the patient undergoing a laparoscopic operation are the same as those required for the comparable open operation. A patient who is undergoing an elective colonic procedure and needs preoperative bowel preparation should be admitted before the operation for this purpose. Patients with sickle cell disease who require laparoscopic procedures should be transfused to a hemoglobin of 10 g/dL. Preoperative admission for hydration of these patients is not believed to be as necessary as it was in the past, but transfusion continues to be a mainstay of the preoperative preparation.

GENERAL PRINCIPLES

Although for thoracoscopy, it is possible to effect collapse of the ipsilateral lung through a variety of measures, insufflation is necessary to create an adequate working space in the abdomen. I have used inflating pressures of 12 to 15 mm Hg in numerous infants without deleterious effects. The primary reason to reduce this pressure is the presence of underlying heart or lung disease. If there is underlying lung disease, an elevated pressure may raise the hemidiaphragms, which can be followed by a corresponding reduction in tidal volume, ventilation, and oxygenation. In an infant with chronic heart disease who is volume dependent, the higher inflating pressures may reduce venous return to the heart, with a corresponding reduction in cardiac output. Other than these two areas, insufflation of 12 to 15 mm Hg has been used routinely in all patients at my institution. A final caveat centers on the lack of an adequate working space despite a high intra-abdominal pressure and adequate flow. In such an instance, the surgeon should evaluate whether the patient is adequately paralyzed. If the patient is not paralyzed, it may not be possible to create an adequate working space despite high flows and high inflating pressures.

Angled telescopes are essential for safety and adequate visualization. There are currently very few indications for a 0-degree telescope. A 0-degree telescope may be used for a laparoscopic cholecystectomy and for initial diagnostic laparoscopy. However, to see around the corners of the abdominal viscera, use of an angled telescope is paramount. For most of the operations at my institution, either a 45-degree angled 5-mm telescope or a 70-degree angled 5-mm telescope is used. For fundoplication or cholecystectomy, a 45-degree angled telescope is employed. For a pyloromyotomy, a splenectomy, a laparoscopic pull-through, or an appendectomy, a 70-degree angled telescope is employed. In addition, for evaluation of the contralateral inguinal region in a child with a known unilateral inguinal hernia, a 70-degree angled telescope is essential for adequate visualization of the contralateral inguinal ring. Although some authors feel that a 3-mm telescope can be useful, there is no advantage to using the smaller telescope in the umbilicus. A 5-mm port results in the same cosmetic appearance as a 3-mm port inserted in the center of the umbilicus, as the umbilicus is scar and heals quite nicely. Therefore, in my mind, there is no advantage to using a 3-mm telescope, even in infants. A disadvantage of using a 3-mm cannula and telescope is that there is often inadequate space in the cannula around the telescope to allow adequate insufflation.

Over the past 10 years, a couple of vessel-sealing devices have been developed. The Harmonic Scalpel (Ethicon Endosurgery, Cincinnati, OH) was developed in the late 1990s. Coagulation occurs when the blade, vibrating at 55,000 Hz, couples with protein and denatures it to form a coagulum that seals small vessels. The Ligasure (Covidien, Mansfield, MA) has been developed over the past 5 years and is useful as well for ligation and division of mesenteric vessels or short gastric vessels in older patients requiring fundoplication. It works by melting the collagen and elastin in the vessel wall and re-forming it into a permanent seal. Moreover, these instruments are also helpful for splenectomy and for thoracic procedures. Both of them come as 5-mm instruments and are well suited for pediatric application.

As a general statement, the largest and usually the initial cannula is placed in the umbilicus. Again, the reasoning is that the umbilicus is composed mainly of scar and it is quite easy to hide a large incision at this site. For children undergoing laparoscopic appendectomy or splenectomy at my institution, a 12-mm port is placed in the umbilicus and the resulting scar is quite pleasing.

Finally, my colleagues and I use a stab incision technique in infants and young children almost exclusively. With this approach, an initial cannula is placed in the umbilicus and insufflation achieved through this cannula. A stab incision using a #11 Bard Parker (Becton-Dickinson, Franklin Lakes, NJ) blade is then used to create the tract through which instruments are passed (Fig. 2-1). This stab incision technique is employed for all operations in infants and young children and can even be applied to some adolescents. As an example, for a fundoplication, one 5-mm cannula is placed in the umbilicus and four stab incisions are used. For a laparoscopic splenectomy, a 12-mm port is placed in the umbilicus and a 5-mm port is placed in the midline epigastrium. Two stab incisions are then used (Fig. 2-2A). For a laparoscopic cholecystectomy, the two right-sided instruments are usually placed through stab incisions rather than ports unless the patient is extremely hefty (see Fig. 2-2B). In general, this technique is ideal for instruments that do not need to be exteriorized and then reinserted on a regular basis. The only operation in which this stab incision technique is not used currently is an appendectomy, for which a 12-mm port is

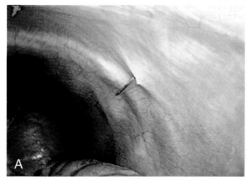
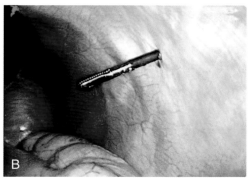

Figure 2-1.   The stab incision technique can be used to introduce instruments in infants and young children. **A,** A stab incision using a #11 blade is used to create the tract through which the instrument is passed. **B,** After removal of the knife, the instrument is passed through the skin and soft tissue tract.

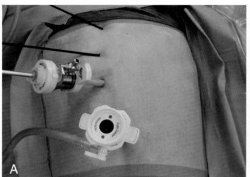
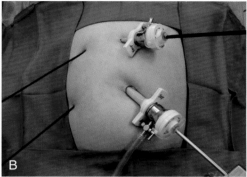

Figure 2-2. The stab incision technique can be used for many operations, including some in older children with relatively thin abdominal walls. **A,** For a laparoscopic splenectomy, a 12-mm port is placed in the umbilicus and a 5-mm port is placed in the midline epigastrium where the telescope is inserted. Two stab incisions are then used cephalad to the 5-mm cannula. **B,** For a laparoscopic cholecystectomy, the two right-sided instruments can often be placed through stab incisions rather than ports unless the patient is extremely hefty. In general, this technique is ideal for instruments that do not need to be exteriorized and then reinserted on a regular basis for the operation.

Table 2-1   Savings to the Patient and to the Hospital, Realized by Using Stab Incision Technique

Procedure (No.)	Cannulas Used per Patient	Cannulas Saved per Patient	Savings with Step System ($)		Savings with Ethicon System ($)	
			Patient	Institution	Patient	Institution
Nissen (209)	1	4	117,040	51,832	76,912	34,276
Nissen (adolescent) (14)	2	3	5,880	2,604	3,864	1,722
Appendectomy (102)	2	1	14,280	6,324	9,384	4,182
Pyloromyotomy (77)	1	2	21,560	9,548	14,168	6,314
Cholecystectomy (31)	2	2	8,680	3,844	5,704	2,542
Splenectomy (21)	2	2	5,880	2,604	3,864	1,722
Pull-through (20)	2	1	2,800	1,240	1,840	820
Ligation of testicular vessels (AT) (15)	1	2	4,200	1,860	2,760	1,230
Esophagomyotomy (7)	2	3	2,940	1,302	1,932	861
Adrenalectomy (6)	2	2	1,680	744	1,104	492
Varicocele (5)	1	2	1,400	620	920	410
Ovarian (2)	1	2	560	248	368	164
Meckel diverticulum (2)	2	1	280	124	184	82
511 operations	714	1324	$187,180	$82,894	$123,004	$54,817

AT, abdominal testis.

placed in the umbilicus and two 5-mm cannulas are introduced in the left mid abdomen and left lower quadrant.

Our group recently looked at the financial implications of the stab incision technique in 511 operations. If the stab incision technique was used, a savings of $187,000 in patient charges and $82,894 in institutional charges were realized if the Step cannula system (Covidien, Mansfield, MA) was used. The savings were $123,004 to the patient and $54,817 to the institution if Ethicon cannulas were used (Table 2-1). Moreover, these are small incisions and are usually closed only with Steri-Strips. Finally, only one patient has returned with a possible complication related to the stab incision technique. In this patient, there was concern that a piece of omentum might have herniated into the incision tract. However, this soft tissue enlargement resolved with observation.

SAFETY AND CONCERNS FOR CHILDREN

Because of the small size of the pediatric patient, a number of safety considerations are peculiar to this age group. Insertion of a urinary catheter is not generally required unless a prolonged procedure is anticipated. However, operations in which bladder decompression is helpful include laparoscopic pull-through for Hirschsprung's disease and for imperforate anus. For other operations, it is quite easy to manually empty the bladder in children if bladder decompression is required. Gastric decompression with an orogastric tube remains important for upper abdominal procedures.

Because the child's abdominal cavity is much smaller than an adult patient's cavity, it is important to widely space the ports and instruments to allow adequate working space. An efficient procedure is not possible if the instruments are situated too close together. This can be especially true when performing an advanced laparoscopic procedure in an infant.

The abdominal wall of young children, and especially infants, is very pliable. When introducing cannulas or a Veress needle with an attached expandable sleeve, it is very important to watch for inadvertent injury to the underlying viscera. Once the sharp trocar of the cannula or Veress needle has pierced the peritoneum, the trocar

or needle should be directed transversely across the abdominal cavity and not toward the underlying viscera (Fig. 2-3). With this technique, injury to underlying structures should be minimized.

For most operations, the initial cannula is introduced in the umbilicus. We prefer the cutdown approach although others use the Veress needle technique. With the cutdown technique, a vertical incision is made in the center of the umbilicus and carried down to the fascia. The fascia is then incised with the cautery and the Step cannula system is used. However, instead of introducing the Veress needle and expandable sleeve directly in the abdominal cavity, only the expandable sleeve is introduced gently into the abdominal cavity, followed by insertion of the cannula with a blunt-tip stylet through the expandable sleeve (Fig. 2-4). In this way, it is extremely unlikely that the underlying viscera will be injured with the blunt-tip trocar. Often, especially in young children, there is an umbilical hernia, so this approach can be quite easy. Again, when introducing the blunt-tip cannula and trocar, it is important to try to insert the trocar and cannula away from the underlying viscera so as not to injure them.

Another important consideration centers on the use of endoscopic retrieval bags. Although these are required for entrapment and subsequent morcellation of solid

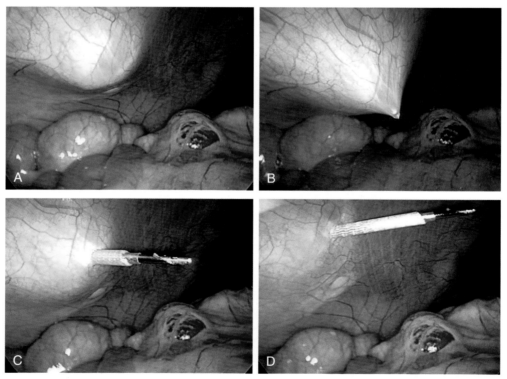

Figure 2-3. The abdominal wall of young children, and especially infants, is very pliable. When introducing cannulas with sharp trocars or a Veress needle with an attached expandable sleeve, it is important to watch for inadvertent injury to underlying viscera. After identification of the site for introduction of the cannula (**A**), the sleeve and Veress needle pierce the peritoneum (**B**). Once the trocar or needle has pierced the peritoneum, it should be directed transversely across the abdominal wall and not toward the underlying viscera (**C** and **D**). With this technique, injury to the underlying structures should be minimized.

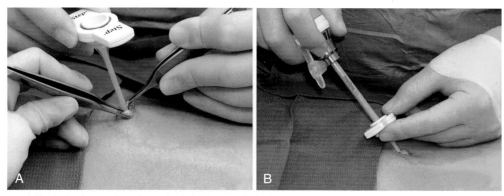

Figure 2-4. The umbilical site is usually where the initial cannula is introduced. We prefer the Step cannula system because of its safety; with this system, a vertical incision is made in the umbilical skin and carried down to the fascia. After incision in the peritoneum with the cautery, the expandable sleeve is introduced without the Veress needle (**A**). In this way, it is extremely unlikely that underlying viscera will be injured when the blunt-tipped trocar and cannula are inserted (**B**).

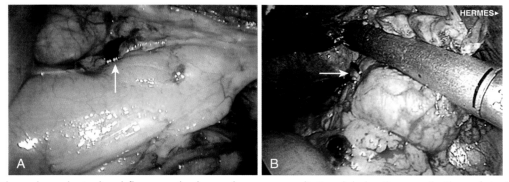

Figure 2-5. If the endoscopic staple misfires, massive hemorrhage may result. To minimize the complications of stapler malfunction during a laparoscopic splenectomy, we clip the splenic artery early in the operation (**A**). If there is stapler malfunction when it is fired across the hilum (**B**), bleeding should be from the splenic vein and should be more readily controllable than from the divided splenic artery. The *arrows* point to the clips on the splenic artery.

organs such as the spleen, they are also useful for removing malignant lesions to prevent seeding of the tract and for infectious etiologies such as acute appendicitis. Regarding acute appendicitis, if the specimen cannot be extracted intact through the umbilical port, then an endoscopic retrieval bag is usually introduced, and the specimen and bag are exteriorized through the umbilical fascial incision after removal of the port. When morcellation of the specimen in the bag is required, it is important not to morcellate too vigorously, as rupture of these bags with subsequently spillage of the contents has been described. The endoscopic stapler is often used in advanced minimally invasive surgical operations and is useful for ligation and division of the mesoappendix and the appendix when performing an appendectomy, and for ligation and visualization of the splenic hilum when performing a splenectomy. However, malfunction of these staplers has occurred in this latter setting with subsequent rapid hemorrhage. To minimize the complications of stapler malfunction, we clip the splenic artery early in the course of the laparoscopic splenec-

tomy (Fig. 2-5). There are two advantages to early clipping of the splenic artery. First, the spleen should decrease in size because of autotransfusion through the splenic vein. Second, if there is a stapler malfunction, the bleeding is from the splenic vein and should be more readily controllable than from the divided splenic artery.

A final concern regards closure of the fascial incisions. With the use of the Step cannula system with radial expansion of the abdominal wall muscles as the cannula and blunt trocar are inserted, most 3- and some 5-mm fascial incisions (other than the umbilicus) do not need closure. However, with a thin patient, we usually close the anterior sheath of the 5-mm incisions. Ten-mm incisions (especially in thin patients) should always be closed to prevent fascial herniation.

Complications with introduction of the Veress needle and cannulas have markedly diminished over the past 15 years. However, some abdominal wall vessels, especially the inferior epigastric vessels, can be injured if they are pierced by either a sharp trocar, a Veress needle, or a #11 blade. In a thin patient, these vessels can often

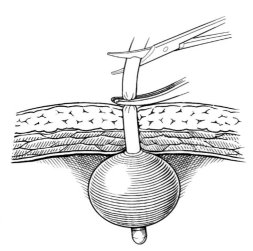

Figure 2-6. During insertion of a cannula with a sharp trocar, bleeding can develop from laceration of abdominal wall vessels. In more obese patients, it can be difficult to visualize these vessels. To help control hemorrhage, a deflated Foley catheter can be inserted through the cannula and the cannula withdrawn over the catheter. The inflated balloon is then lifted up against the abdominal wall and the tubing is clamped at the skin level with a hemostat.

be visualized through the abdominal wall, secured with a hemostat, and suture ligated. In more obese patients, it can be difficult to visualize these vessels. A useful technique of placing a deflated Foley catheter through the cannula, withdrawing the cannula over the catheter, and inflating the balloon has been described. The balloon is then lifted up against the abdominal wall, and the tubing is clamped at the skin level with a hemostat (Fig. 2-6). It can remain clamped for up to 24 hours if necessary. However, occasionally there is massive bleeding from these vessels, and laparotomy may be required for vascular control.

3
Laparoscopic Nissen Fundoplication

George W. Holcomb III

Gastroesophageal reflux is a frequently seen condition in infants and children. In fact, in premature and young infants, it can be normal until the lower esophageal sphincter (LES) matures. With maturation of the LES, these symptoms often resolve spontaneously. In other infants and children, medical management is effective in relieving symptoms, but medical management is not likely to yield long-term results after several years of age. Laparoscopic fundoplication provides a very effective treatment for the long-term cure of this condition and its associated complications.

INDICATIONS FOR WORKUP AND OPERATION

Infants with gastroesophageal reflux who are feeding well and growing nicely do not usually require laparoscopic fundoplication, as the condition often resolves spontaneously with medical management in this very young age group. Indications for surgical intervention in young infants includes acute life-threatening events secondary to aspiration, failure to thrive with associated weight loss, and the need for placement of a gastrostomy in neurologically impaired infants. In older patients, indications for intervention include failure of medical therapy, esophagitis, and reactive airway disease secondary to gastroesophageal reflux. Also included in this older group are the neurologically impaired children who cannot protect their airway and require placement of a gastrostomy for enteral alimentation.

The standard workup centers on a pH study to objectively document the presence of gastroesophageal reflux. However, the pH study is only about 90% sensitive, so for a patient with symptoms suggestive of gastroesophageal reflux but a normal pH study, either a second pH study or endoscopy with biopsy should be performed. Preoperative gastroparesis is often improved after a laparoscopic fundoplication and, for this reason, a preoperative gastric emptying study is useless in the initial evaluation of these patients. Similarly, an upper gastrointestinal contrast study is only 70% sensitive and usually does not contribute additional information.

OPERATIVE TECHNIQUE

The patient is placed supine on the operating room table, and general endotracheal anesthesia is administered. Infants and young children are positioned at the foot of the bed in a frogleg position (Fig. 3-1A). The foot of the bed is dropped so that the surgeon and assistant can stand at the end of the bed (see Fig. 3-1B). For older children, the legs are placed in stirrups. An orogastric tube is introduced to decompress the stomach, but a urinary catheter is not routinely inserted. If a gastrostomy is needed, this incision is marked prior to insufflation. This site will also be one of the working incisions for the laparoscopic fundoplication. A single monitor is positioned over and slightly cephalad to the patient's head.

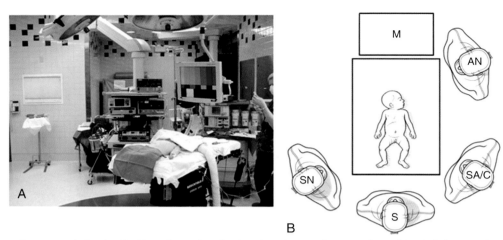

Figure 3-1. For a laparoscopic fundoplication, the patient is placed supine on the operating table. **A,** Infants and young children are positioned at the foot of the bed in a frogleg position, and the foot of the bed is dropped. **B,** The surgeon (S) and surgical assistant/camera holder (SA/C) stand next to the patient at the end of the bed. The surgical assistant is to the right of the surgeon and the scrub nurse (SN) is to the surgeon's left. A single monitor (M) is used and is positioned over and cephalad to the patient's head. AN, anesthesiologist.

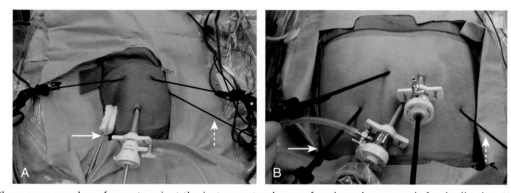

Figure 3-2. There are a number of ways to orient the instruments when performing a laparoscopic fundoplication. With our technique, the 45-degree angled 5-mm telescope is introduced after insertion of the 5-mm umbilical cannula. The liver retractor is introduced in the patient's right subcostal region (*solid arrow*). The two main working ports are in the left and right epigastrium. The main working port for the surgeon is the one in the patient's left epigastric region. It is through this incision that dissecting instruments, needle holder, and suture are introduced. The instrument used by the surgical assistant is in the patient's left subcostal region (*dashed arrow*). The stab incision technique can be used for both infants (**A**) and adolescents (**B**).

After the preparation and draping, a vertical 5-mm incision is made in the center of the umbilicus, and dissection is continued through the umbilical fascia with cautery. An umbilical hernia is often present, especially in infants and young children, providing easy access to the peritoneal cavity. Using the Step system (Covidien, Mansfield, MA), an expandable sheath is inserted carefully into the peritoneal cavity. A 5-mm cannula with a blunt-tipped trocar is then introduced through the expandable sheath, and CO_2 insufflation is initiated with a flow rate of 3 to 5 L/min and a maximal pressure of 12 to 15 mm Hg. A 5-mm, 45-degree angled telescope is introduced through the umbilical cannula and diagnostic laparoscopy is performed.

After a brief diagnostic laparoscopy, four accessory stab incisions are made (see Chapter 2). The first incision is created in the patient's right subcostal region,

which is the site for introduction of the liver retractor. We prefer the flexible 3-mm or 5-mm liver retractor made by Snowden-Pencer for this purpose, and we secure it to the operating room table with the Thompson instrument holder (Thompson Surgical Instruments, Traverse City, MI). The two main working sites for the operation are to the right and left of the midline in the upper epigastrium. In the left hand, the surgeon uses an atraumatic grasper that has been inserted through the stab incision in the patient's right epigastrium. The incision in the patient's left epigastrium is the surgeon's primary working site. Through this incision, dissecting instruments and the needle holder (and harmonic scalpel, if used) are introduced. The final stab incision is in the patient's left lateral subcostal region, through which an atraumatic forceps is introduced for retraction purposes by the assistant surgeon (Fig. 3-2).

The initial operative step is to ligate and divide the short gastric vessels. This dissection starts at a point one-third the way down the greater curvature of the stomach (Fig. 3-3). In infants and children up to the age of 5 years, this ligation and division is performed with the Maryland dissecting instrument connected to cautery. For children older than 5 years, the harmonic scalpel (Ethicon Endosurgery, Cincinnati, OH) is preferred for this purpose. (In these older children, instead of a stab incision in the left epigastrium, a 5-mm cannula is used.) Dissection along the greater curvature is carried to the esophageal hiatus, where the hiatus is carefully inspected. If an adequate intra-abdominal esophagus is present, as little dissection as possible is performed to help prevent transmigration of the fundoplication wrap through an enlarged esophageal hiatus (Fig. 3-4). However, if there is no visual evidence of a significant amount of intra-abdominal esophagus, the peritoneum overlying the left aspect of the esophagocrural junction is incised to allow mobilization of the distal esophagus

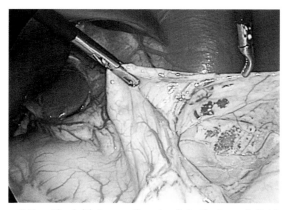

Figure 3-3. The initial operative step is to ligate and divide the short gastric vessels. This dissection starts at a point a third of the way down the greater curvature of the stomach. The Maryland dissecting instrument attached to cautery is used for this purpose. The harmonic scalpel can be used in older children.

down into the abdominal cavity. After assessment of the esophageal length (and esophageal mobilization if required), the retroesophageal space is opened from the patient's left side (see Fig. 3-4).

After creation of this adequate retroesophageal window, attention is turned to the right side of the esophagus for further mobilization if needed. In almost every case, either an enlarged esophageal hiatus is present or one has been created posteriorly. Therefore, the crura are approximated posteriorly with a single 2-0 suture on an RB needle in infants, or with an 0-silk on an SH needle in adolescents. The length of this suture is approximately 11 cm. The suture is secured with an intracorporeal knot-tying technique. On occasion, because of the size of the hiatus, a second suture is needed. So as to not angulate the esophagus too much posteriorly, this second suture is usually placed anterior to the esophagus and incorporates a portion of the anterior esophageal wall with the crural closure. Again, 2-0 or 0-silk suture is used for this purpose.

Next, the esophagus is secured to the crura circumferentially with interrupted 3-0 silk sutures on an RB-1 needle. Usually, these sutures are placed at the 7-, 11-, 1-, and 5-o'clock positions and are tied intracorporeally as well (Fig. 3-5). The purpose of these esophagocrural sutures is twofold. First, it is to secure the esophagus in an intra-abdominal position to reduce the incidence of gastroesophageal reflux. Second, the sutures are designed to obliterate the space between the esophagus and the crura and, it is hoped, to prevent transmigration of the fundoplication wrap into the lower mediastinum.

At this point, having closed the crura and secured the esophagus to the crura, attention is turned toward the fundoplication. The telescope is reoriented so that it is easy to visualize the retroesophageal space from the patient's right side of the esophagus. The gastric fundus is grasped with the atraumatic grasping forceps in the surgeon's left hand and delivered through the retroesophageal space (Fig. 3-6A). It is then oriented appropriately to ensure that there is no twisting of the fundus

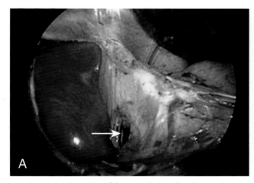
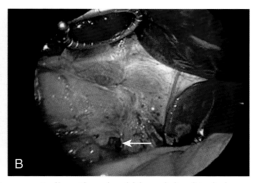

Figure 3-4. If an adequate length of intra-abdominal esophagus is present, dissection should be minimal to help prevent migration of the fundoplication wrap through an enlarged esophageal hiatus. As described in Pearls, the phreno-esophageal ligament is kept intact on both the patient's right side of the esophagus (**A**) and the patient's left side of the esophagus (**B**). Note creation of the retroesophageal window has been initiated (*arrows*).

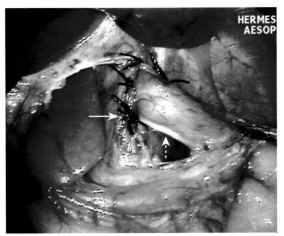

Figure 3-5.   After closure of the hiatus with a 2-0 silk suture placed posterior to the esophagus (*solid arrow*), esophagocrural sutures are placed at the 7-, 11-, 1-, and 5-o'clock positions around the esophagus. The purpose of these sutures is to secure the esophagus in an intra-abdominal position to reduce the incidence of postoperative reflux. In addition, they are designed to obliterate the space between the esophagus and the crura in an effort to prevent transmigration of the fundoplication wrap into the lower mediastinum. The posterior vagus nerve is also visualized (*dotted arrow*).

as it is brought through the retroesophageal space (see Fig. 3-6B). The fundus is then returned through the retroesophageal space, and a bougie is introduced orally by the anesthesiologist (see Fig. 3-6C). In infants and young children, the appropriate size of the bougie depends on the patient's weight (Table 3-1). A great deal of care must be taken to ensure that the bougie is carefully guided into the stomach and does not inadvertently perforate the esophagus or stomach.

Table 3-1 Recommended Bougie Size for Esophageal Calibration	
Weight (kg)	**Bougie Size (Fr)**
2.5-4.0	20-24
4.0-5.5	24-28
5.5-7.0	28-32
7.0-8.5	32-34
8.5-10.0	34-36
10.0-15.0	36-40

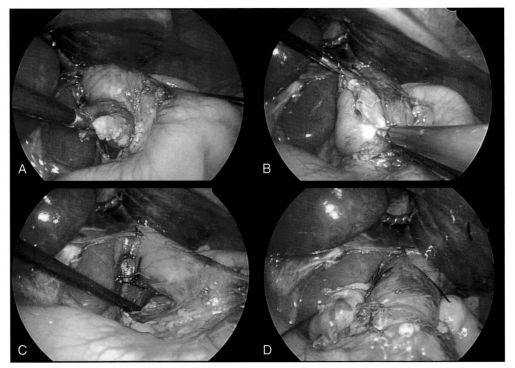

Figure 3-6.   After crural closure and approximation of the esophagus to the crura, the telescope is oriented for improved visualization through the retroesophageal space. The gastric fundus is visualized and is brought through the retroesophageal space (**A**) and oriented appropriately to ensure there is no evidence of twisting of the fundus (**B**). Once it is correctly oriented, the fundus is returned through the retroesophageal space and a bougie is introduced by the anesthesiologist (**C**). Care must be taken to ensure that the bougie is carefully guided into the stomach and does not inadvertently perforate the esophagus or stomach. Three sutures are used to create the fundoplication wrap. The most cephalad suture also incorporates a portion of the anterior esophagus (**D**).

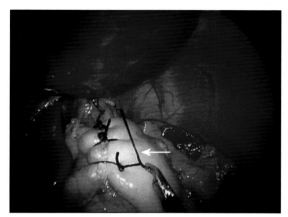

Figure 3-7. The fundoplication length is always measured and should approximate 2 cm in infants and young children and 2.5 cm in adolescents. The silk suture (*arrow*) that is being used to measure the fundoplication length has been cut to 2 cm in length.

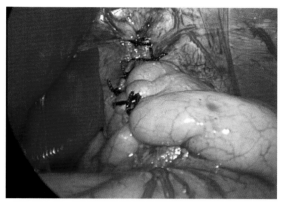

Figure 3-8. Ideally, the fundoplication should be oriented at approximately 10- or 11-o'clock when viewing it from the midline. Such orientation indicates that more of the fundoplication wrap is brought anteriorly over the esophagus rather than under the esophagus, which might lead to dysphagia.

Once the bougie has been introduced into the stomach, the fundus is brought back through the retro-esophageal space and sewn to itself in a standard Nissen fundoplication technique. Silk sutures (2-0) on an RB-1 needle in infants and young children and 0-silk sutures on an SH needle in adolescents are used to secure the fundoplication. Usually, three sutures are placed, with the most cephalad suture also incorporating the anterior wall of the esophagus (see Fig. 3-6D). The length of the first silk suture is 12 cm, and the remaining ones are 8 to 10 cm. The posterior and anterior vagus nerves are both incorporated within the wrap. The fundoplication length is always measured and should approximate 2 cm in infants and young children and 2.5 cm in adolescents (Fig. 3-7). At this point, the bougie is removed, the instruments are withdrawn, and the stab incisions are approximated with Steri-Strips. The umbilical fascia is closed with absorbable suture and the umbilical skin approximated with 5-0 plain catgut suture. Sterile dressings are then applied and anesthesia is terminated.

POSTOPERATIVE CARE

The patients are admitted after the operation and allowed to drink clear liquids or formula approximately 8 hours after the operation at a low volume and low concentration. The volume and concentration can be advanced over 24 hours. Over 80% of our patients are ready for discharge the day after the operation, and the remaining 20% are discharged on the second postoperative morning. We have not had a patient who was admitted the day of the operation require hospitalization longer than 48 hours.

In children older than 1 or 2 years, it is extremely important to institute a mechanical soft diet for 3 weeks, as there is swelling that occurs at the level of the fundoplication. This is especially true for adolescents, in whom moderate bites of meat, toast, or the like become lodged at the fundoplication wrap early in the postoperative course. With these feeding instructions, only one patient in 400 has required postoperative dilation by the author.

PEARLS

1. If gastrostomy is to be performed as well, mark the site in the left epigastrium (LUQ) before insufflation, and use this site as one of the stab incisions.
2. If the LUQ stab incision is not to be used as the site for the gastrostomy, close the fascia with a 5-0 absorbable suture (or 4-0 suture in older patients), as this fascial incision tends to dilate with introduction or removal of instruments and can lead to entrapment of omentum. The other stab incisions can be closed with Steri-Strips.
3. Do not incise the phreno-esophageal membrane around the esophagus if there is adequate esophagus already in the abdomen. Integrity of this peritoneal attachment may be important in preventing transmigration of the wrap postoperatively.
4. There is no way to achieve a tension-free, loose, "floppy" Nissen fundoplication without taking down the short gastric vessels.
5. When the Nissen fundoplication has been completed, the suture line should lie at the 10- or 11-o'clock position (Fig. 3-8). If the suture line lies to the viewer's right of 11-o'clock, there may be too much wrap posterior to the esophagus, which may lead to dysphagia.
6. If the liver is large, position the umbilical cannula and telescope under it, as this helps elevate the liver and improves visualization.

PITFALLS

1. Avoid overly aggressive hiatal dissection, if possible.
2. Avoid entering the mediastinum, if possible.
3. Watch for injury to the stomach or colon during takedown of the short gastric vessels.
4. Watch for an aberrant left hepatic artery.
5. Know where the left gastric artery is and be sure you are cephalad to it when creating the retroesophageal space.
6. Remain cognizant of the vagus nerves.

RESULTS

Between January 2000 and December 2004, I performed 249 laparoscopic Nissen fundoplications (St. Peter, Valusek, Calkins 2007). In the first 130 patients (January 2000 to March 2002), extensive esophageal mobilization was performed and the esophagus was not secured to the crura. In this group, no patient required postoperative esophageal dilation for dysphagia. However, transmigration of the fundoplication wrap occurred in 15 (12%) of the patients.

From April 2002 through December 2004, 119 patients underwent fundoplication with minimal esophageal mobilization (as described in this chapter) as well as placement of esophagocrural sutures. Only six patients (5%) have developed transmigration of the fundoplication wrap in this group ($P = .072$). The relative risk of transmigration with extensive mobilization and without the esophagocrural sutures was 2.29.

In this second group of patients, initially only two esophagocrural sutures were placed in the first 20 patients. Four (25%) of these patients developed transmigration of the wrap. In the next 43 patients, three esophagocrural sutures were used, and only 2 (4.6%) of these patients developed wrap transmigration. In the last 56 patients undergoing fundoplication in this group, four esophagocrural sutures were employed and no

Table 3-2 Minimal Esophageal Dissection: Effectiveness of Esophagocrural Sutures

Esophagocrural Sutures	Patients	Wrap Transmigration	
		Incidence	No. of Patients
2	20	25%	4
3	43	4.6%	2
4	56	0%	0

patient has developed transmigration clinically. These results can be seen in Table 3-2.

SELECTED REFERENCES

1. Boix-Ochoa J, Canals J: Maturation of the lower esophagus. J Pediatr Surg 11:749-756, 1976
2. DeMeester TR, Wernly JA, Bryant GH, et al: Clinical and in vitro analysis of determinants of gastroesophageal competence. Am J Surg 137:39-46, 1979
3. Werlin SL, Dodds WJ, Hogan WJ, et al: Mechanisms of GER in children. J Pediatr 97:244-249, 1980
4. Chung DW, Georgeson KE: Fundoplication and gastrostomy. Semin Pediatr Surg 7:213-219, 1998
5. Ostlie DJ, Holcomb GW III: Laparoscopic fundoplication and gastrostomy. Semin Pediatr Surg 11:196-201, 2002
6. Ostlie DJ, Miller KA, Holcomb GW 3rd: Effective Nissen fundoplication length and bougie diameter size in young children undergoing laparoscopic Nissen fundoplication. J Pediatr Surg 37:1664-1666, 2002
7. Ostlie DJ, Holcomb GW III: The use of stab incisions for instrument access in laparoscopic operations. J Pediatr Surg 38:1837-1840, 2003
8. Rothenberg SS: The first decade's experience with laparoscopic Nissen fundoplication in infants and children. J Pediatr Surg 40:142-147, 2005
9. St. Peter SD, Valusek PA, Calkins CM, et al: Use of esophagocrural sutures and minimal esophageal dissection reduces the incidence of postoperative transmigration of laparoscopic Nissen fundoplication wrap. J Pediatr Surg 42:25-29, 2007

4
Laparoscopic Thal Fundoplication

Klaas (N) M. A. Bax

Gastroesophageal reflux (GER) is a common problem in children, and even more common in the neurologically impaired population. Although medication can often alleviate the negative impact of acid reflux on the esophagus and airways, non–acid reflux with poor weight gain or symptoms of pulmonary aspiration may still persist. An open approach for surgical management of reflux has become obsolete. All antireflux operations can now be performed endoscopically. After much debate about the best procedure, it is generally thought that all are effective, provided the surgeon has experience in the technique.

INDICATIONS FOR WORKUP AND OPERATION

Symptomatic GER not responding to medical treatment or recurring after medication withdrawal is an indication for operation. There is no consensus regarding the ideal method to diagnose pathologic gastroesophageal reflux. Most pediatric surgeons agree that the history is very important in making this diagnosis. It is helpful when a pH study confirms the clinical diagnosis of pathologic reflux, but the history is not always concordant with the results of the pH study. Pathologic reflux is not necessarily acid reflux. To detect non–acid reflux, impedance measurement and ultrasonography can be diagnostic, but the literature on these diagnostic tools in children is scant. A barium swallow excludes anatomic abnormalities such as a hiatal hernia or gastric outlet or duodenal obstruction. Esophagoscopy should be performed when esophagitis is suspected to document the degree of this complication, and it should be repeated to check the response to medical treatment. Currently, there is not a sensitive test to prove a causal relationship between pulmonary symptoms and GER. The issue of delayed gastric emptying causing pathologic gastroesophageal reflux is a difficult one, as normal values in children are not available and as delayed gastric emptying may improve after fundoplication. In neurologically impaired children in need of a gastrostomy, concomitant antireflux surgery has been advocated. Gastrostomy feedings in such children without concomitant antireflux surgery, however, may improve the nutritional state of these children, and this may have a positive effect on GER. There is no hard evidence that a gastrostomy initiates GER. The decision to carry out antireflux surgery in neurologically impaired children in need of a gastrostomy should be staged: first a gastrostomy, and then antireflux surgery if symptoms of GER persist or occur de novo.

Preoperatively, all patients receive an enema to empty the colon, as a feces- or gas-loaded colon interferes with optimal visualization.

OPERATIVE TECHNIQUE

General anesthesia supplemented with low thoracic epidural analgesia is preferred. Full muscle relaxation is maintained throughout the procedure.

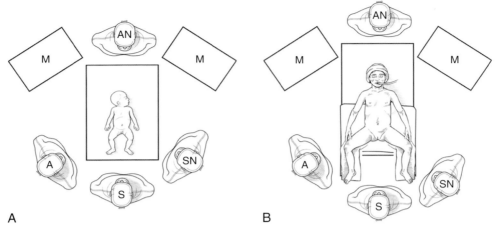

Figure 4-1. The position of the patient, operating personnel, and equipment for a laparoscopic Thal fundoplication. **A,** Small children are placed in a frogleg position at the lower end of the operating table. **B,** Larger children are placed supine at the lower end of the table with their legs abducted on leg supports. The surgeon (S) stands at the foot of the bed with the assistant (A) to the surgeon's left. AN, anesthesiologist; M, monitor; SN, scrub nurse.

Depending on the size of the child, a nasogastric tube (26 to 28 or 30 Fr) is positioned in the stomach. The tube is used for emptying of the stomach, for identification of the distal esophagus, and for avoiding narrowing of the hiatus when applying the posterior crural suture. A urinary catheter is inserted because of the epidural analgesia and maintained as long as the epidural analgesia is administered, which is usually until the next morning.

Small children are placed in a frogleg position at the lower end of the operating table (Fig. 4-1). The legs are enveloped with the sheet that covers the table to avoid the child's slipping off the table when the table is put in a reverse Trendelenburg position. Larger children are placed supine at the lower end of the table with their legs abducted on leg supports. The legs are wrapped to the leg supports for the reason just mentioned. The surgeon stands at the lower end of the operating table or in between the legs. The camera person, when right-handed, stands to the left of the surgeon, the scrub nurse to the right. Two monitors at either side of the head of the patient are used. The use of two screens in all types of endoscopic surgery is standard, but in anti-reflux surgery, one will suffice. When the child is severely scoliotic and spastic, the patient's position has to be adapted accordingly. It is advantageous to imagine where the hiatus in such a patient is located and to mark were the telescope and other ports should be inserted. Once this is done, it becomes obvious where the surgeon, the camera person, and the scrub nurse should be positioned. The final position of the secondary ports is decided after the telescope has been inserted and the patient's anatomy is seen.

All cables, usually seven (camera, light cable, CO_2 tube, suction, irrigation, internal monopolar high-frequency electrocautery [HFE], and external HFE), come from the same side. No other energy-applying systems are needed.

Only reusable cannulas and instruments are used. All cannulas have a siliconized sleeve. A 6-mm cannula is introduced in an open way through the infraumbilical fold (Fig. 4-2). The umbilical opening is made so small that the cannula with the blunt trocar dilates the opening, which helps avoid a gas leak. The cannula is secured in place with a 2-0 Vicryl (Ethicon, Inc., Somerville, NJ) suture that incorporates the skin and fascia and is tied to the stopcock on the cannula to keep the cannula from pulling out. A 5-mm 30-degree telescope is used. After verification that the cannula is in the peritoneal cavity, CO_2 pneumoperitoneum is started at a preset pressure of 8 mm Hg and a flow of 2 L/min in small children and 5 L/min in older children. Next, a 3.8-mm sleeved cannula is inserted in the patient's right hypochondrium for the surgeon's left-hand 3.5-mm instruments. Symmetrically, in the patient's left hypochondrium, a 6-mm cannula is inserted for the surgeon's right-hand instruments. The covering cap is replaced with a cap for 3.5-mm instruments, which allows for the introduction of 3-0 Ethibond (Ethicon, Inc., Somerville, NJ) sutures on a V-5 needle with a 3.5-mm needle grasper. Such a needle can be introduced through the cannula without the need for straightening it. Another sleeved 3.8-mm cannula is inserted subcostally at the anterior axillary line on the left for a fenestrated forceps with ratchet, which is used to grasp the stomach. This grasper is held by the scrub nurse.

Finally, an appropriate-size blade of a Nathanson (Mediflex Surgical Products, Islandia, NY) retractor is introduced directly below the xiphoid process and is positioned under the left lobe of the liver, thus exposing

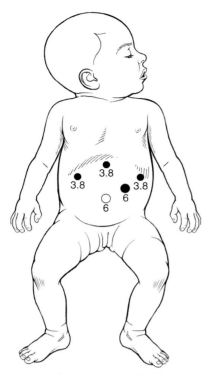

Figure 4-2. The position of the cannulas for a laparoscopic Thal fundoplication. The umbilical port is 6 mm in size and is introduced through an incision in the infraumbilical fold. A 3.8-mm sleeved cannula is inserted in the patient's right epigastric region for the surgeon's left-hand 3.5-mm instruments. Symmetrically, in the patient's left epigastrium, a 6-mm cannula is inserted for the surgeon's right-hand instruments. A 3.8-mm sleeved cannula is inserted subcostally in the anterior axillary line on the patient's left. A grasper placed through this port is held by the scrub nurse. In the subxiphoid port (shown as 3.8 mm), a 3.5-mm endoscopic grasper is inserted to retract the liver in small children. In larger children, an appropriate-sized Nathanson retractor is introduced at this site and positioned under the left lobe of the liver.

the anterior hiatus (Fig. 4-3). The blade is secured to the supporting device, which is mounted on the rail of the operating table. Alternatively, in small children, a 3.5-mm Allis-type endoscopic grasper is inserted through a subxiphoidal 3.8-mm cannula. The grasper is positioned under the left lobe of the liver and is secured to the anterior edge of the hiatus. This grasper does not need any support.

The cardioesophageal area is put under tension by grabbing and pushing the anterior stomach inferiorly. The dissection is started by incising the hepatogastric ligament close to the right crus longitudinally with scissors (Fig. 4-4A). The hepatic branches of the vagus nerve are not divided. If there is an aberrant left hepatic artery, it usually runs at the junction of the hard and flaccid parts of the hepatogastric ligament. Next, the loose ligaments fixing the fundus to the diaphragm are detached,

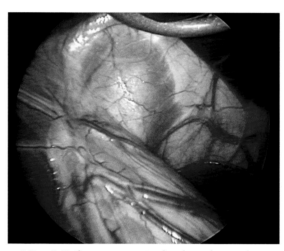

Figure 4-3. A Nathanson retractor has been inserted underneath the left lobe of the liver, which exposes the hiatal area beautifully.

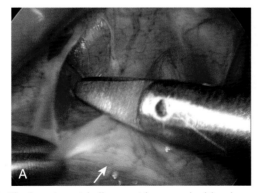

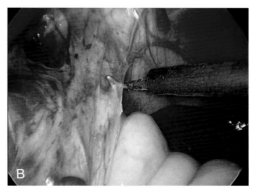

Figure 4-4. **A,** The hepatogastric ligament is opened with scissors above the hepatic branches of the anterior vagus nerve (*arrow*). **B,** The anterior phreno-esophageal ligament is being incised from the patient's left side.

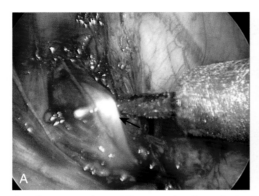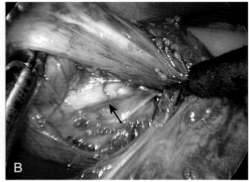

Figure 4-5. **A,** The phreno-esophageal ligament has been incised anteriorly, and the anterior vagus nerve is seen (*arrow*). **B,** A window posterior to the esophagus and posterior vagus nerve (*arrow*) has been created.

again using hook diathermy, while the grabbing instrument pushes the stomach inferiorly and to the right. In this way, the lateral part of the left crus comes into view. The anterior phreno-esophageal ligament is incised with the hook electrocautery from left to right, taking care not to injure the anterior vagus nerve (see Fig. 4-4B). The anterior part of the hiatus is opened bluntly and the anterior vagus nerve is identified (Fig. 4-5A). Next, the groove between the esophagus and the left crus is dissected using blunt dissection and hook electrocautery. Opening of the crus itself should be avoided, and the thin fascial layer covering the crura should be left intact. Next, the stomach is pushed inferiorly and to the left, and the groove between the esophagus and the right crus is dissected free using blunt dissection and electrocautery. The pars flaccida is opened, and the peritoneum between the right crus and the stomach is opened up. The groove between the esophagus and the right crus is dissected farther until the posterior part of the hiatus comes into view. The esophagus with the nasogastric tube in situ is elevated with the surgeon's left-handed instrument. The retroesophageal space is bluntly dissected with identification of the posterior vagus nerve, which may or may not lie somewhat separate from the esophagus (Fig. 4-5B). Once the vagus nerve is identified, the nerve is lifted up together with the esophagus and the retroesophageal space is created until the left subdiaphragmatic space is reached. The direction of the dissection of the retroesophageal space is rather transverse. One should not dissect obliquely into the hiatus, as this may injure the left mediastinal pleura or the left crus. It may be advantageous during the dissection of the retroesophageal space to pull the nasogastric tube back into the esophagus. A vessel loop is inserted through the 6-mm cannula in the left hypochondrium and positioned around the distal esophagus above the hepatic branches of the anterior vagus nerve. The ends of the vessel loop are clipped together anteriorly with two metal clips using a nondisposable instrument (Fig. 4-6). The grasping forceps introduced subcostally now grabs the ends of the vessel loop distal to the clips. By

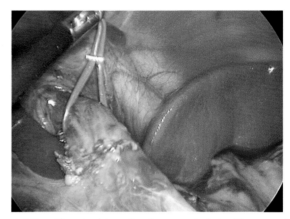

Figure 4-6. The esophagus has been encircled with a vessel loop.

pulling on the vessel loop, further mobilization of the distal esophagus is easily accomplished using blunt and hook electrocautery dissection. The short gastric vessels are not divided.

The posterior hiatus is closed with one 3-0 Ethibond suture introduced with a 3.5-mm needle holder through the 6-mm cannula in the left hypochondrium. This can be started from the right or from the left side of the esophagus. A portion of the left crus is taken that includes the thin fascial layer rather than the muscle fibers. Next, a portion of posterior esophagus is secured and finally a bite of the right crus, again taking the fascial layer rather than the muscle fibers (Fig. 4-7). The suture is then tied while the nasogastric tube is in the stomach to avoid narrowing of the esophagus. Next, an anterior fundoplication is performed with two rows of three interrupted 3-0 Ethibond sutures (Fig. 4-8A). The first row starts on the left. A portion of stomach is taken at the greater curvature at a distance of about 1 cm from the angle of His. Next, a bite of esophagus is taken on the left about halfway down the intra-abdominal part of the esophagus. This suture is then tied. The second suture takes the anterior gastric wall in the middle, about 1 cm distal to the fat pad, and is secured to the anterior esophageal wall about halfway down its intra-abdominal length. Care is taken not to include the anterior vagus nerve. The third suture secures the anterior gastric wall on the right, again 1 cm below the fat pad, as well as the esophageal wall on the right, halfway down its intra-abdominal length. The vessel loop is now removed and a second row of three sutures is inserted (see Fig. 4-8B). The first suture approximates the anterior gastric wall on the left, close to the greater curvature about 1 cm cephalad to the previous suture, to the left esophageal wall, close to the diaphragm and upper left crus. A bite of adjacent diaphragm is incorporated as well. The second suture secures the anterior gastric wall, about 1 cm cephalad to the middle suture of the first row, to the anterior esophageal wall close to and including part of the diaphragm. The final suture approximates the anterior gastric wall on the right, about 1 cm cephalad to the third suture of the first row, to the esophageal wall on the right, close to and including the diaphragm or upper right crus.

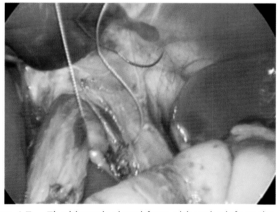

Figure 4-7. The hiatus is closed from either the left or the right, depending on the surgeon's preference, incorporating part of the posterior esophagus with this suture.

If a gastrostomy is needed, the anesthesiologist is asked to inflate the stomach with 50 mL of air, which rotates the greater curvature slightly anteriorly and allows the surgeon to decide where the gastrostomy should be positioned, which is usually at the junction of the fundus and the corpus. This region is grasped and brought to the anterior abdominal wall. The shortest distance is chosen, but the linea alba is avoided. Usually a position in the mid epigastrium, but slightly to the patient's left of the middle line, is identified. Undue traction is avoided. A stab incision is made, through which the stomach is grasped and exteriorized. Four 5-0 Vicryl sutures attach the seromuscular gastric wall to the skin, taking only very small bites of skin. Next, the stomach is punctured with a needle, and a guidewire is inserted through the hole. An appropriate peel-away sheath and catheter is then inserted into the stomach. This process is watched under laparoscopic control. The cannulas are removed under vision. The 6-mm cannula sites are closed with Vicryl to the fascia and Steri-Strips (3M Co., St. Paul, MN) to the skin. The nasogastric tube is then removed.

POSTOPERATIVE CARE

Postoperatively, epidural analgesia supplemented with paracetamol suppositories is given. The next morning, the epidural analgesia is discontinued but the paracetamol is continued for another day. Liquid feeding is started the next morning, and when this goes well, normal oral feeding is started. The patient is usually discharged the second day after surgery. Occasionally there is dysphagia. When this occurs, liquid feeding is continued at home for 2 to 3 weeks.

In patients who have been fed by a nasogastric tube preoperatively, gastrostomy feeding is started the morning after surgery. The first day, half the requirements are given, and full requirements the second postoperative day.

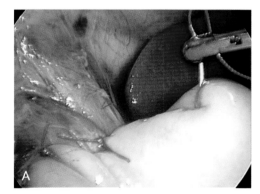
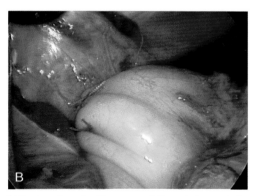

Figure 4-8. **A,** The anterior stomach, about 1 cm below the angle of His, is sutured with a row of three interrupted sutures to the esophagus, halfway down its intra-abdominal length. **B,** A second row of three interrupted sutures secures the anterior stomach wall to the esophagus and adjacent diaphragm.

PEARLS

1. Do not jeopardize the operation by not having good port position. An extra port is better than a difficult operation.
2. In larger children, it may be advantageous to insert the telescope cannula halfway between the xiphoid process and the umbilicus.
3. Good retraction of the left lobe of the liver makes hiatal surgery much easier. A Nathanson retractor achieves this goal.
4. For the Thal fundoplication, there is no need to divide the hepatic branches of the anterior vagal nerve or the short gastric vessels.
5. Encircling the distal esophagus with a vessel loop allows dissection of the esophagus, insertion of the posterior hiatal suture, and placement of the first row of three fundoplication sutures relatively easily.
6. Having a large nasogastric tube in place when tying the posterior hiatal suture avoids narrowing of the esophagus.

PITFALLS

1. Be aware for an aberrant left hepatic artery.
2. The anterior vagus nerve lies close to both the phreno-esophageal ligament and the esophagus. Early identification is imperative. The posterior vagal nerve lies at a distance from the esophagus and is easier to identify.
3. The location of the gastrostomy should be dictated by intraoperative evaluation, especially in view of the fact that the anterior gastric wall has been used for creation of the fundoplication. Be aware that too distal an insertion can cause retching and vomiting.

RESULTS

Between 1993 and 2002, 149 children underwent 157 laparoscopic antireflux procedures. Nearly half of the children were neurologically impaired. The median follow-up has been 4.5 years. Nineteen children died; none of the deaths was related to the antireflux surgery. The results were good in 120 children (80.5%), but the results were less than optimal in 29 children (19.5%). Eight children underwent reoperation (5.4%). None of the children with a follow-up longer than 5 years have developed symptoms related to GER. The Thal fundoplication is a safe procedure with favorable long-term results, even in the neurologically impaired group.

SELECTED REFERENCES

1. Hament JM, Bax NM, van der Zee DC, et al: Complications of percutaneous endoscopic gastrostomy with or without concomitant antireflux surgery in 96 children. J Pediatr Surg 36:1412-1415, 2001
2. van der Zee DC, Bax KN, Ure BM, et al: Long-term results after laparoscopic Thal procedure in children. Semin Laparosc Surg 9:168-171, 2002
3. Esposito C, van der Zee DC, Settimi A, et al: Risks and benefits of surgical management of gastroesophageal reflux in neurologically impaired children. Surg Endosc 17:708-710, 2003
4. Ludemann R, Watson DI, Jamieson GG, et al: Five-year follow-up of a randomized clinical trial of laparoscopic total versus anterior 180 degrees fundoplication. Br J Surg 92:240-243, 2005

5
Laparoscopic Esophagomyotomy

Girolamo Mattioli, Alessio Pini Prato, and Vincenzo Jasonni

E sophageal achalasia (EA) is a rare functional disorder of the esophagus characterized by abnormal motility of the esophageal body (nonperistaltic waves) associated with incomplete, delayed, or absent relaxation of the lower esophageal sphincter (LES). The incidence is about 0.3 to 11 per million population per year, with a prevalence of about 80 per million population. Only 5% of the patients suffering from this disease are younger than 15 years of age.

Although EA is usually considered an acquired esophageal motility disorder, several studies have suggested that genetic background may play a role in its development, especially in children. Although the etiology and pathogenesis remain controversial, the abnormal esophageal motility in EA seems to result from defects in or imbalance between the excitatory and inhibitory neuromuscular transmitters.

Many different treatments have been proposed including pharmacologic agents (calcium blockers, sildenafil, or isosorbide dinitrate), pneumatic dilation, removable self-expanding metal stents, and injection of botulin toxin. However, the results are transitory, and repeated treatments are frequently required. The only means to definitively relieve symptoms is esophagomyotomy. In 1914, Heller described an anterior–posterior esophageal myotomy. Later, Zaaijer and colleagues proposed an anterior myotomy alone for the same purpose. These techniques should be associated with a fundoplication, aimed at avoiding postoperative gastroesophageal reflux and protecting the esophageal mucosa. A partial anterior fundoplication (the Dor procedure) is the most effective in reducing the risk of stenosis or recurrence of achalasia and in preventing gastroesophageal reflux (GER). A laparoscopic modified Heller-Dor procedure is therefore the treatment of choice for EA.

INDICATIONS FOR WORKUP AND OPERATION

The onset of symptomatic EA is variable. Almost all patients present with fluid dysphagia ("paroxysmal dysphagia"), retention, and regurgitation of undigested food. Chest pain is described in up to 40% of patients. Pulmonary inhalation, failure to thrive, and halitosis are associated symptoms.

In any case of suspected EA, the patient should undergo a barium contrast study, a 24-hour esophageal pH study, esophageal manometry, and esophagogas-troduodenoscopy. The contrast study usually shows a dilated esophagus (megaesophagus) that funnels to a stricture of the distal esophagus ("mouse tail" or "bird beak" sign) (Fig. 5-1). The 24-hour esophageal pH monitoring excludes the presence of concomitant gastroesophageal reflux disease. The esophagogastroduodenoscopy should demonstrate the absence of any stricture or mucosal abnormality. Finally, the diagnosis is reached with esophageal manometry that demonstrates the absence of normal esophageal motility (nonperistaltic waves) and of post-deglutitive LES relaxation. Operative intervention is recommended after diagnostic confirmation.

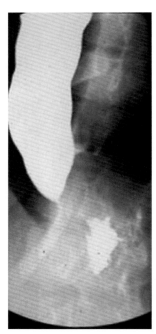

Figure 5-1. The typical appearance of achalasia is seen on this esophagram. The esophagus is dilated above the constricted lower esophageal sphincter.

PREOPERATIVE PREPARATION

Three days before surgery, the patients are fed only fluids to allow the distal esophagus to empty and to prevent retained food in the distal esophagus at the time of the procedure. The day before surgery, the patients are kept in a fasting state. Enemas are administered both the day before and early in the morning of surgery to reduce colonic distention.

Once in the operating room, a nasogastric tube is introduced when the patient is still awake to evacuate and decompress the dilated esophagus and stomach and to reduce the risk of aspiration during tracheal intubation. A clean esophagus is mandatory to minimize spill of contents in the event of inadvertent mucosal perforation.

OPERATIVE TECHNIQUE

The patient is placed supine in the lithotomy and reverse Trendelenburg position, and general endotracheal anesthesia is administered. Skin preparation with meticulous scrubbing of the umbilicus is performed. The operative field should include the whole abdomen from the pubis to the sternum and laterally to the anterior axillary lines in case conversion to an open operation is required.

The surgeon stands between patient's legs. The assistant holding the telescope is on the patient's right and the assistant surgeon is on the patient's left. The monitor

is positioned on the right of the patient at the head of the table (Fig. 5-2A). A five-port technique is used. We prefer to use 5-mm ports in younger children and to use 10-mm ports in adolescents (see Fig. 5-2B). The first cannula (5 or 10 mm) is inserted in the umbilicus. CO_2 insufflation is used to create a pneumoperitoneum up to 12 mm Hg. Similarly, as in all laparoscopic hiatal procedures, four additional cannulas are inserted in a semicircular pattern: (a) left paraumbilical (5 mm) for the retraction of the stomach during dissection, (b) left subcostal (5 mm) and (c) right subcostal as working ports, and (d) epigastric or subxiphoid (5 or 3 mm) for retraction of the liver.

The anterior gastric wall is grasped to retract the esophagus downward. The esophageal wall is grasped on each side of the planned site of the myotomy, and the muscle fibers are bluntly spread to expose the submucosa (Fig. 5-3A). A Maryland dissecting instrument is then used to create a plane between the submucosa and muscle fibers (see Fig. 5-3B). Using either the hook cautery or an ultrasonic scalpel, the esophageal muscle fibers are incised and coagulated cephalad into the lower mediastinum (Fig. 5-4). The myotomy then is directed caudally through the circular esophageal fibers at the LES (Fig. 5-5). The length of the myotomy is established by intraoperative manometry or by resorting to specific landmarks. Our landmark for the proximal end of the dissection is the proximal dilated esophagus where it is crossed by the anterior vagal nerve that moves from the left esophageal side to the anterior wall. The distal landmark is the transverse esophageal vessel, which crosses the esophagogastric junction (Fig. 5-6). A complete myotomy is demonstrated by mucosal herniation (Fig. 5-7). Mucosal integrity is checked by insufflating air inside the esophagus through the nasogastric tube. Mucosal herniation is protected using an anterior 180-degree anterior gastric fundoplication (Dor). The anterior face of the stomach is initially fixed to the left muscular edge of the esophageal myotomy and left crus, then to the right side of the myotomy, and finally to a portion of the right crus using nonabsorbable, interrupted synthetic sutures (Fig. 5-8).

Clear fluids and broad-spectrum short-term antibiotic prophylaxis (piperacillin) are administered intravenously during the first 24 hours postoperatively. The patients are fed on postoperative day 1 after a water-soluble esophageal contrast study is performed to detect leakage or incomplete myotomy.

PEARLS

1. We suggest dissecting only the anterior esophageal wall and mediastinum to reduce the risk of GER.
2. It is mandatory to perform a high myotomy in the mediastinum (up to the dilated esophagus or to the previously described landmark) and low onto the

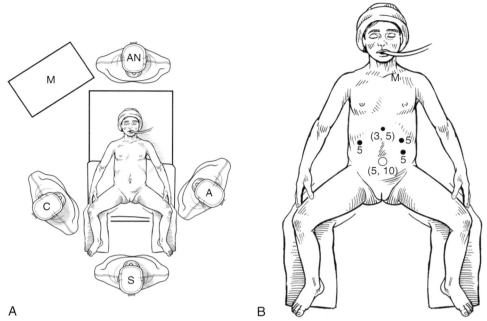

Figure 5-2. The patient is positioned supine and in stirrups. **A,** The surgeon (S) stands between the patient's legs for optimal ergonomics. The camera holder (C) is on the patient's right and the assistant surgeon (A) is on the patient's left. The monitor is positioned to the right of the patient at the head of the operating table. **B,** A five-port technique is employed. The first cannula is inserted in the umbilicus. A 5- or 10-mm angled telescope is introduced through this umbilical port. Four additional cannulas are inserted in a semicircular pattern. Left and right subcostal ports are used as working ports for the surgeon. An epigastric or subxiphoid port (5 or 3 mm) is used for introduction of the liver retractor. A 5-mm left paraumbilical site is used by the assistant for retraction of the stomach during dissection. AN, anesthesiologist.

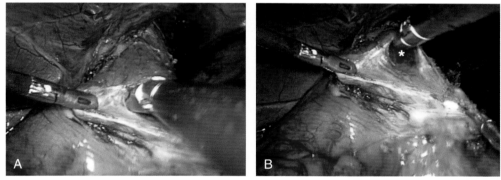

Figure 5-3. **A,** The esophageal wall is grasped on each side of the planned myotomy, and the muscle fibers are spread bluntly using the Maryland dissector to expose the submucosa. **B,** The plane between the submucosa (*asterisk*) and overlying muscle fibers is then entered and enlarged.

stomach (down to the transverse vessels previously described) (Figs. 5-4 through 5-7).

3. The myotomy should be carried out with a hook diathermy pulling the muscle fibers far from the mucosa to avoid mucosal burns or perforation. Alternatively, the ultrasonic scalpel with the "hot" side anteriorly can also be used.

4. The anterior fundoplication is performed to reduce the development of GER and to minimize leakage in case of mucosal perforation. It should always be performed in association with a modified Heller procedure (Fig. 5-8).

5. Immediately before re-alimentation, each patient should undergo a water-soluble contrast study to exclude recurrence, residual disease, perforation, and GER.

PITFALLS

1. Pneumatic dilation of the esophagus should be avoided, as this treatment carries a high risk of complication and makes it harder to perform a subsequent Heller-Dor procedure.

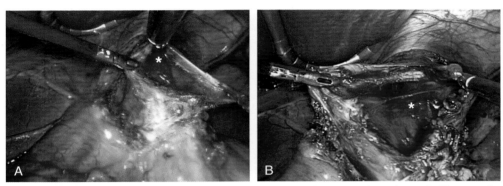

Figure 5-4. **A,** Using the hook cautery (or ultrasonic scalpel in this photograph), the esophageal muscle fibers are incised and coagulated cephalad into the lower mediastinum. **B,** The plane between the submucosa (*asterisk*) and the longitudinal muscle fibers is well visualized.

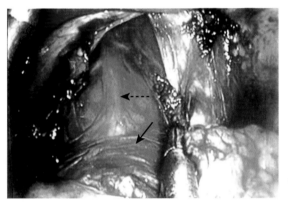

Figure 5-5. Caudally, the myotomy proceeds through the circular esophageal fibers (*solid arrow*) at the level of the LES. Note the anterior vagus nerve as it courses over the submucosa (*dotted arrow*).

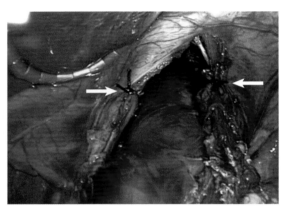

Figure 5-7. The upper portion of the completed esophagomyotomy. The edges of the myotomy have been sutured to the left and right crura (*arrows*) to prevent re-apposition of the muscular edges.

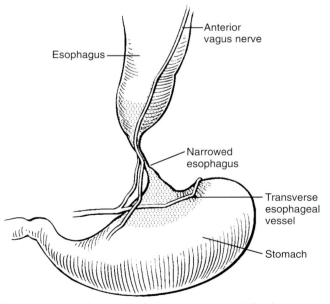

Figure 5-6. Our landmarks for the proximal and distal extent of the dissection (*stippled area*) are the proximal dilated esophagus where it is crossed by the anterior vagus nerve that moves from the left side of the esophagus to an anterior position. Distally, our landmark is the transverse esophageal vessel at the esophagogastric junction.

RESULTS

Since January 1994, 17 children have undergone the operation. The mean age at operation was 10 years (range, 5 to 14) and the mean weight was 45 kg (25 to 72). Four patients were female and 13 were male. All the procedures were accomplished laparoscopically. The mean operative time was 125 minutes (range, 90 to 180). In no patient did we experience a mucosal perforation. Bleeding from an esophageal vessel occurred in one case, and clip positioning was required. No patient needed transfusion or reoperation.

The nasogastric tube was removed soon after awakening in 11 of 17 patients and on postoperative day 1 in the remaining six children. No patient was found to have a leak on the esophageal contrast study. All patients were fed by mouth on postoperative day 1 with fluid meals and were sent home with full oral feeding by postoperative day 3.

All the patients were seen and examined postoperatively to detect early postoperative complications and followed to identify recurrence of symptoms resulting

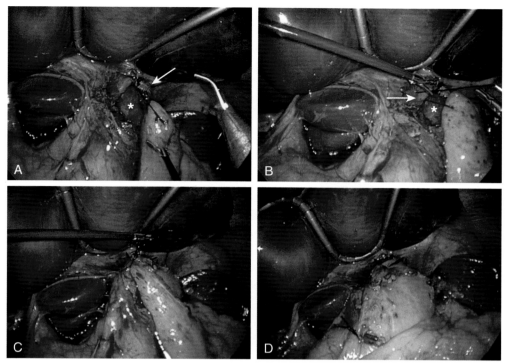

Figure 5-8.   A Dor fundoplication is performed after the esophagomyotomy. **A,** The anterior portion of the stomach is initially fixed to the muscular edge of the myotomy (*arrow*) and crus on the patient's left side. **B,** It is then secured to the muscular edge of the myotomy and crus (*arrow*) on the right side. In both **A** and **B**, the submucosa of the esophagus is marked with an *asterisk*. **C,** The anterior stomach is then secured to the lateral portion of the patient's right crus to keep it in an anterior position. **D,** Finally, the anterior stomach is sutured to the right border of the stomach to take tension off the other sutures.

from stricture or the appearance of gastroesophageal reflux. The Visick symptoms score was used to evaluate postoperative outcome: 1, no symptoms; 2, better than before surgery; 3, no modifications; 4, new symptoms or complications.

The mean follow-up was 50 months (range, 6 to 102). The postoperative clinical score was Visick 1 in 14 cases and Visick 2 in three cases. In one of these three children, symptoms reappeared 6 months after surgery and completely disappeared after one esophageal dilation. Another patient was neurologically impaired and required parental care for feeding. The final patient developed dysphagia but did not have a recurrence or a stricture as evaluated by esophageal barium meal and endoscopy. No patient developed gastroesophageal reflux on postoperative pH monitoring.

SELECTED REFERENCES

1. Heller E: Extramukose cardioplastik beim chronischen Cardiospasmus mit dilatation des Ösophagus. Mitt Grenzgeb Med Chir 27:141-145, 1914
2. Nihoul Fekete C, Bawab F, Lortat Jacob J, et al: Achalasia of the esophagus in childhood: Surgical treatment in 35 cases, with special reference to familial cases and gluco-corticoid deficiency association. Hepatogastroenterology 38:510-513, 1991
3. Myers NA, Jolley SG, Taylor R: Achalasia of the cardia in children: A worldwide survey. J Pediatr Surg 29:1375-1379, 1994
4. Bortolotti M, Mari C, Lopilato C: Effects of sildenafil on esophageal motility of patients with idiopathic achalasia. Gastroenterology 118:253-257, 2000
5. Hurwitz M, Bahar RJ, Ament ME: Evaluation of the use of Botulin toxin in children with achalasia. J Pediatr Gastroenterol Nutr 30:509-514, 2000
6. Mayberry JF: Epidemiology and demographics of achalasia. Gastrointest Endosc Clin N Am 11:235-248, 2001
7. Mehra M, Bahar RJ, Ament ME: Laparoscopic and thoracoscopic esophagomyotomy for children with achalasia. J Pediatr Gastroenterol Nutr 33:466-471, 2001
8. Paterson WG: Etiology and pathogenesis of achalasia. Gastrointest Endosc Clin N Am 11:249-266, 2001
9. Patti MG, Albanese CT, Holcomb GW III, et al: Laparoscopic Heller myotomy and Dor fundoplication for esophageal achalasia in children. J Pediatr Surg 36:1248-1251, 2001
10. Watanabe Y, Ando H, Seo T, et al: Attenuated nitrergic neurotransmission to interstitial cells of Cajal in the lower esophageal sphincter with esophageal achalasia in children. Pediatr Int 44:145-148, 2002
11. Mattioli G, Esposito C, Pini Prato A, et al: Results of the laparoscopic Heller-Dor procedure for pediatric esophageal achalasia. Surg Endosc 17:1650-1652, 2003

6
Laparoscopic Gastrostomy

Michael V. Tirabassi and Keith E. Georgeson

Creation of a gastrostomy is one of the procedures most frequently performed by a pediatric surgeon. The three most common options for surgical gastrostomy are open Stamm gastrostomy, percutaneous endoscopic gastrostomy (PEG), and laparoscopically assisted gastrostomy. Stamm gastrostomy, the most invasive of these options, requires a laparotomy. This technique offers the security of suture fixation of the stomach to the abdominal wall and a purse-string suture around the gastrostomy tube as it penetrates the gastric wall. Percutaneous endoscopic gastrostomy, the least invasive, fails to allow the surgeon visualization of the tube's pathway within the peritoneal space. PEG also fails to provide any suture fixation of the stomach to the abdominal wall. Appropriate siting of the gastrostomy within the stomach is possible, but less precise, using the PEG technique. Laparoscopically assisted gastrostomy affords the safety of both temporary suture fixation of the stomach to the abdominal wall and visualization of the gastrostomy button's path through the peritoneal space during placement. Additionally, the site of penetration through the stomach wall can also be carefully selected.

INDICATIONS FOR WORKUP AND OPERATION

Feeding gastrostomy is needed in children who have failure to thrive or swallowing difficulties. Failure to thrive may be secondary to inadequate caloric intake, inadequate absorption, an increased metabolic state, or defective caloric utilization. Gastroesophageal reflux disease (GERD) may contribute to failure to thrive. GERD should be considered in any child referred for feeding gastrostomy, because a child with failure to thrive and GERD may be a candidate for concurrent fundoplication at the time of the gastrostomy. The underlying mechanisms for failure to thrive should be carefully considered before a decision is made to insert a gastrostomy tube or button.

OPERATIVE TECHNIQUE

General anesthesia is used for most laparoscopic gastrostomy procedures. Some children referred for feeding gastrostomy have chronic pulmonary or cardiac disease. Preoperative evaluation of the child should include assessment of cardiac and respiratory status. Additionally, the procedure should not be performed while a child has signs or symptoms of an acute illness, a skin infection near the operative site, or suboptimal treatment of a chronic disease.

Small infants and children are positioned supine at the end of the table in a frogleg position and secured with tape to the operating table (Fig. 6-1A). The surgeon stands on the patient's left side and the camera holder is at the foot of the bed. A single monitor is placed above the head of the patient (Fig. 6-1B). Larger children are positioned supine with their legs together and extended. A single 3- or 5-mm cannula is inserted through the umbilicus for introduction of the telescope or camera. This location for the telescope allows good visualization of the gastric wall and the peritoneal space between the abdominal wall and the stomach. Before insufflation, an appropriate site for the gastrostomy should be marked in the left upper abdomen, taking care to stay away from the subcostal margin. This site will be the location for insertion of the instrument to grasp the stomach and bring it to the anterior abdominal wall (Fig. 6-2).

After establishing a pneumoperitoneum to a pressure of 10 to 12 mm Hg through the umbilical cannula, a

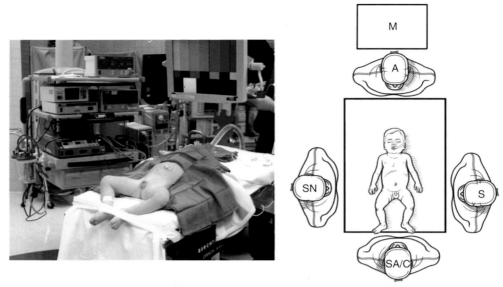

Figure 6-1. Infants and small children are positioned supine at the end of the table in a frogleg position and secured with tape to the operating table. Personnel positioning is shown in the diagram. The surgeon (S) stands on the patient's left side, with the surgical assistant/camera holder (SA/C) positioned at the foot of the bed. A single monitor (M) is placed above the head of the patient. The scrub nurse (SN) is usually across from the surgeon. A, anesthesiologist.

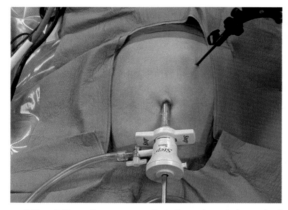

Figure 6-2. A 3- or 5-mm cannula is introduced through the umbilicus, and an adequate pneumoperitoneum is created. A stab incision is made in the patient's left upper quadrant at the site of the gastrostomy and a 3-mm grasping instrument is introduced at this site.

30- or 45-degree telescope is inserted and directed toward the left upper quadrant. The stomach is insufflated with 30 to 60 cc of air through a red rubber catheter inserted into the stomach by the anesthesiologist (Fig. 6-3A). Insufflating the stomach should help prevent the back wall from being incorporated with the stay stitches. A locking grasper is then inserted through the premarked site in the left upper quadrant and is used to grasp the anterior wall of the stomach at the location selected for the gastrostomy site (Fig. 6-3B). This site is approximately two thirds of the distance from the gastroesophageal junction to the pylorus and

should not be too close to the pylorus or fundus. Care should be taken to avoid injury to the gastroepiploic vessels.

The gastrostomy site on the stomach is grasped with the jaws of the grasper at right angles to the visual plane between the scope and the grasper. Using 2-0 monofilament, U-stitches are passed through the abdominal wall parallel to the axis of the telescope, taking at least a 1-cm bite of gastric wall. The U-suture is then passed back through the abdominal wall (Fig. 6-4). The four ends of the two U-stitches should form a square, with the left upper quadrant instrument in the middle of the square. A variety of sutures can be utilized as the U-stitches. Monofilament suture seems to work best. For most infants, 0-PDS on a CT-1 needle (Ethicon, Inc., Somerville, NJ) works well. For infants in the intensive care nursery, a 2-0 PDS on an SH needle is used. For adolescents and patients with a large amount of subcutaneous tissue, a 1 PDS or a 2 Prolene (Ethicon, Inc.) is needed.

The stomach grasper is then removed. The Cook vascular dilator set (Cook, Inc., Bloomington, IN) is used for this operation. A needle from the Cook set is inserted into the stomach through the left upper quadrant stab incision. This needle pierces the stomach in the middle of the square formed by the U-sutures (Fig. 6-5). Entrance into the lumen of the stomach is marked by the sudden release of the air previously introduced into the stomach by the anesthesiologist through the orogastric tube. A J-tipped guidewire from the Cook set is advanced through the needle into the stomach. The needle is then removed. Sequential dilation of the abdominal wall

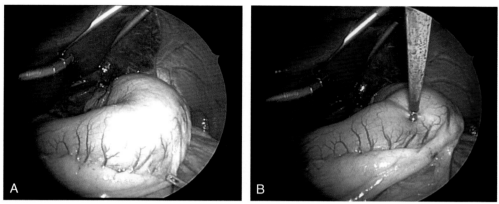

Figure 6-3. A, The stomach has been inflated with 60 cc of air that was introduced through a red rubber catheter positioned in the stomach by the anesthesiologist. Insufflating the stomach should help prevent the back wall of the stomach from being incorporated with the U-stitches. **B,** The locking grasper has been inserted through the left upper quadrant and is being used to grasp the anterior wall of the stomach at the selected location for the gastrostomy.

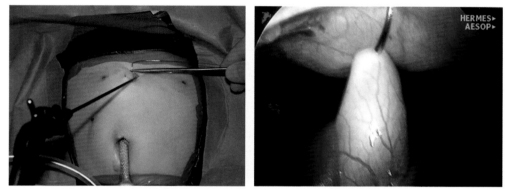

Figure 6-4. The patient undergoing the laparoscopic gastrostomy has also undergone a laparoscopic fundoplication (note incisions). A locking grasper has been inserted through the left upper abdominal working port and secured to the stomach at the site for the gastrostomy. With the anterior wall of the stomach delivered near the anterior abdominal wall, two monofilament U-stitches are passed through the abdominal wall parallel to the axis of the telescope, taking at least a 1-cm bite of the stomach. The U-suture is then passed out through the abdominal wall.
(Reprinted with permission from Holcomb GW III: Gastroesophageal reflux disease in infants and children. In Fischer FE [ed]: Mastery of Surgery [ed 5]. Philadelphia, Lippincott Williams & Wilkins, pp 650-661, 2007.)

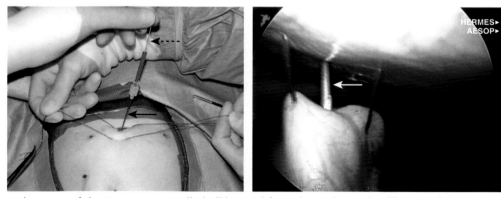

Figure 6-5. After placement of the U-sutures, a needle (*solid arrows*) from the Cook vascular dilator set is introduced through the incision on the anterior abdominal wall and into the stomach. The U-sutures are placed on tension for ease of placing the needle through the center of the square formed by the U-stitches. A guidewire (*dotted arrow*) is then introduced through the needle into the stomach.
(Reprinted with permission from Holcomb GW III: Gastroesophageal reflux disease in infants and children. In Fischer FE [ed]: Mastery of Surgery [ed 5]. Philadelphia, Lippincott Williams & Wilkins, pp 650-661, 2007.)

tract and gastrotomy is performed over the guidewire using the 8, 12, 16, and 20 French dilators in the Cook set. The tract can be dilated by spreading a hemostat if needed. The tract is dilated up to size 20 Fr for either a 12 or 14 Fr button (Fig. 6-4C). The 20 Fr dilator is passed only through the abdominal wall but is not pushed into the stomach. The 8 Fr dilator is then inserted through the lumen of a Mic-Key gastrostomy button (Ballard Medical Products, Draper, UT), and both are advanced over the guidewire into the stomach (Fig. 6-6). The balloon of the button is slowly inflated with care to make certain that the balloon does not inflate outside the stomach and push the stomach away from the abdominal wall. Also, the angled telescope can be used to look around the stomach to be sure the button has not been placed outside the stomach. The two U-sutures are tied snugly over the wings of the gastrostomy button externally (Fig. 6-7). Feedings are initiated in 6 to 12 hours.

POSTOPERATIVE CARE

The U-sutures should be cut and removed 48 to 72 hours after performing the gastrostomy to avoid pain and strangulation of the tissue inside the U-stitches. Although it rarely occurs, a significant management challenge is early gastrostomy button displacement. If the button becomes dislodged within the first few weeks after its insertion, the gastrostomy tract can usually be carefully navigated with an 8 Fr dilator. Once the dilator is introduced into the stomach, a guidewire is passed through the dilator and the tract is dilated by introducing progressively larger dilators over the guidewire as in the original gastrostomy technique. The gastrostomy button is then reintroduced over the guidewire with the 8 Fr dilator within the lumen of the button. The intraluminal position of the gastrostomy button should be verified with injection of contrast material using fluoroscopic visualization.

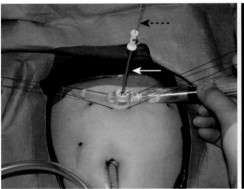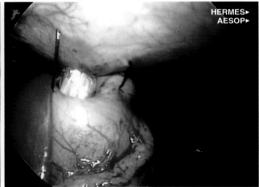

Figure 6-6. After serial dilation of the abdominal wall tract and gastrotomy with the vascular dilator set, the 8 Fr dilator (*arrow*) is inserted through the lumen of the Mic-Key gastrostomy button. Both are advanced over the guidewire (*dotted arrow*) and into the stomach.
(Reprinted with permission from Holcomb GW III: Gastroesophageal reflux disease in infants and children. In Fischer FE [ed]: Mastery of Surgery [ed 5]. Philadelphia, Lippincott Williams & Wilkins, pp 650-661, 2007.)

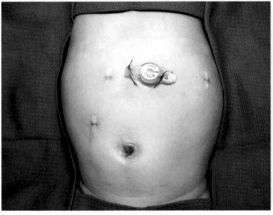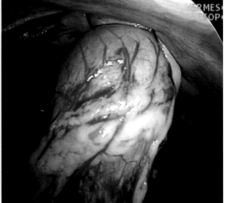

Figure 6-7. Extracorporeally, the U-stitches are tied over the wings of the gastrostomy button. The other incisions used for the laparoscopic fundoplication have been closed with Steri-Strips. In the internal view on the *right*, note that the stomach has been distended with inflation of the balloon on the button and that the U-stitches closely approximate the stomach wall to the anterior peritoneum.
(Reprinted with permission from Holcomb GW III: Gastroesophageal reflux disease in infants and children. In Fischer FE [ed]: Mastery of Surgery [ed 5]. Philadelphia, Lippincott Williams & Wilkins, pp 650-661, 2007.)

7
Laparoscopic Pyloromyotomy

Mark L. Wulkan

Hypertrophic pyloric stenosis (HPS) is the most common surgical disease in infants. Most children present between the ages of 2 and 8 weeks with nonbilious projectile vomiting. They are often dehydrated with a hypochloremic, hypokalemic metabolic alkalosis. Because of the trend toward earlier diagnosis with ultrasound, the degree of dehydration and electrolyte imbalance is not as dramatic as in the past. The disease is caused by progressive hypertrophy of the pyloric muscle. Since Ramstedt described the first successful pyloromyotomy in 1912, treatment has been operative pyloromyotomy. In selected high-risk patients, atropine has been used with some success. Since the first laparoscopic pyloromyotomy was described by Alain in 1991, this approach has become more widely used and is the preferred technique by many pediatric surgeons.

INDICATIONS FOR WORKUP AND OPERATION

Infants with HPS typically present with progressive nonbilious emesis. The emesis typically occurs just after feeding and is often projectile in nature. The infants may be hungry after the emesis. The symptoms can be very similar to those seen with gastroesophageal reflux disease (GERD). A thorough history and physical exam-ination can help distinguish GERD from HPS. It is not uncommon for the infant to have had several formula changes prior to presentation. On physical examination, the infants often appear dehydrated. An experienced pediatric surgeon can palpate the hypertrophied pylorus the majority of the time; however, most patients present to the pediatric surgeon with an ultrasound demonstrating HPS. During the abdominal examination, the stomach must be emptied and the infant satiated with a pacifier dipped in sugar or a bottle of a sugar or electrolyte solution. Once the olive is palpated, no further diagnostic workup is necessary. Preoperative electrolytes should be checked to guide resuscitation. Objective measurements used to determine HPS on ultrasound are a thickness greater than 3.5 to 4 mm and a length greater than 16 to 17 mm. The diagnosis may also be made by an upper gastrointestinal series contrast study.

Prior to operation, it is imperative to correct the dehydration and any electrolyte abnormalities. Preoperative orogastric decompression is optional. In our institution, resuscitation is started with D5 $\frac{1}{2}$ NS plus 30 meq KCl/L at 150 mL/kg/24 hr. The infant is given a bolus of 10 to 20 cc/kg normal saline as needed. Electrolytes are rechecked every 6 to 8 hours to monitor the resuscitation. The urine output is also closely monitored. The endpoints of resuscitation are adequate urine output and normalization or near normalization of the electrolytes. The dextrose concentration may be increased to 10% to maintain glucose delivery as fluid requirements decrease.

OPERATIVE TECHNIQUE

After induction of general anesthesia and endotracheal intubation, the patient is placed transverse on the operating room table (Fig. 7-1A). The monitor is positioned across the table from the surgeon and assistant, cephalad to the patient (Fig. 7-1B). The initial cannula is inserted using a modified Veress technique. If the umbi-

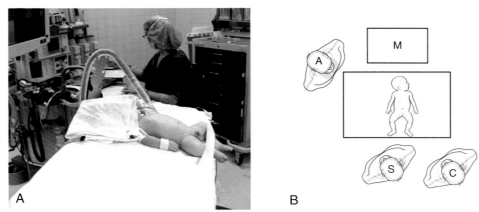

Figure 7-1. **A,** The patient is positioned transversely across the operating table. A red rubber catheter has been inserted to distend the stomach after the myotomy. **B,** The surgeon (S) stands at the foot of the patient. The camera holder (C) is usually positioned to the surgeon's right. The monitor (M) is above the patient. A, anesthesiologist.

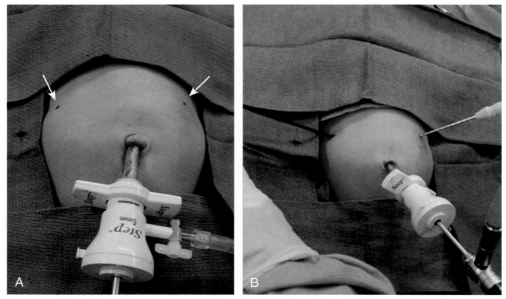

Figure 7-2. **A,** The umbilical cannula and telescope have been introduced. The sites for insertion of the instruments in the epigastrium are marked (*arrows*). **B,** The instruments have been inserted using the stab incision technique.

licus is dry, a vertical stab incision is made with a #11 blade through the center of the umbilicus. There is usually a small umbilical hernia present, through which the Veress needle is placed. If the umbilicus is still "wet," a transverse infraumbilical crease incision is made. Care is taken to ensure that the Veress needle is inserted into the peritoneal cavity. The needle should not be directed cephalad, as it may inadvertently cannulate the umbilical vein. A 4.2-mm reusable cannula and trocar are inserted and a 4-mm 30-degree laparoscope is introduced. Alternatively, a 5-mm port and a 5-mm laparoscope may be used as well. The abdomen is insufflated to 10 to 12 mm Hg of CO_2. Stab incisions are then made with a #11 or #15 scalpel in the right and left epigastrium, followed by insertion of 3-mm instruments

(Fig. 7-2). A bowel grasper is used in the surgeon's left hand, and an arthrotomy knife (Linvatec, Largo, FL) is used in the right hand.

An incision is made on the anterior surface of the pylorus beginning just proximal to the junction with the duodenum (near the vein of Mayo) and is curved onto the antrum of the stomach (Fig. 7-3A). One of the pitfalls is making the incision too superficial. Remember, if the patient truly has hypertrophic pyloric stenosis, the muscular wall thickness should be at least 4 mm thick. The knife is then retracted into the sheath and is slid into the incision to begin the myotomy. The sheathed knife is then twisted 60 to 90 degrees to begin breaking the muscular wall (Fig. 7-3B). This maneuver deepens the initial incision and makes it easier to insert the

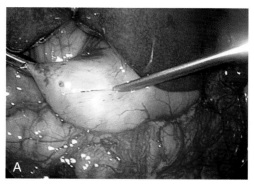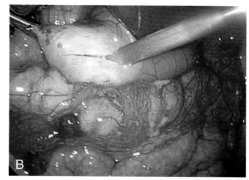

Figure 7-3. **A,** The duodenum is grasped with the atraumatic grasping forceps in the surgeon's left hand and an incision is made with an arthrotomy knife on the anterior surface of the pylorus just proximal to the vein of Mayo and extended to the pyloric–antrum junction. **B,** The knife blade is then withdrawn into the sheath. The sheathed knife is then pushed into the myotomy and twisted to deepen the initial incision so that the pyloric spreader can be introduced.

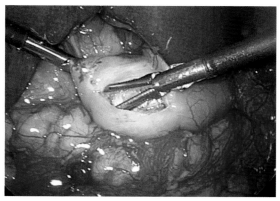

Figure 7-4. A pyloric spreader is then introduced to gently spread the hypertrophied pyloric musculature.

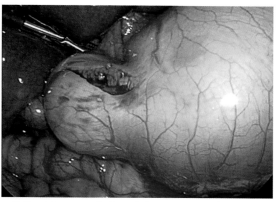

Figure 7-5. After completion of the myotomy, the stomach is insufflated with 60 cc of air introduced through the red rubber catheter to be sure there is no evidence of an occult mucosal perforation.

pyloric spreader (Fig. 7-4). The myotomy is extended distally to the junction of the stomach and the duodenum, and proximally onto the antrum of the stomach. Remember that perforations usually occur distally, and inadequate myotomies are usually caused by incomplete muscular division proximally. An adequate proximal extent of the myotomy is determined by visualization of the oblique muscular fibers seen in the antrum. Care is taken distally not to enter the fold of duodenal mucosa at the gastroduodenal junction.

Once the myotomy is completed, the stomach is inflated with air (Fig. 7-5) The anesthetist inserts a 14 Fr suction catheter in the stomach with a stopcock. A 60-mL syringe is attached to the stopcock. The stomach is inflated under direct visualization while the duodenum is obstructed with the instrument in the surgeon's left hand. The myotomy site is then carefully inspected to make sure that there is no occult perforation. The air is then evacuated from the stomach and the catheter is removed. Omentum can be placed over the myotomy if desired (Fig. 7-6). Next, the instruments are removed. The gas is allowed to escape through the umbilical cannula, which is done to prevent "stove piping" of

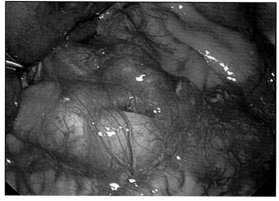

Figure 7-6. Omentum has been placed over the myotomy in this patient to help with hemostasis.

omentum out the abdominal stab wounds. The umbilical fascia is closed with 3-0 monofilament absorbable suture, and the umbilical skin is closed with interrupted 5-0 plain catgut suture. The epigastric stab incisions are closed with Steri-Strips (3M Company, St. Paul, MN) (Fig. 7-7).

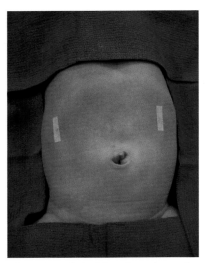

Figure 7-7. The epigastric incisions have been closed with Steri-Strips. The umbilical fascia and skin have been closed with absorbable sutures.

POSTOPERATIVE CARE

All patients are monitored for apnea postoperatively. One ounce of clear liquid is given 3 hours postoperatively. If the clear liquid is tolerated, the infant is advanced to formula or breast milk. Nursing mothers are allowed to nurse ad libitum, whereas infants on formula are restricted by increasing each feeding by 1 ounce to a maximum of 3 ounces. The parents are reassured that some postoperative emesis is normal. The intravenous fluids are discontinued when the child is tolerating 2 ounces of formula or nursing for 10 to 15 minutes at a time. The child may be discharged when tolerating adequate intake and after an age-appropriate postanesthesia observation period.

PEARLS

1. Be definitive with the seromuscular incision with the arthrotomy knife. A shallow cut through the serosa can lead to difficulty getting the pyloric spreader into the incision.
2. Do not allow omentum to follow your instruments out of the abdomen. It can be difficult to reduce and may lead to incisional herniation postoperatively.
3. You do not need to back off the feeding regimen if the patient vomits postoperatively. Instruct the parents and the nurses that the baby will spit up and may even vomit postoperatively, just not as much as was occurring preoperatively. In general, the earlier and faster the infants are fed, the faster they are ready to go home.

PITFALLS

1. An inadequate myotomy occurs proximally. Be sure to extend the myotomy proximally onto the antrum where the oblique muscular fibers can be seen.
2. Perforations occur distally. As I have gained more experience, I am less aggressive distally.
3. Grasp the duodenum definitively. Use the length of the grasper to distribute the force evenly. A partial grasp of the duodenum can lead to inadvertent duodenal perforation.
4. If the child looks ill and has persistent postoperative emesis, a study to evaluate for an occult perforation may be warranted.

RESULTS

I have attempted 105 and completed 104 laparoscopic pyloromyotomies. The average age at operation was 37 days. Most of the patients were discharged on the first postoperative day. There were two perforations. The first occurred in the third patient. The perforation developed during aggressive distal spreading when the pyloric spreader slipped under the muscle, causing perforation that was easily visualized. The perforation was repaired through a small right upper quadrant incision with a U-stitch and omental patch. The second perforation occurred proximally with the initial pyloric incision with the arthrotomy knife. This perforation was repaired laparoscopically with a U-stitch and omental patch. (This complication occurred in the 62nd patient in the series.) Both patients had uneventful postoperative courses and were discharged with no long-term sequelae.

Recently, a prospective randomized trial comparing laparoscopic and open pyloromyotomy was completed. One hundred patients were evaluated in each arm. There were no incomplete myotomies in either group, and one perforation occurred in the open group (St. Peter et al. 2006).

SELECTED REFERENCES

1. Alain JL, Grousseau D, Terrier G: Extramucosal pyloromyotomy by laparoscopy. Surg Endosc 5:174-175, 1991
2. Campbell BT, McLean K, Barnhart DC, et al: A comparison of laparoscopic and open pyloromyotomy at a teaching hospital. J Pediatr Surg 37:1068-1071, 2002
3. Hall NJ, Ade-Ajayi N, Al-Roubaie J, et al: Retrospective comparison of open versus laparoscopic pyloromyotomy. Br J Surg 91:1325-1329, 2004
4. van der Bilt JD, Kramer WL, van der Zee DC, Bax NM: Laparoscopic pyloromyotomy for hypertrophic pyloric stenosis: Impact of experience on the results in 182 cases. Surg Endosc 18:907-909, 2004

5. Yagmurlu A, Barnhart DC, Vernon A, et al: Comparison of the incidence of complications in open and laparoscopic pyloromyotomy: A concurrent single institution series. J Pediatr Surg 39:292-296, 2004

6. Kim SS, Lau ST, Lee SL, et al: Pyloromyotomy: A comparison of laparoscopic, circumumbilical, and right upper quadrant operative techniques. J Am Coll Surg 201:66-70, 2005

7. St. Peter SD, Holcomb GW III, Calkins CM, et al: Open versus laparoscopic pyloromyotomy for pyloric stenosis: A prospective, randomized trial. Ann Surg 224:363-370, 2006

8
Laparoscopic Antroplasty

Keith E. Georgeson

Many children with chronic gastroesophageal reflux also have delayed gastric emptying. Although the practice is controversial, some pediatric surgeons perform a gastric drainage procedure at the time of fundoplication for the purpose of improving gastric emptying. The most commonly performed procedure for improving gastric emptying is pyloroplasty. Fonkalsrud (1992) has popularized the antroplasty, which he has stated is equivalent to pyloroplasty in improving gastric emptying. Antroplasty is easier to perform laparoscopically than pyloroplasty. Further studies are needed to document the efficacies of pyloroplasty and antroplasty to improve gastric emptying.

INDICATIONS FOR WORKUP AND OPERATION

The primary indication for antroplasty is delayed gastric emptying. This delay in emptying is usually diagnosed with a thorough history and documented by a radionuclide scintiscan. Upper gastrointestinal (GI) radiography and upper GI endoscopy are also helpful in excluding other causes of gastric outlet obstruction, such as an antral web.

OPERATIVE TECHNIQUE

There are no unique anesthesia issues for this procedure. General endotracheal intubation is employed in all patients. The patient is positioned with the legs folded or in stirrups at the end of the table. The operator works from a position at the end of the operating table or between the patient's legs (Fig. 8-1). Ports are placed in positions similar to those used for pyloromyotomy. A 5-mm cannula is inserted through the umbilicus for the endoscope. Ports are placed on either side of the umbilicus in the left and right upper quadrants and are the working sites for the operator. A fourth cannula is placed laterally in the anterior axillary line in the right epigastrium to hold a retractor to elevate the liver (Fig. 8-2). A U-stitch placed extracorporeally around the falciform ligament and tied over a bolster can also be used instead of a liver retractor. A 30- to 45-degree telescope through the umbilical port gives an excellent view of the antrum and pylorus.

The proximal duodenum is grasped just distal to the pylorus with a grasper held in the surgeon's left hand; the grasper is inserted through the patient's right upper abdominal port. An L-tip cautery is employed to deliver cutting current to open the longitudinal and circular muscle fibers beginning just proximal to the vein of Mayo in the pylorus (Fig. 8-3). Alternatively, an arthroscopy knife can be used. The seromuscular incision in the pylorus is continued proximally for a distance of 2.5 cm. Care should be taken to avoid injury to the underlying mucosa. The muscle fibers are then spread with a pyloric spreader until the mucosa pouts through the incision (Fig. 8-4). This dissection should be continued distally a few millimeters onto the duodenum. A laparoscopic Maryland dissecting instrument is also useful to separate the muscle fibers from the mucosa. When the pyloromyotomy has been completed by the cutting and spreading of the muscle fibers, a 2-0 silk suture is placed between the proximal end of the linear muscle splitting incision and attached to the middle of the distal end of the linear incision. When the suture is tied, it converts the linear incision into a transverse closure in a manner similar to the Heineke-Mikulicz pyloroplasty. Two or three more transverse sutures are employed to complete the transverse closure of the antroplasty (Fig. 8-5). Feeding can be initiated 12 hours postoperatively.

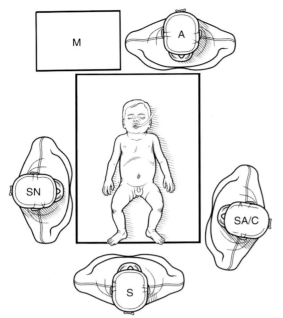

Figure 8-1.   For a laparoscopic antroplasty, the patient is positioned supine on the operating table. Infants are placed in a frogleg position at the end of the table, and the legs are taped securely. Stirrups, if needed, can be used for an older patient. The surgeon (S) is positioned at the foot of the table or between the legs (if stirrups are used). The surgical assistant/camera holder (SA/C) is to the right of the surgeon, and the scrub nurse (SN) is to the surgeon's left. A single monitor (M) is used, positioned to the right of the anesthesiologist (A). If two monitors are used, one is placed on either side of the patient's head.

PEARLS

1. The cannula arrangement for fundoplication works very well for laparoscopic antroplasty.
2. Small cautery burns to the submucosa are not a problem, as they will be covered by muscle after transverse closure of the pyloromyotomy
3. The linear seromuscular incision in the pyloric muscle should be extended several millimeters onto the duodenum for best results.
4. A hole in the antral mucosa should be repaired and then covered with muscle during transverse closure.

PITFALLS

1. Antroplasty may lead to postoperative dumping.

RESULTS

I have performed antroplasty in 57 patients for delayed gastric emptying (Sampson et al. 1998). In all patients, the antroplasty was coupled with a fundoplication. Ten of these patients had a postoperative gastric emptying study that documented, on average, a 50% improvement in gastric emptying. However, I suspect that the fundoplication had much to do with the improved gastric emptying.

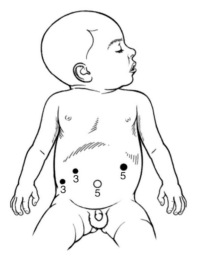
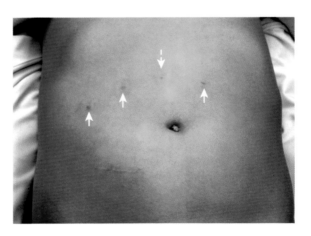

Figure 8-2.   The diagram and the operative photo show placement of ports or instruments for laparoscopic antroplasty (*solid arrows*). The port positions are similar to those used for pyloromyotomy. A telescope attached to a camera is introduced through a 5-mm cannula inserted through the umbilicus. The ports or stab incisions placed on either side of the midline in the right and left upper quadrants are the working sites for the operator. If a fourth cannula or instrument is needed for retraction of the liver, it is placed laterally in the right upper abdomen in the anterior axillary line. In the photograph, the *dotted arrow* depicts a small mark in the skin made by a U-stitch placed extracorporeally around the falciform ligament.

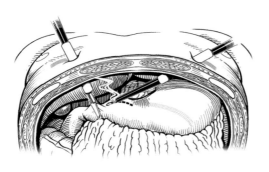
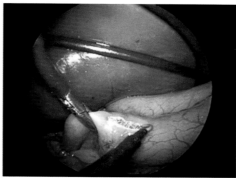

Figure 8-3.   A hook or L-tip cautery is used to deliver cutting current to outline the planned incision in the longitudinal and circular muscles of the pylorus. This dissection is continued distally a few millimeters onto the duodenum. The duodenum is secured distally with an instrument in the surgeon's left hand.

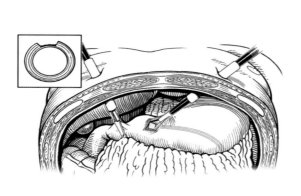
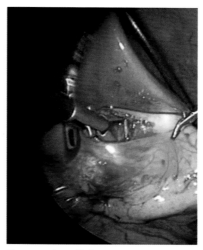

Figure 8-4.   After the serosal incision, the muscle fibers of the pylorus are gently spread until the mucosa pouts through the incision. Unlike in a baby with pyloric stenosis, the pyloric muscle is not hypertrophied in these patients, so a little more bleeding occurs with the myotomy here.

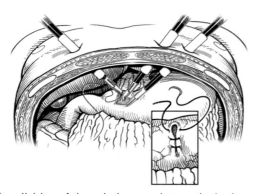
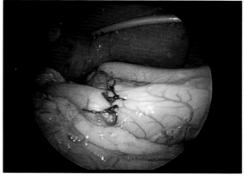

Figure 8-5.   After division of the pyloric musculature, the horizontal seromuscular incision is closed transversely as is done in a Heineke-Mikulicz pyloroplasty. Three transverse sutures are usually needed to complete the transverse closure of the antroplasty.

SELECTED REFERENCES

1. Byrne WJ, Kangarloo H, Ament ME, et al: Antral dysmotility: An unrecognized cause of chronic vomiting during infancy. Ann Surg 193:177-183, 1981
2. McCallum RW, Berkowitz DM, Lerner E: Gastric emptying in patients with gastroesophageal reflux. Gastroenterology 80:285-291, 1981
3. Papaila JG, Wilmot D, Grosfeld JL, et al: Increased incidence of delayed gastric emptying in children with gastroesophageal reflux. Arch Surg 124:933-936, 1989
4. Fonkalsrud EW, Ament ME, Vargas J: Gastric antroplasty for the treatment of delayed gastric emptying and gastroesophageal reflux in children. Am J Surg 164:327-331, 1992
5. Brown RA, Wynchank S, Rode H, et al: Is a gastric drainage procedure necessary at the time of antireflux surgery? J Pediatr Gastroenterol Nutr 25:377-380, 1997
6. Sampson LK, Georgeson KE, Royal SA: Laparoscopic gastric antroplasty in children with delayed gastric emptying and gastroesophageal reflux. J Pediatr Surg 33:282-285, 1998

9
Laparoscopic Repair of Duodenal Atresia and Stenosis

Klaas (N) M. A. Bax

There are few reports on laparoscopic procedures in neonates. This may be related to the low incidence of most abdominal conditions in neonates (except for hypertrophic pyloric stenosis), the limited working space in the neonate (making complicated surgery such as the correction of duodenal atresia difficult), the often associated congenital (including cardiac) abnormalities, and the metabolic, ventilatory, and hemodynamic consequences of CO_2 insufflation. When the child has incomplete duodenal obstruction, as is the case in duodenal stenosis, it may present later, making laparoscopic correction easier as the abdominal working space is larger. Moreover, there is less discrepancy between the diameter of the lumina of the proximal and distal duodenum. This chapter discusses the laparoscopic correction of duodenal atresia, duodenal web, and duodenal stenosis.

INDICATIONS FOR WORKUP AND OPERATION

The diagnosis of complete duodenal obstruction is easy. There is usually polyhydramnios, and the dilated stomach as well as the dilated upper duodenum are easily seen antenatally on ultrasound or postnatally on a plain abdominal radiograph (Fig. 9-1). After birth, there is usually bilious vomiting. If the proximal duodenum is not markedly dilated and air is seen distally, malrotation with volvulus should be immediately excluded by an upper gastrointestinal contrast study. Duodenal atresia and intestinal malrotation may coexist, and a high proportion of patients with intrinsic duodenal lesions have trisomy 21. Also, concomitant congenital abnormalities should be sought.

Before taking the child to the operating room, any electrolyte or acid–base disturbances should be corrected. In complete duodenal obstruction, prophylactic antibiotics should be administered.

OPERATIVE TECHNIQUE

General anesthesia, in combination with regional analgesia, is employed. A urinary catheter is inserted and remains in as long as epidural analgesia is given. A nasogastric tube is introduced as well.

The child is placed in frogleg position at the lower end of the operating table. The legs should be enveloped to prevent the patient from slipping off the table when the table is put in reversed Trendelenburg. The surgeon stands at the caudal end of the table, with the camera person to the right-handed surgeon's left and the scrub nurse to the right. Two monitors are used, one to the right and one to the left of the head of the patient

(Fig. 9-2A). All cables, seven in total, come off one side of the table. No cable lies on the child.

All cannulas and instruments are nondisposable. Four ports are usually needed (Fig. 9-2B). All cannulas have a siliconized sleeve. In neonates, a 24-cm-long, 5-mm, 30-degree telescope and 20-cm-long, 3.5-mm instruments are used. The 6-mm sleeved telescope cannula is inserted in an open technique through an incision in the infraumbilical fold. The incision in the linea alba and peritoneum is made as small as possible, after which the 6-mm cannula with a blunt trocar is

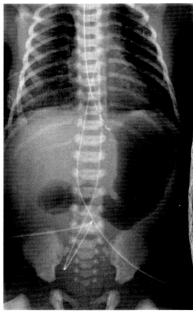

Figure 9-1.   The typical "double bubble" sign is seen in this newborn with duodenal atresia.

pushed inside, thus obtaining tight closure to help prevent escape of CO_2. The interior part of the cannula is lifted up and to the left, and a 2-0 Vicryl (Ethicon, Inc., Somerville, NJ) suture is placed through the skin and fascia and tied to the stopcock of the cannula. Care is taken not to insert too much of the cannula inside the abdomen, as this will reduce the already limited working space. By pulling on the cannula, the abdominal working space can be increased to a certain extent. Before insufflating, the telescope is inserted to make sure that the cannula tip is inside the peritoneum. The pneumoperitoneum pressure is set to 8 mm Hg and the flow at 1 L/min in the neonate. A temporary increase in pressure to 10 mm Hg is advantageous when inserting the secondary cannulas. A 3.8-mm cannula is inserted pararectally on both the right and left at the level of the umbilicus. All cannulas are secured to the abdominal wall with 2-0 Vicryl sutures tied around the stopcock. The liver can be pulled upward by inserting a 2-0 Vicryl suture underneath the falciform ligament (Fig. 9-3). If this does not retract the liver enough, a 3.5-mm Diamond-Flex (Snowden-Pencer, Tucker, GA) liver retractor is inserted through a subxiphoidal 3.8-mm port. Alternatively, an Allis-type grasper with ratchet can be introduced through the same subxiphoidal cannula. The grasper is then put under the right lobe of the liver and secured to the lateral peritoneum on the right (Fig. 9-3). The liver rests on this forceps. Support for this forceps is usually not needed.

ATRESIA OR STENOSIS

The dilated upper duodenum is easily visualized and is freed from the surroundings. Next, the small distal duo-

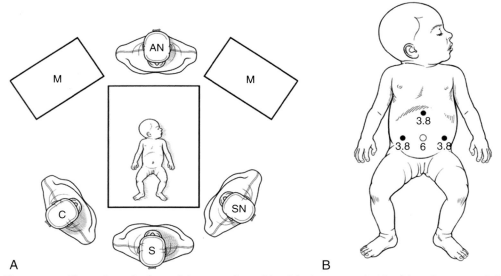

A   B

Figure 9-2.   **A,** The surgeon (S) stands at the foot of the operating table with the camera holder (C) to the surgeon's left and scrub nurse (SN) to the right. The infant is positioned at the end of the operating table. AN, anesthesiologist; M, monitor. **B,** The location and size (in millimeters) of the four ports.

cannula increases the working space, which is very limited in duodenal atresia.

2. Duodenal stenosis is easier to deal with, as the child is usually somewhat older and as there is less difference in caliber between the segments.

3. Concomitant intestinal malrotation should be corrected first.

4. Do not make the enterotomies with diathermy, as injury to the edges may jeopardize anastomotic healing.

5. Convert when you are not happy.

RESULTS

Before 2000, four children with intrinsic duodenal obstruction, two with atresia and two with stenosis, underwent exploratory laparoscopy. The duodenum was kocherized in these patients, but the operation was completed through a mini–right upper quadrant laparotomy. Our first real attempt at laparoscopic duodenoduodenostomy in a patient with atresia occurred in January 2000. Since that time, 22 children with intrinsic duodenal obstruction (16 with atresia, 2 with a web, and 4 with stenosis) have had a laparoscopic approach with intention to treat. Twelve of these patients had trisomy 21 and one had the Feingold syndrome. This last patient, who had a combination of esophageal atresia with distal tracheoesophageal fistula and duodenal atresia, both repaired endoscopically, died from sepsis. The anastomoses did not leak.

In our series, there has been a high incidence of concomitant anomalies (four esophageal atresia, one Hirschsprung disease, one atrioventricular septal defect, and one tetralogy of Fallot). Four patients had associated malrotation and one had a dilated upper duodenum without frank stenosis. In the atresia group of 16 infants, there were four conversions, two because of associated malrotation, one because of a very dilated upper duodenum in association with pure esophageal atresia, and one because of a dilated upper duodenum and concern about missing a membrane. Six duodenal anastomoses leaked, one of which occurred in the converted group. In the two patients with a web, one was converted because of difficulties in finding the web after duodenotomy. The second one recovered uneventfully. One of the four children with duodenal stenosis developed a re-stenosis, most likely because electrocautery was used to create the enterotomies.

SELECTED REFERENCES

1. Bax NM, Ure BM, van der Zee DC, et al: Laparoscopic duodenoduodenostomy for duodenal atresia. Surg Endosc 15:217, 2001

2. Gluer S, Petersen C, Ure BM: Simultaneous correction of duodenal atresia due to annular pancreas and malrotation by laparoscopy. Eur J Pediatr Surg 12:423-425, 2002

3. Rothenberg SS: Laparoscopic duodenoduodenostomy for duodenal obstruction in infants and children. J Pediatr Surg 37:1088-1089, 2002

4. Nakajima K, Wasa M, Soh H, et al: Laparoscopically assisted surgery for congenital gastric or duodenal diaphragm in children. Surg Laparosc Endosc Percutan Tech 13:36-38, 2003

5. Steyaert H, Valla JS, Van Hoorde E: Diaphragmatic duodenal atresia: Laparoscopic repair. Eur J Pediatr Surg 13:414-416, 2003

10
Laparoscopic Ladd Procedure

Christopher R. Moir

Malrotation refers to a variety of rotation and fixation anomalies of the midgut intestine. These conditions predispose the bowel to obstruction by congenital bands, twisting on a narrow mesenteric root, or internal herniation through peritoneal defects. The goal of malrotation repair is to prevent catastrophic events with loss of the entire midgut. The objectives of a Ladd procedure are to divide the congenital peritoneal bands and widen the mesenteric root. Full abdominal exploration may also identify internal hernias associated with malrotation. Division of these sacs often provides symptomatic relief of a partial obstruction. The laparoscopic approach for malrotation without volvulus has been widely reported. A laparoscopic approach to children with midgut volvulus is not currently recommended.

INDICATIONS FOR WORKUP AND OPERATION

Candidates for an elective laparoscopic Ladd procedure require upper gastrointestinal (UGI) contrast confirmation of a rotational anomaly. Exceptions include children undergoing laparoscopic exploration for concomitant disease or for abdominal pain of uncertain origin. The child who presents with equivocal findings on a UGI series but pain consistent with proximal intestinal obstruction is also a candidate for exploration and repair. This latter indication must be used sparingly in children with chronic abdominal pain.

Computed tomographic (CT) scanning is also being used to identify children with malrotation with or without volvulus. The superior mesenteric artery and vein positions are reversed in children with intestinal nonrotation. Internal herniation can also be identified with this approach. Although I prefer a confirmatory UGI series, it is reasonable to proceed directly to laparoscopy when CT findings are certain. False-positive scans are rare, but the false-negative rate is 25%. Similarly, contrast enemas can diagnose malrotation with certainty; however, the false-negative rate approaches 40%.

Intestinal midgut volvulus is a relative contraindication to laparoscopy. Selected candidates for laparoscopic exploration include children with a nonobstructive volvulus presenting on an intermittent basis. Conversion to an open procedure is recommended whenever gastrointestinal compromise is encountered, or when manipulation of the bowel for detorsion is problematic.

Reduction of internal hernias and excision of the hernia sac are technically well within the skill of most laparoscopic surgeons and usually result in almost immediate relief of long-term partial obstructive symptoms. The procedure is straightforward and well tolerated.

Age is not a contraindication to laparoscopy. The procedure has been successfully performed in patients ranging in age from infants to middle-aged adults.

OPERATIVE TECHNIQUE

Under general anesthesia, the child is placed supine on the operating table with the arms tucked. The stomach and bladder are decompressed. The surgeon is usually positioned to the right of the patient and the surgical assistant or camera holder is to the patient's left (Fig. 10-1A). For older children, it may be advantageous to

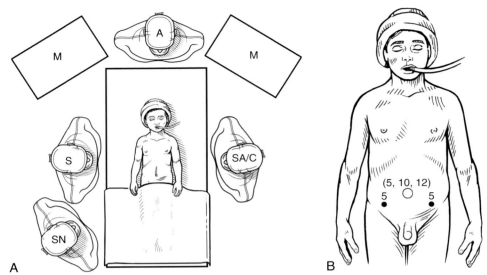

Figure 10-1.   A, Personnel placement for a laparoscopic Ladd procedure. The child is placed supine on the operating table. The surgeon (S) usually stands to the patient's right and the surgical assistant/camera holder (SA/C) is usually positioned opposite the surgeon. The scrub nurse (SN) is positioned to the surgeon's right. For older patients, the lithotomy position may be preferred. In this situation, the surgeon is usually positioned between the patient's legs. A, anesthesiologist; M, monitor. **B,** Port placement for a laparoscopic Ladd procedure. A 5- or 10- to 12-mm umbilical port is selected based on the patient's size and intentions to perform a transumbilical appendectomy. Two 3- or 5-mm instruments are placed through the anterior abdominal wall to triangulate the operative field. These incision sites are typically located in the right flank or suprapubic region and left abdomen.

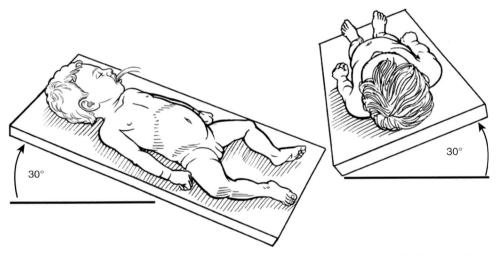

Figure 10-2.   After insertion of the ports and instruments, the patient is placed in reverse Trendelenburg position and tilted about 30 degrees to the left.

place the patient in lithotomy position, with the surgeon between the patient's legs. After preparation and draping, a vertical intraumbilical skin incision is made and the abdomen opened through the midline. A 5- or 10- to 12-mm port is selected based on patient size and whether the intention is to perform a transumbilical appendectomy. The abdomen is insufflated with carbon dioxide to a pressure of 11 to 15 mm Hg, depending on the age and size of the child. After general exploration, two 5-mm or smaller instruments are placed through the anterior abdominal wall to triangulate the operative

field. Incision sites are typically located in the right flank or suprapubic positions and left abdomen (Fig. 10-1B). The patient is tilted about 30 degrees to the left and in reverse Trendelenburg position (Fig. 10-2).

The first obligation of the surgeon is to identify whether intestinal malrotation is present. Even if a radiographic contrast study has indicated the likely presence of malrotation, this needs to be confirmed in each instance. First, the location of the cecum and the location of the ligament of Treitz are important landmarks in identifying whether malrotation is present. If the cecum is in the left lower quadrant (Fig. 10-3A) and the ligament of Treitz appears to have developed normally (Fig. 10-3B), it is evident that the patient does not have malrotation and further exploration is not needed.

In a child with classic nonrotation, the congenital bands are identified beneath the liver, crossing between the duodenum and jejunum to the cecum and terminal ileum (Fig. 10-4). In older children with long-standing partial obstruction or herniation, the Ladd bands may have been molded into a cocoon-like deformity (Fig. 10-5). In all cases, the Ladd bands are grasped and elevated for division using sharp dissection (Fig. 10-6). It is unnecessary to kocherize the duodenum. In children with partial rotation, the duodenum may be tortuous, requiring traction and counter-traction on the paraduodenal bands for adequate visualization and dissection. As the bands are divided, the cecum and ascending colon are gently retracted to the patient's left to continue tension on the remaining tissue. Final dissection continues well down onto the ileocecal mesentery. The goal is to separate the cecum and colon to the left and widen the mesentery as much as possible (Fig. 10-7). Once all bands are divided, the appendix is grasped and elevated through the umbilicus for extracorporeal appendectomy (Fig. 10-8). The mesentery is clamped and tied. Stump inversion is at the surgeon's discretion. The cecum is returned to the abdomen and hemostasis checked. The ports, if used, are removed under direct vision and the umbilicus is closed in layers with absorbable suture.

POSTOPERATIVE CARE

Children begin clear fluids the day of surgery and are discharged home in 1 to 2 days, depending on

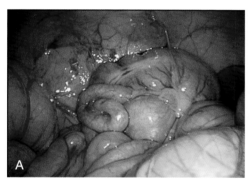 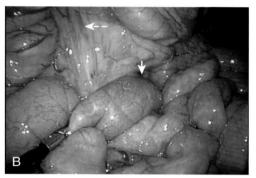

Figure 10-3.   When the diagnosis is not certain, exploration of the abdominal cavity is mandatory to identify whether the patient has intestinal malrotation. If the cecum is in the right lower quadrant (**A**) and the ligament of Treitz (**B**) is normal, the patient does not have malrotation and does not need a Ladd procedure. Note the middle colic vessels (*dotted arrow*) and the ligament of Treitz (*solid arrow*) in **B**.

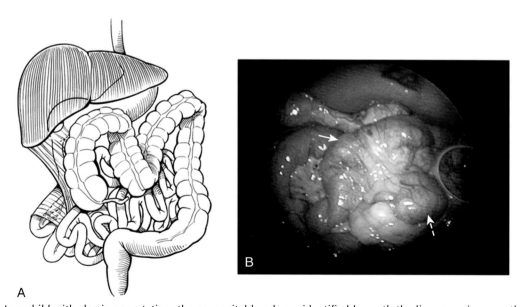

Figure 10-4.   In a child with classic nonrotation, the congenital bands are identified beneath the liver, crossing over the duodenum and attaching to the cecum. In the operative photo on the right, the duodenum is identified with a *solid arrow* and the cecum with a *dotted arrow*.

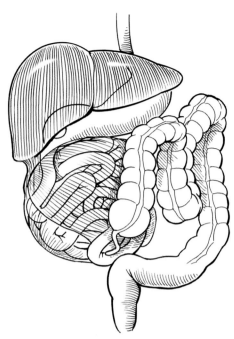

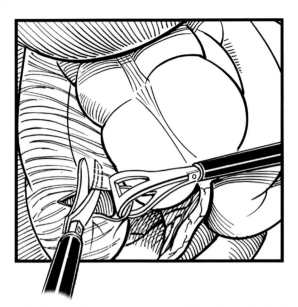

Figure 10-6.   In all cases, the peritoneal bands are divided sharply so as not to cause cautery injury to the intestine.

Figure 10-5.   In older children with long-standing partial obstruction or internal herniation, the Ladd bands may cause the bowel to form into a cocoon-like deformity.

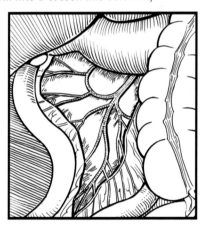

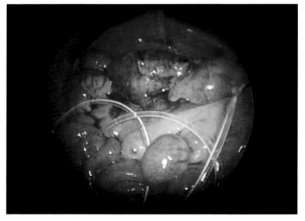

Figure 10-7.   Once the Ladd bands have been divided, allowing mobilization of the cecum and ascending colon, the goal is to widen the mesentery and position the cecum as far to the patient's left as possible. In the operative photograph, notice the widened small bowel mesentery. The cecum has been placed far to the patient's left and is not visible on the photograph. This patient also had an indwelling ventriculoperitoneal shunt.

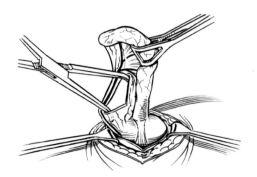

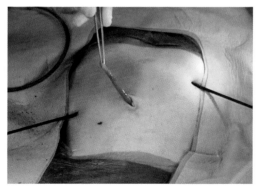

Figure 10-8.   Extracorporeal appendectomy is possible and eliminates the need for a large port for the endoscopic stapler. The appendix is grasped with one of the intracorporeal instruments and brought into view through the umbilicofascial defect, where it is grasped and exteriorized.

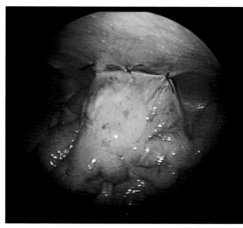

Figure 10-9. To secure the cecum and ascending colon to the patient's left, cecopexy can be performed by tacking the taenia of the cecum to the left lateral peritoneum, as shown in this photograph.

reestablishment of gastrointestinal activity. With extensive mobilization of the bowel, hospitalization may be necessary for another 1 or 2 days. Antibiotics are not routinely administered. The child is allowed to ambulate without restriction.

PEARLS

1. The less air in the intestine, the better. For elective procedures, a bowel preparation improves mobilization of the colon by reducing stool burden.
2. Allow enough room for extensive instrument manipulation by placing the port sites at a distance from the congenital bands. In some cases, it can be advantageous to position both instruments in the patient's left abdomen.
3. Some surgeons advocate an open operation to create a certain amount of adhesion formation, which might prevent recurrent volvulus. At laparoscopy, the widened mesenteric root is preserved by placing the free small bowel over the site of the congenital band excision. This may prevent re-adhesion of the cecum to the duodenum. Additionally, a cecopexy can be performed along the left lateral abdominal wall to secure the cecum to the right and widen the mesentery (Fig. 10-9).
4. The laparoscopic learning curve involves complete division of the Ladd bands. Take extra time to ensure that all bands are divided from the proximal duodenum to the cecum and terminal ileum.
5. For small children, the distances are short and the bands thin and relatively avascular. Use of cautery could damage intestine. Sharp dissection or the ultrasonic scalpel is a preferred alternative.
6. Transumbilical appendectomy is easy in patients with a mobile mesentery. It is generally less expen-

sive than an intracorporeal procedure. The umbilical incision and port position are performed in anticipation of an open appendectomy. When necessary, intracorporeal appendectomy can also be accomplished.

PITFALLS

1. Handling of infant bowel may produce serosal tears and postoperative small bowel obstruction. It is generally unnecessary to grasp the bowel. All traction can be placed on the bands or appendix.
2. Laparoscopic detorsion of volvulus should be done only under exceptional circumstances. Although possible in patients with chronic intermittent torsion, the amount of manipulation necessary and the potential damage to swollen bowel is not worth the benefit of maintaining a laparoscopic approach.
3. Internal herniation can be repaired by a laparoscopic approach. Persistence in identifying the defect and excising the sac will provide excellent outcomes without the need to convert. The finding of a hernia is not an indication for an open procedure; rather, further exploration and changes in patient position will help the defect to be visualized and the repair to be completed.
4. Constipation is a frequent consequence of malrotation. Where possible, preoperative bowel preparation and postoperative laxatives may speed recovery.

RESULTS

In a combined review of published and unpublished data from the Mayo Clinic of 51 patients undergoing a laparoscopic malrotation procedure, full oral intake was achieved 1 day earlier and length of hospitalization was 40% less than in those undergoing an open operation. Day 1 narcotic use was reduced 10-fold. Of 18 patients available for follow-up study, 16 reported full resolution of symptoms and two were much improved. No patient has returned with recurrent volvulus or severe symptoms (Matzke et al. 2005).

SELECTED REFERENCES

1. Bass KD, Rothenberg SS, Chang JH: Laparoscopic Ladd's procedure in infants with malrotation. J Pediatr Surg 33:279-281, 1998
2. Prasil P, Flageole H, Shaw KS, et al: Should malrotation in children be treated differently according to age? J Pediatr Surg 35:756-758, 2000
3. Gluer S, Petersen C, Ure BM: Simultaneous correction of duodenal atresia due to annular pancreas and malrotation by laparoscopy. Eur J Pediatr Surg 12:423-425, 2002

4. Matzke GM, Moir CR, Dozois EJ: Laparoscopic Ladd procedure for adult malrotation of the midgut with cocoon deformity: Report of a case. J Laparoendosc Advan Surg Tech 13:327-329, 2003

5. Tsumura H, Ichikawa T, Kagawa T, et al: Successful laparoscopic Ladd's procedure and appendectomy for intestinal malrotation with appendicitis. Surg Endosc 17:657-658, 2003

6. Antedomenico E, Singh NN, Zagorski SM, et al: Laparoscopic repair of a right paraduodenal hernia. Surg Endosc 18:165-166, 2004

7. Kalfa N, Zamfir C, Lopez M, et al: Conditions required for laparoscopic repair of subacute volvulus of the midgut in neonates with intestinal malrotation: 5 cases. Surg Endosc 18:1815-1817, 2004

8. Matzke GM, Dozois EJ, Larson DW, et al: Surgical management of intestinal malrotation in adults: Comparative results for open and laparoscopic Ladd procedures. Surg Endosc 19:1416-1419, 2005

11
Laparoscopic Jejunostomy

Keith E. Georgeson

Jejunostomy is not commonly performed in children. Most pediatric surgeons prefer gastrostomy as an enteral feeding option. Gastrostomy provides a more versatile feeding port because it allows both bolus and drip feedings to be administered, whereas only continuous feedings can be given through a jejunostomy. Two types of jejunostomy are used. A simple tube jejunostomy is most often used for children needing a short-term enteral feeding of less than 4 weeks. A laparoscopic Roux-en-Y jejunostomy is preferred for long-term jejunal feeding. Children with gastroparesis, uncorrectable gastroesophageal reflux, or severe chronic retching with intragastric feeds are the primary candidates for this Roux-en-Y approach.

INDICATIONS FOR WORKUP AND OPERATION

Temporary simple jejunostomy is indicated whenever a short-term need for enteral nutrition is desired. Jejunostomy is selected over gastrostomy if there is concern about gastroesophageal reflux or if upper gastrointestinal suture lines need to be protected. As mentioned, Roux-en-Y jejunostomy is selected for patients with a chronic need for enteral nutrition who are not suitable candidates for gastrostomy.

OPERATIVE TECHNIQUE

There are no unique anesthesia issues for performing a laparoscopic jejunostomy. Endotracheal intubation and general anesthesia are used. Care is taken to avoid inflating the stomach and small intestine with air during induction. The patient is placed in a supine position and secured to the operating table by taping the legs to the frame of the table. The patient can then be moved into either a lateral or a Trendelenburg position without danger of sliding off the table. The surgeon and camera operator are positioned on the patient's left side (Fig. 11-1A). Three ports are inserted along the anterior axillary line on the patient's left side (Fig. 11-1B). Two of the three ports are located in the left upper quadrant, and the lowest port is located in the left lower quadrant of the abdomen. The most cephalad and caudal ports can be 3 mm in diameter. The port for the telescope is 4 or 5 mm in diameter. A 30- or 45-degree telescope is optimal.

TUBE OR BUTTON JEJUNOSTOMY

The technique for the tube or button jejunostomy is almost identical to that described for a laparoscopic gastrostomy (see Chapter 6). A pneumoperitoneum is developed through a very small umbilical incision, and a Veress needle is inserted. Once the pneumoperitoneum is created, a 5-mm cannula is inserted in the left mid-abdomen and the telescope or camera is introduced through this port. The other two ports are then inserted as illustrated in Figure 11-1. The patient is placed in reverse Trendelenburg position and tilted to the right.

The ligament of Treitz is identified by lifting the transverse colon and identifying the most proximal jejunum. A point on the jejunum is selected about 15 cm distal

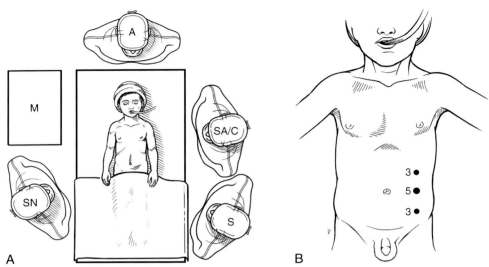

A   B

Figure 11-1. **A,** A child undergoing a laparoscopic jejunostomy is placed in the supine position on the table and secured to the operating table by taping the legs to the frame of the table. The patient can then be moved into a lateral or a Trendelenburg position without sliding off the operating table. The surgeon (S) and the surgical assistant/camera holder (SA/C) are positioned on the patient's left. The scrub nurse (SN) is situated according to the surgeon's preference. The monitor (M) should be across the patient so that the working site is between the surgeon and the monitor. A, anesthesiologist. **B,** A pneumoperitoneum is created by using a Veress needle inserted through a very small umbilical incision, and then three ports are inserted on the left side of the patient along the anterior axillary line. The most cephalad and caudal ports can be 3 mm in diameter. The cephalad 3-mm port is the site for insertion of the catheter into the jejunum. Stab incisions work well for these two sites. The telescope port is either 4 or 5 mm in diameter. A 30- or 45-degree telescope works best.

to the ligament of Treitz for insertion of the jejunal catheter. This site is brought to the anterior abdominal wall with a grasping clamp inserted through the left lower port. Using a large round needle, a U-stitch is passed extracorporeally through the abdominal wall and through the jejunum at the site selected on the anterior abdominal wall (Fig. 11-2). The needle is then brought back through the abdominal wall forming a U. The U-stitch is tied snugly over a bolster on the skin's surface. A needle is inserted beginning laterally in the midclavicular line of the left upper abdomen pointing toward the bowel attached to the abdominal wall. The needle is passed through the muscle layers of the abdominal wall and is carefully advanced extraperitoneally under laparoscopic surveillance for about 3 cm. The peritoneum is then penetrated at the point of the tethered jejunum (Fig. 11-3A). The needle is advanced until it penetrates into the jejunal lumen. A guidewire is inserted through the needle and advanced into the jejunum. The needle is then removed. A dilator and a peel-away vascular catheter introducer are passed over the guidewire into the jejunal lumen. The dilator is removed along with the guidewire, and the jejunostomy catheter is inserted through the catheter introducer into the jejunum for a distance of at least 10 cm (Fig. 11-3B).

A cuffed Broviac (Bard Access, Salt Lake City, UT) catheter works well for this type of feeding jejunostomy. The cuff should be left less than 1 cm outside of the

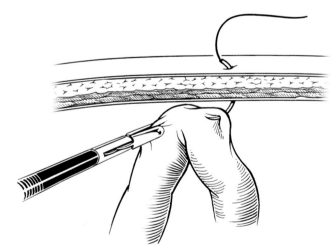

Figure 11-2. A point on the jejunum is selected about 15 cm distal to the ligament of Treitz. This piece of jejunum is brought to the abdominal wall with a grasping forceps which has been inserted through the left lower port. Using a large round needle, a U-stitch is passed extracorporeally through the abdominal wall and through the jejunum at the point selected on the anterior abdominal wall. The needle is then brought back through the abdominal wall forming a U.

abdominal wall. The cuff is very useful for securing the catheter to the abdominal wall. The catheter introducer is then peeled away, leaving the jejunostomy tube in place. Two more U-stitches are passed through the abdominal wall and jejunum under laparoscopic

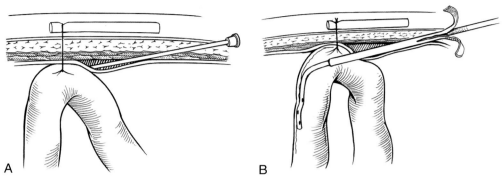

Figure 11-3. **A,** After approximation of the jejunum to the anterior abdominal wall, a needle is inserted beginning laterally in the midclavicular line of the left upper quadrant pointing toward the bowel attached to the abdominal wall. This needle is passed through the muscle layers of the abdominal wall and is carefully advanced extraperitoneally under laparoscopic surveillance for about 3 cm. The peritoneum is then penetrated at the point of the tethered jejunum. **B,** A guidewire is introduced through the needle and advanced into the jejunum. A dilator and peel-away sheath are then passed over the guidewire, the dilator is removed along with the guidewire, and the jejunostomy catheter is inserted through the peel-away sheath into the jejunum for a distance of at least 10 cm. The sheath is then peeled away, keeping the catheter in the jejunum. In both **A** and **B**, the U-stitch holding the jejunum next to the abdominal wall has been tied externally over a bolster.

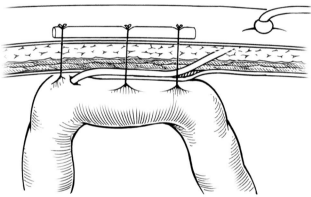

Figure 11-4. The cuff of the vascular catheter is left outside the abdominal wall and is useful for securing the catheter to the abdominal wall. Two more U-stitches are then passed through the abdominal wall and jejunum under laparoscopic surveillance, proximal to the original U-stitch. These additional U-sutures are also tied externally over a bolster and help prevent volvulus of the jejunum by broadening the length of the bowel tethered to the abdominal wall.

surveillance proximal to the original U-stitch, to buttress the jejunum against the extraperitoneal jejunostomy tube as illustrated in Figure 11-4. These sutures help to prevent rotation and a volvulus of the jejunum by broadening the length of the bowel tethered to the abdominal wall. Feedings may be initiated within 24 hours of placement of the jejunostomy catheter.

ROUX-EN-Y JEJUNOSTOMY

A fourth port is needed to perform a laparoscopic Roux-en-Y jejunostomy. A 12-mm cannula is inserted through the patient's umbilicus. The transverse colon is lifted up against the abdominal wall to identify the most proximal jejunum just distal to the ligament of

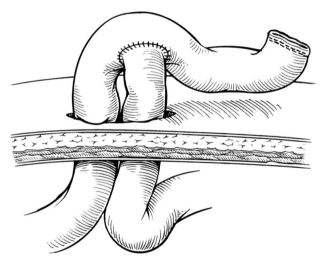

Figure 11-5. For a Roux-en-Y jejunostomy, a point is selected 15 to 20 cm distal to the ligament of Treitz. The jejunum is divided at this point using an endoscopic stapler inserted through the 12-mm umbilical port. After removing the umbilical port, the proximal and distal jejunal segments are exteriorized through the umbilical fascial defect, which sometimes needs to be enlarged. An end-to-side anastomosis is performed extracorporeally, leaving 15 cm of distal jejunum as the Roux limb.

Treitz. A point is selected 15 to 20 cm distal to the ligament of Treitz. The jejunum is divided at this point using an endoscopic stapler inserted through the 12-mm umbilical port. After removing the umbilical port, the proximal and distal ends of the jejunum are exteriorized through the umbilical fascial defect, which sometimes needs to be enlarged. An end-to-side anastomosis is performed extracorporeally, leaving 15 cm of distal jejunum as a Roux limb (Fig. 11-5). The jejunal anastomosis is returned to the abdominal cavity and the umbilical port site is closed with fascial and skin sutures. The stapled end of the Roux limb is attached to the abdominal wall using two U-sutures as previously described. A small incision is made in the skin over the end of the Roux-en-Y limb.

At this point, the operation is almost identical to a laparoscopic gastrostomy (see Chapter 6). The Cook vascular dilator set (Cook, Inc., Bloomington, IN) works well for this part of the operation. A needle is passed through a small incision in the abdominal wall and into the lumen of the jejunum at the site for insertion of the button. A J-tipped guidewire is passed through the needle into the jejunal lumen. The tract is serially dilated over the guidewire, and a 12-French Mic-Key button (Ballard Medical Products, Draper, VT) is passed over the guidewire into the lumen of the jejunum. An 8-Fr dilator is used to stiffen the stem of the gastrostomy button during its insertion into the jejunum. The Roux limb is then attached to the anterior abdominal wall with several internal sutures or several U-sutures to stabilize this jejunal segment so that it will not volvulize (Fig. 11-6). The defect in the mesentery is closed with silk sutures to prevent an internal hernia.

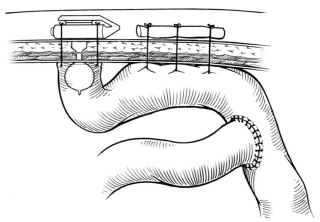

Figure 11-6. The stapled end of the Roux limb is then attached to the abdominal wall using two U-sutures. A small incision is made over the skin at the end of the Roux limb. At this point, a 12-French button is introduced into the end of the Roux limb in a technique identical to a laparoscopic gastrostomy. Again, the Roux limb is attached to the anterior abdominal wall with several internal or several extracorporeal U-sutures (as seen) to stabilize this limb and to prevent volvulus.

PEARLS

1. The 6.6 Broviac catheter is an excellent catheter choice for simple jejunostomy. The catheter can be introduced with an appropriately sized vascular introducer kit. The Dacron cuff on the catheter can be secured to the skin just outside the skin tunnel with a monofilament suture.
2. The Roux-en-Y jejunostomy button can be changed easily after about 6 weeks.

PITFALLS

1. Failure to obtain a broad-based attachment of the jejunum to the anterior abdominal wall can lead to volvulus of the Roux limb.

RESULTS

We have performed only a few laparoscopic jejunostomies. These few jejunostomies have functioned satisfactorily and were completed as described in this chapter.

SELECTED REFERENCES

1. Curet-Scot M, Shermeta DW: A comparison of intragastric and intrajejunal feedings in neonatal piglets. J Pediatr Surg 21:552-555, 1986
2. Georgeson KE: Laparoscopic versus open procedures for long-term enteral access. Nutri Clin Pract 12(Suppl 1):S1-2, 1997

12
Laparoscopic Ileocolectomy for Crohn's Disease

Steven S. Rothenberg

The advent of minimally invasive surgical techniques has allowed resection of small bowel lesions and conditions without the need for a major laparotomy. Numerous reports in the literature have described successful laparoscopic resection of diseased bowel in patients with Crohn's disease. These reports have shown a trend toward shorter hospital stay, decreased pain and postoperative ileus, smaller incisions, reduced cost, and fewer complications with the laparoscopic approach than with open resection. The diseased segment can be mobilized laparoscopically followed by either a resection (extracorporeal or intracorporeal) or an anastomosis. For the patient with chronic pain or with a fixed obstruction, laparoscopy is another safe and effective treatment option.

INDICATIONS FOR WORKUP AND OPERATION

Patients with Crohn's disease who present with chronic abdominal pain and with evidence of partial or complete obstruction, and who have failed to improve with medical therapy, should be considered for surgical intervention. Malnutrition (failure to thrive), abscess, fistula, and a palpable abdominal mass are also indications. The workup for all patients should consist of a small-bowel contrast study to demonstrate the presence of fixed strictures. In most cases, the diseased bowel involves the terminal ileum extending to and including the ileocecal valve. Occasionally, a computed tomographic scan is helpful in identifying an inflammatory mass, abscess, or the suggestion of a fistula. In some cases, colonoscopy may be useful for diagnostic purposes and to evaluate the ileocecal valve. Because most of these patients are at least partially obstructed, a formal bowel preparation is generally not tolerated. If the procedure is not being done for an acute total obstruction, then a 2- to 3-day preparation with clear liquids can be used.

OPERATIVE TECHNIQUE

The patient is positioned supine on the operating table. The left arm is tucked to the patient's side, and both the surgeon and assistant are on the patient's left side (Fig. 12-1). The viewing monitor is placed on the right side of the table at the level of the right iliac crest. A routine skin preparation is performed, a nasogastric tube is inserted, and the bladder is emptied with a Credé maneuver. Using a Veress needle, a pneumoperitoneum is established through an umbilical ring incision. A 12-mm cannula is placed through this incision. This port will be used for the telescope, for access with the endoscopic stapler (ES), and for removal of the specimen. Three additional ports are then introduced (Fig. 12-1): two 5-mm operating ports are positioned in the mid-epigastric and suprapubic areas, and a 5-mm retraction port is situated in the right upper quadrant. A brief survey of the abdomen is performed, and the small

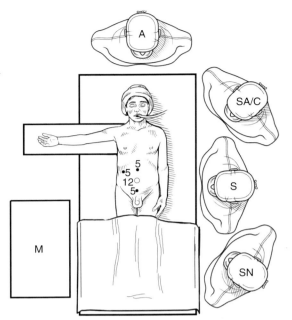

Figure 12-1. For a laparoscopic ileocolectomy for Crohn's disease, the patient is placed supine on the operating table. The surgeon (S) and surgical assistant/camera holder (SA/C) are positioned on the patient's left side. The viewing monitor (M) is positioned to the right of the patient at the level of the iliac crest. The scrub nurse (SN) is positioned according to the surgeon's preference. Usually, a 12-mm cannula is introduced through the umbilicus, which will be the initial port for the telescope, for access for the endoscopic stapler, and for removal of the specimen if an intracorporeal anastomosis is performed. Three additional ports are then inserted. Two 5-mm operating ports are positioned, one in the mid-epigastric area and the other in the suprapubic area. In addition, a 5-mm retraction port is usually placed in the patient's right upper abdomen. A, anesthesiologist.

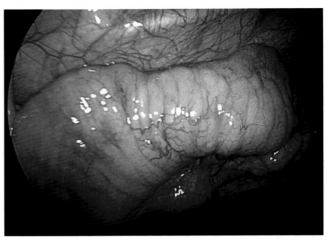

Figure 12-2. This photograph shows the typical creeping fat of diseased ileum seen at the time of laparoscopic ileocolectomy for Crohn's disease.

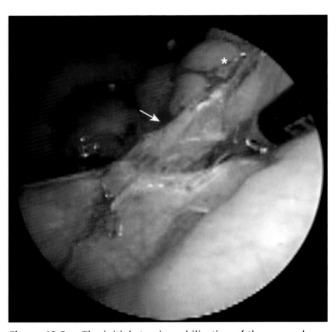

Figure 12-3. The initial step is mobilization of the cecum by detaching the lateral peritoneal attachments to the cecum (*arrow*), with separation of the inflammatory adhesions. The cecum has been marked with an *asterisk*.

bowel should be examined from the ligament of Treitz to the ileocecal valve to identify the diseased areas of the bowel (Fig. 12-2). The extent of ileocecal disease is determined, and the length of the bowel to be resected is identified. This portion of bowel is mobilized using sharp and blunt dissection, including detachment of the cecal-peritoneal attachments and separation of inflammatory adhesions (Fig. 12-3). The bowel is then divided at the proximal resection margin using the ES (Fig. 12-4).

Division of the mesentery can be accomplished by a number of methods depending on the surgeon's preference, the equipment available, and the degree of inflammation and thickening of the mesenteric leaf (Fig. 12-5). Mesenteric division can be performed using the ES, ultrasonic scissors, cautery, or the Ligasure (Covidien, Mansfield, MA). Usually, more than one modality is used for each patient. Dissection of the mesentery is carried out as close to the bowel wall as possible. This line of division allows the surgeon to avoid potential injury to other structures, such as the ureter, that may

have been involved with the inflammatory response. With mesenteric dissection complete, the distal resection line (which is usually distal to the cecum) is divided with a second application of the ES. The specimen is then placed out of the way in the pelvis.

After ensuring adequate mobilization of the distal and proximal intestinal segments, an intracorporeal anastomosis is performed. To accomplish this, the bowel segments are aligned side to side with 5 to 6 cm of overlap, and stay sutures are placed. The segments are stabilized by placing tension on the upper stay suture with an instrument inserted by the assistant through the

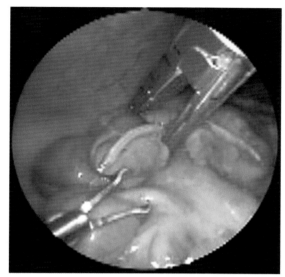

Figure 12-4.   The proximal extent of the ileocolectomy has been identified, and division of the bowel at this site has been performed with the endoscopic stapler.

right upper quadrant port. Enterotomies measuring 1 cm are made in each bowel limb at the proximal end of the overlap (Fig. 12-6A). Quick placement of a suction device will prevent any significant spillage of bowel content, even in cases of complete obstruction. With traction on the upper stay suture and countertraction on the lower stay suture, an ES is inserted through the 12-mm port, and each arm of the device is directed into the enterotomies (see Fig. 12-6B). Firing of the stapler results in a 3- to 4-cm functional side-to-side anastomosis. After removal of the ES, the staple line is examined for bleeding and integrity (Fig. 12-7A). The remaining 1.5- to 2-cm enterotomy is closed with a running suture of 2-0 Vicryl or Ethibond (Ethicon, Inc., Somerville, NJ) (Fig. 12-7B). The mesenteric defect is closed with interrupted sutures. An end-to-end sutured anastomosis can also be performed if the surgeon prefers, but this requires resection of the occluding staple lines and increases the risk of significant peritoneal contamination with no added benefit.

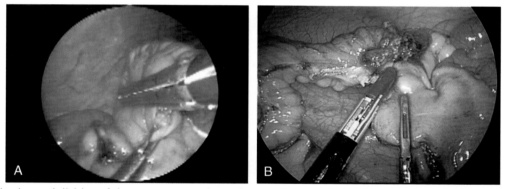

Figure 12-5.   Ligation and division of the mesentery can be performed with a variety of instruments. Often, more than one instrument is used. **A,** The endoscopic stapler is used to ligate and divide the mesentery. **B,** The Ligasure is used for the same purpose in a different patient.

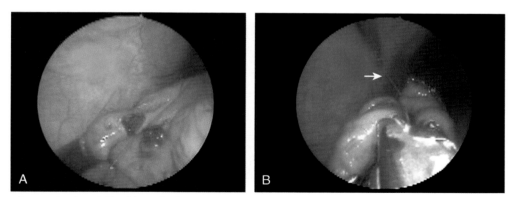

Figure 12-6.   **A,** The proximal and distal intestinal segments have been aligned side by side with 5 to 6 cm of overlap. Enterotomies measuring approximately 1 cm have been made in each bowel limb for insertion of the endoscopic stapler. **B,** With traction on the stay suture (*arrow*), each arm of the endoscopic stapler has been directed through the enterotomies and into the lumen of the two segments.

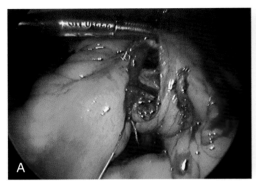 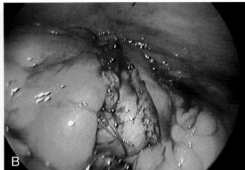

Figure 12-7. **A,** The intraluminal staple line is being examined for bleeding and integrity after removal of the endoscopic stapler. **B,** The remaining 1.5- to 2-cm enterotomy has been closed with a running 2-0 Ethibond suture.

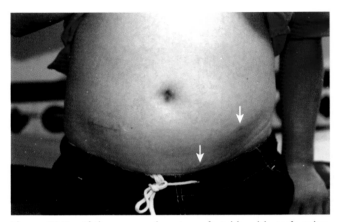

Figure 12-8. If the surgeon is not comfortable with performing an intracorporeal anastomosis, another option is to make a 4- to 5-cm right lower abdominal incision and perform the anastomosis extracorporeally. In this patient, the 12-mm umbilical port has been nicely hidden. Note the two left-sided, 5-mm cannula sites (*arrows*).

After completion of the anastomosis, the resected segment is retrieved using a specimen bag that has been introduced through the umbilical cannula. This sometimes requires piecemeal removal of the specimen with atraumatic clamps. Occasionally, it is necessary to enlarge the umbilical incision, but the maximal incision size should be 3 cm. This larger incision can easily be hidden in the contours of the umbilical skin fold. The fascial and skin incisions are closed with absorbable suture. If the surgeon is not comfortable with performing an intracorporeal anastomosis, another option is to make a small (approximately 5-cm) right lower quadrant muscle-sparing incision and perform the anastomosis extracorporeally (Fig. 12-8). The specimen can then be removed through this incision.

POSTOPERATIVE CARE

A nasogastric tube is usually left overnight, and perioperative antibiotics are continued for 24 to 48 hours. Generally, liquids are started on the first postoperative day unless the patient had a significant preoperative ileus or obstruction, or if a large abscess is encountered during the procedure. Most patients are discharged in 2 to 3 days, and immunosuppressive therapy can be tapered on an outpatient basis.

PEARLS

1. The laparoscopic approach is best used for isolated ileocolic disease. If there is a large phlegmon or there are multiple matted loops of bowel, it can be extremely difficult to dissect the mesentery safely.
2. If it is difficult to insert the endoscopic stapler into the two enterotomies, another stay suture can be placed at the apex of the two holes, thereby bringing them together. This "tag" can then be held by the assistant to stabilize the bowel while the stapler is inserted. A second tag can be placed at the lower end if necessary.
3. When trying to save the ileocecal valve, it is usually better to perform an end-to-end, hand-sewn anastomosis.
4. If the bowel is thickened and difficult to manipulate, it is helpful to add a fifth port to manipulate the bowel.
5. While closing the enterotomy with a running suture, it is helpful to place a stay suture at the bottom of the suture line to provide countertension. This suture may also be used to tie the running suture.

PITFALLS

1. The mesentery is often more thickened and diseased than was apparent. Stay relatively close to the bowel wall and maintain meticulous hemostasis during the dissecting process. Be aware that any device may fail to provide complete hemostasis.
2. Inadequate mobilization of the right colon can make it difficult to properly align the two bowel segments to perform the side-to-side anastomosis.

3. There may be other severely affected segments of bowel in addition to the terminal ileum. Be sure to run the bowel and carefully look for areas of partial obstruction.
4. Trying to save the ileocecal valve at all cost can result in a recurrent stricture or failed anastomosis. If there is not at least 6 cm of nondiseased ileum proximal to the ileocecal valve, it is advisable not to attempt to spare it.

RESULTS

Since 1994, I have seen 38 patients, aged 10 to 18 years, with ileocolic strictures from Crohn's disease that have required resection. Partial obstruction was present in all 38 patients; chronic abdominal pain was the primary symptom in 18, and 8 presented with acute obstruction. Two patients had more than one stricture. Laparoscopic resection was successful in 37 of 38 patients. One patient had a giant phlegmon with multiple loops of matted bowel that required conversion to an open operation. The one postoperative leak was treated conservatively with intravenous antibiotics and bowel rest for 5 days, with complete resolution. Two patients required a second surgery, both performed laparoscopically, one for a recurrent stricture at the anastomotic site 14 months after the initial resection and one for a new stricture 3 years after the first resection. Five patients presented with signs and symptoms of partial obstruction or pain, but their symptoms resolved with nonoperative management.

SELECTED REFERENCES

1. Alabaz O, Iroatulam AJN, Nessin A, et al: Comparison of laparoscopic assisted and conventional ileocolic resection in Crohn's disease. Eur J Surg 166:213-217, 2000
2. Diamond IR, Langer JC: Laparoscopic-assisted versus open ileocolic resection for adolescent Crohn disease. J Pediatr Gastroenterol Nutr 33:543-547, 2001
3. Hamel CT, Hildebrandt U, Weiss EG, et al: Laparoscopic surgery for inflammatory bowel disease. Surg Endosc 15:642-645, 2001
4. Milsom JW, Hammerhofer KA, Bohm B, et al: Prospective, randomized trial comparing laparoscopic versus conventional surgery for refractory ileocolic Crohn's disease. Dis Colon Rectum 44:1-8, 2001
5. Tabet J, Hong D, Kim CW, et al: Laparoscopic versus open bowel resection for Crohn's disease. Can J Gastroenterol 4:237-242, 2001
6. Rothenberg SS: Laparoscopic segmental intestinal resection. Semin Pediatr Surg 11:211-216, 2002
7. Dutta S, Rothenberg SS, Chang J, Bealer J: Total intracorporeal laparoscopic resection of Crohn's disease. J Pediatr Surg 38:717-719, 2003

13
Laparoscopic Management of Ileocolic Intussusception

Keith E. Georgeson

I leocolic intussusception is diagnosed by a characteristic history and confirmed by ultrasound or contrast enema. Contrast enema with air, saline, or barium is usually successful in reducing the intussusception in the majority of cases. Surgical exploration is necessary to complete the reduction in approximately 10% to 20%. Laparoscopy offers an excellent approach for surgical evaluation and management of intussusception. In most cases, the intussusception in infants and young children can be completely reduced using the laparoscopic approach. The remaining patients usually require bowel resection because of infarcted bowel. Bowel resection can be performed laparoscopically, but it is more commonly completed by using a small incision over the point of intended resection and anastomosis.

INDICATIONS FOR WORKUP AND OPERATION

The primary indication for laparoscopic reduction of an ileocolic intussusception is failure of the contrast or air enema to completely reduce the intussusception. A second indication for laparoscopic reduction is the presence of a jejunoileal or ileoileal intussusception. The child should be adequately hydrated preoperatively and is usually given broad-spectrum antibiotics. Children whose abdomens are massively distended are not suitable candidates for laparoscopic exploration.

OPERATIVE TECHNIQUE

The patient should be fully hydrated before induction of anesthesia. The child's stomach should be emptied using a nasogastric tube to avoid vomiting and aspiration during induction. General endotracheal intubation and a general anesthetic are used.

The patient is positioned supine. The legs and thighs should be taped to the table so that the child can be moved into many different positions during the operation to aid the surgeon in exploring the abdomen. The surgeon and the assistant/camera holder stand on the patient's left side (Fig. 13-1). Three ports are usually required for reduction of the intussusception (Fig. 13-2). The abdomen is initially entered using a vertical incision through the umbilicus. A Veress needle surrounded by an expandable sheath is passed through the umbilical defect into the peritoneal cavity under direct vision. A 5- or 10-mm cannula with a blunt tip is advanced through the sheath, which is left in place after removing the Veress needle. The pneumoperitoneum is developed after inserting the umbilical cannula through the sheath. A second port is positioned to the left of the rectus muscle in the left lower quadrant. This port is used for a 4-mm, 30-degree telescope to monitor the reduction of the intussusception. A third 3-mm instrument is inserted suprapubically. A cannula can be used, but the stab incision technique works well at this site. The second and third ports are placed using endoscopic surveillance via the umbilical cannula. These port positions can be modified depending on the location of the

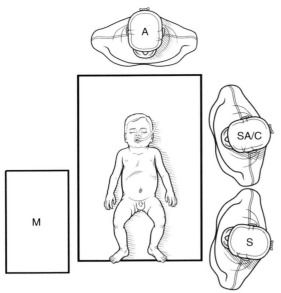

Figure 13-1. For laparoscopic reduction of an ileocolic intussusception, the patient is positioned supine. The patient is secured to the operating table so that the table can be moved into several positions during the operation, thus aiding the surgeon's exploration of the abdomen. The surgeon (S) and a surgical assistant/camera holder (SA/C) stand on the patient's left side. The monitor (M) is positioned across from the surgeon on the patient's right side, so that the area of dissection is in line between the telescope attached to the camera and the monitor. A scrub nurse can be positioned at the discretion of the surgeon. A, anesthesiologist.

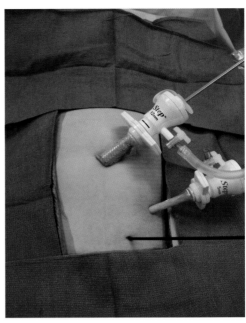

Figure 13-2. Placement of ports and instruments for intussusception reduction. First, an umbilical cannula is placed and a pneumoperitoneum is created. The telescope is introduced through this port, and then the secondary ports in the left lower abdomen (5-mm) and suprapubic region (3-mm instrument introduced via a stab incision) are inserted. The telescope is rotated toward the 5-mm lower abdominal port; the working ports are the umbilical and suprapubic ports. It is often helpful to place a larger, atraumatic grasping forceps through the umbilical port, in which case a 10-mm umbilical port may be advantageous.

intussusception. For a jejunoileal or an ileoileal intussusception, the cannulas and instruments should be oriented toward the upper portion of the abdomen or the right lower quadrant, respectively.

The primary operative principle in laparoscopic reduction of an ileocolic intussusception is to distract the intussuscepted small bowel out of the colon. Although surgeons have been taught not to pull the intussusception apart, this technique works well if precautions are taken not to tear the wall of the small bowel or the colon during operative distraction. A 5- or 10-mm Babcock or small-bowel clamp is passed through the umbilical port site. A 3-mm small-bowel grasper is used in the surgeon's left hand. The small bowel is grasped with the Babcock or small-bowel clamp placed over the bowel wall and clamped onto the mesentery of the small intestine. The cecum is pushed or grasped with the intestinal grasper in the surgeon's left hand. Distracting tension is then applied to the intussusception (Fig. 13-3). An ileocolic intussusception should be treated like an incarcerated inguinal hernia. By pulling gently but firmly on the small bowel and stabilizing the colon, the edema in the wall of the intussuscepted small intestine is slowly squeezed out, allowing reduction of the intussusception (Fig. 13-4). Usually, once this edema has dissipated, the reduction of the remainder of the

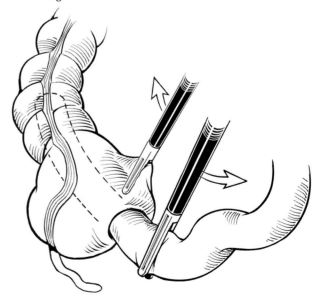

Figure 13-3. The small bowel is grasped with a Babcock or small-bowel clamp. It is best to completely grasp the entire segment of the small bowel that is intussuscepted into the colon, so that the bowel is not torn in the attempt to distract the intussusception. A larger clamp in the umbilicus is therefore often advantageous. The cecum is then pushed away from the small bowel with an intestinal grasping forceps in the surgeon's left hand.

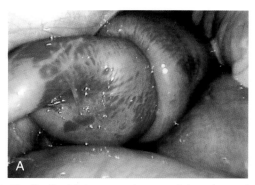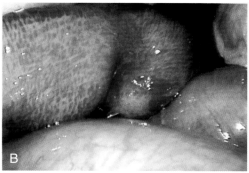

Figure 13-4.   A, The ileoileal intussusception remaining after reduction of the ileum from the colon. **B,** The ileoileal portion has been completely reduced. Note the edema and induration in the wall of the small bowel in both photographs.

small bowel and colon is quite easy, even in long-segment intussusception. The small intestine is reduced sequentially until the intussusception is completely resolved. The appendix is usually left in situ unless it appears to be gangrenous. The ileocecal valve should be inspected circumferentially to ensure complete reduction of the intussusception.

If after 15 or 20 minutes of firm distraction, no progress has been made toward reduction of the intussusception, a transverse incision is made over the right mid-abdomen. A bowel resection should not be performed laparoscopically without first attempting to manually reduce the intussusception. If the bowel cannot be reduced without major linear tears in the seromuscular wall of the colon or small intestine, the involved intestine should be resected and an ileocolostomy performed.

POSTOPERATIVE CARE

After laparoscopic reduction, the patients are not fed for 12 hours, at which time liquids are initiated. The patients are usually advanced to a regular diet over 24 hours and are discharged when ready. For patients who have undergone an open operation requiring intestinal resection, the surgeon should follow usual management practices. Parents are cautioned to return to the hospital should similar signs or symptoms develop.

PEARLS

1. Firm but gentle traction on the small bowel while pushing on the cecum should be used for at least 15 minutes before abandoning laparoscopic reduction of the intussusception.
2. Resection of the involved bowel should not be performed until open, manual reduction of the intussusception has been attempted.
3. Squeezing the colon at the site of the leading edge of the intussusceptum for a few minutes with a 5-mm

small-bowel grasping clamp sometimes helps reduce the intussusception. However, distraction is always required to reduce the intussuscepted bowel laparoscopically.
4. The patient with a recurrent intussusception should be investigated for a lead point.

PITFALLS

1. Grasping only small portions of the bowel wall can result in disastrous tears of the bowel wall. Thus, try to use a large (5- or 10-mm) clamp to securely grasp the ileum to pull on the intussusceptum.
2. Abandoning the laparoscopic reduction after only a minute or two of distraction considerably reduces the frequency of success.

RESULTS

Laparoscopic reduction of an idiopathic ileocolic intussusception has been attempted in 18 patients at the Children's Hospital of Alabama. In 15 patients, the intussusception was successfully reduced laparoscopically without recurrence or other complications. In the three patients in whom the laparoscopic approach was not successful, all required a bowel resection through a right mid-abdominal laparotomy.

SELECTED REFERENCES

1. Cuckow PM, Slater RD, Najmaldin AS: Intussusception treated laparoscopically after failed air enema reduction. Surg Endosc 10:671-672, 1996
2. Davis CF, McCabe AJ, Raine PA: The ins and outs of intussusception: History and management over the past fifty years. J Pediatr Surg 38:60-64, 2003
3. Kia K, Mony V, Drongowski RA, et al: Laparoscopic versus open surgical approach for intussusception requiring operative intervention. J Pediatr Surg 40:281-284, 2005

14
Laparoscopic Appendectomy

Eugene D. McGahren

Appendicitis affects children of all ages. It is one of the first conditions to have been treated with the laparoscopic approach because the procedure is relatively straightforward and does not require intracorporeal suturing. Laparoscopy has also served as a useful technique for teaching the principles of minimally invasive surgery.

A particular benefit of laparoscopy for the treatment of appendicitis is that it allows a full view of the appendix and the surrounding affected area. Also, it allows identification of all areas of purulence that may need to be irrigated and debrided. It allows the use of small incisions, particularly in patients with a generous amount of soft tissue, and this leads to a reduction in wound infections. Finally, it allows a general examination of the entire abdomen, which is particularly useful if laparoscopy is undertaken for suspected appendicitis but the appendix is normal.

INDICATIONS FOR WORKUP AND OPERATION

Appendicitis is one of the most commonly encountered conditions in pediatric surgery. A child typically presents with nonspecific abdominal pain that localizes to the right lower portion of the abdomen over a 24- to 48-hour period. This is often accompanied by some or all of the following: fever, anorexia, a desire to remain still, nausea, vomiting, diarrhea, dysuria. However, the symptoms may be quite nonspecific in smaller children and toddlers. Children of this age group often do not wish to walk and desire comfort from their parents.

Helpful laboratory tests include a leukocyte count with differential, a urinalysis (to exclude the urinary tract as a source of the symptoms), and a pregnancy test in any female of child-bearing age. Historically, these tests and a good history and physical examination have been sufficient to determine whether a child should undergo operation for appendicitis or be observed. Increasingly, imaging studies such as ultrasound, and particularly computed tomography (CT), are being used in evaluating for appendicitis. The CT scan is quite sensitive and specific for appendicitis and has supplanted the ultrasound in most centers. CT is also useful for distinguishing well-formed abscesses from a perforated appendix, or for identifying other causes of the patient's discomfort.

When the diagnosis of appendicitis is suspected or made, operative intervention is indicated for removal of the appendix in most cases. The patient is intravenously hydrated and appropriate antibiotics are administered before operation. If a well-formed abscess is found, appendectomy may be delayed in favor of CT-guided drainage of the abscess combined with antibiotic therapy. Antibiotic therapy alone may be appropriate for such a patient. Laparoscopic appendectomy can then be performed 6 to 8 weeks later.

Laparoscopy can be used in any child who is being operated on for appendicitis, whether as an urgent or an interval procedure. Occasionally, I use an open technique in thin, young boys when the diagnosis of acute, nonperforated appendicitis is certain. Such an operation can be performed with an incision of less than 1 inch, with no difference in postoperative hospital stay or outcome compared with laparoscopy. It also allows training in the open technique. In general, however, laparoscopy is the technique of choice for surgical treatment of appendicitis.

OPERATIVE TECHNIQUE

The patient is placed supine on the operating table, and general endotracheal anesthesia is administered. An orogastric tube is placed by the anesthesiologist for decompression of the stomach. The patient was encouraged to empty the bladder before coming to the operating room, but if that was not accomplished, it can be done via a Credé maneuver or insertion of a urinary catheter after the patient is anesthetized. The abdomen is then prepped and draped widely. Antibiotics are administered if they were not given before the patient's arrival in the operating room. I typically use one monitor placed at the right foot of the table. Cannula positions are in the infraumbilical area (5 mm), right upper lateral area (5 mm), and left lower quadrant (12 mm) of the abdomen (Fig. 14-1). The surgeon manipulates the appendix through the left lower quadrant site, and the assisting surgeon may use the instrument inserted through the right upper quadrant port while controlling the camera. This provides the classic "baseball diamond" orientation of instruments and camera relative to the target organ.

However, depending on the surgeon's preference, other orientations of the ports may be preferred. An orientation with both operating ports on the left side may allow the surgeon to work with both hands while

an assistant controls the camera (Fig. 14-2). Some authors have reported using two, and even one, port to perform the operation.

Local anesthetic (0.2% ropivacaine without epinephrine) is infiltrated into all cannula sites before incision and also before closure. In our preferred technique, an infraumbilical 5-mm skin incision is made. Dissection is then carried down to the midline fascia. Care is taken to provide traction on the fascia with stay sutures or appropriate forceps to avoid injury to underlying structures. A small incision is made in the fascia. I use the Step cannula system (Covidien, Mansfield, MA). The blunt-tipped Veress needle with an expandable sheath is introduced directly through the fascial incision. Once the needle has penetrated the fascia and peritoneum, a glass-tipped syringe with saline is connected to the port of the needle. Aspiration is done to detect any blood or enteric content. If no such findings are encountered, the saline is allowed to drop passively into the abdominal cavity, indicating that the needle is free in the cavity. The abdomen is then insufflated with CO_2 to a pressure appropriate for the size of the child.

If necessary or preferred, a direct opening into the peritoneal cavity can also be created. This is particularly useful if significant inflammation is suspected by preoperative imaging studies. Once the abdomen is insufflated (or the peritoneum is visualized if the opening is direct), a 5-mm cannula with blunt trocar is inserted through the expandable sheath. The blunt trocar is removed and a 30-degree, 5-mm laparoscope is introduced through the cannula.

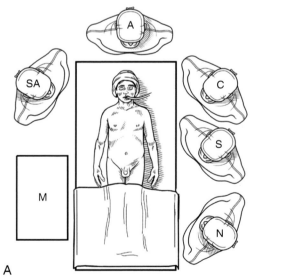

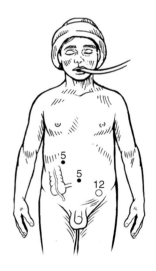

A   B

Figure 14-1.   A, Preferred positioning of personnel for a laparoscopic approach. The surgical assistant (SA) is situated to the patient's right at the level of the right-sided port. The surgeon (S) stands to the patient's left and uses the instrument placed through the 12-mm left lower quadrant port. The camera holder (C) is usually to the right of the surgeon. The scrub nurse (N) stands to the surgeon's left at the foot of the bed. A, anesthesiologist; M, monitor. **B,** Three ports are used with this approach. The assistant uses a retracting grasper through a 5-mm port in the patient's right upper abdomen. The 5-mm camera is inserted through the umbilical port. The surgeon works through the 12-mm left lower abdominal port, through which the stapler is introduced and removed.

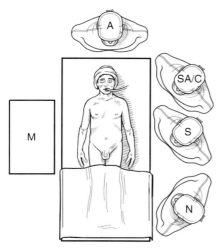
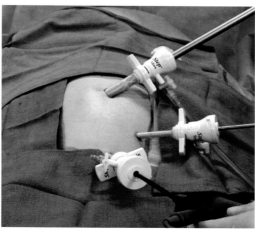

Figure 14-2.   An alternative arrangement of personnel and port placement is seen on the left. The surgeon (S) again stands to the left of the patient. The surgical assistant/camera holder (SA/C) stands cephalad to the surgeon and the scrub nurse (N) is to the surgeon's left. A, anesthesiologist; M, monitor. On the right is a photograph using this port positioning. A 12-mm port is inserted through the umbilicus. This is the port through which the stapler and endoscopic retrieval bag (if used) are introduced and removed. The 5-mm telescope is introduced through the 5-mm left mid-abdominal port. The surgeon works instruments placed through the umbilical port and the left suprapubic port. In this way, a baseball diamond configuration has been accomplished with the camera port at home base, the working ports at first and third base, and the target organ at second base with the monitor in center field.

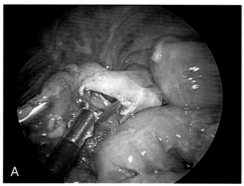
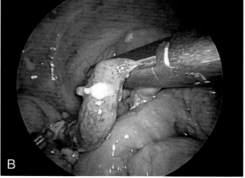

Figure 14-3.   **A,** Once the appendix has been freed from its inflammatory adhesions, a blunt dissecting instrument is used to develop a window in the avascular portion of the mesoappendix near the base of the appendix. **B,** The stapler is then introduced and placed through this window and across the base of the appendix. The appendix is usually ligated and divided first, although sometimes it is easier to initially ligate and divide the mesoappendix.

A general survey of the abdominal cavity is performed to be sure there has not been injury from placement of the initial cannula. The additional ports are then placed under direct visualization. Atraumatic grasping instruments are inserted through the right upper quadrant and left lower quadrant ports. Often there is significant inflammation and adherence of bowel to the appendix. Positioning the patient in Trendelenburg position may facilitate exposure. The bowel, and overlying omentum if present, can usually be swept away rather than grasped. If grasping is necessary to expose the appendix, care must be taken to avoid undue tension and pressure to avoid injury to the intestine or the appendix resulting in spillage of enteric contents. If the appendix is retroperitoneal, care must be taken to avoid injury to the cecum and ureter during dissection.

Attention is paid to identifying the appendix all the way to the base so as not to leave a significant stump. Once the appendix is mobilized, it is lifted to allow dissection to its base. This is sometimes difficult if there is extensive inflammation. By identifying the base, complete removal of the appendix is ensured. In addition, the base is usually relatively healthy and allows for a secure dividing point. In my technique, the appendix or mesoappendix is supported by a grasper through the right upper quadrant port. A blunt dissecting instrument, inserted through the left lower port, is used to dissect through the avascular portion of the mesoappendix next to the base of the appendix (Fig. 14-3A). The appendix and mesoappendix are then sequentially divided using an endoscopic stapler. The stapler is placed through the 12-mm left lower port. (An alternative port arrangement is to have the 12-mm port in the infraumbilical position with a 5-mm port in the left lower quadrant. With this arrangement at the time of stapling, the camera is rotated to the left port. Removal of the specimen with the endoscopic bag is sometimes easier through the more easily stretched infraumbilical site.) It is usually easier to divide the appendix first (Fig. 14-3B). After the stapler is secured, examination is always undertaken to be sure there are no other involved structures before activating the stapler. After the stapler is activated, it is helpful to orient it so that the staple tray is dependent. This helps prevent spillage of unfired staples into the abdomen when the stapler is opened. After ligation and division of the appendix, the meso-appendix is ligated and divided with the stapler and vascular load (Fig. 14-4).

An endoscopic bag is then passed through the 12-mm port and the appendix is dropped into it (Fig. 14-5). The bag with the appendix typically cannot fit through the cannula because of the size of the inflamed appendix. Therefore, the cannula is withdrawn and then the bag is withdrawn directly through the port site. The site may need to be expanded with a clamp to allow passage of the bag. To avoid spillage of the appendiceal contents into the abdomen or the cannula tract, care is taken not to rupture the bag. Once the bag is removed, the cannula is replaced. The pelvis and abdomen are surveyed for any purulent fluid that needs to be removed. The pelvis and suprahepatic space are irrigated and suctioned (Fig. 14-6). The appendiceal stump and the staple line of the mesoappendix are examined for hemostasis. All cannulas are removed under direct vision, and the CO_2 is allowed to express from the abdomen.

The infraumbilical fascia and the fascia of the 12-mm port site are closed with absorbable sutures. If the patient has a thick body wall, a Carter-Thomason device (Inlet Medical, Eden Prairie, MN) is useful to

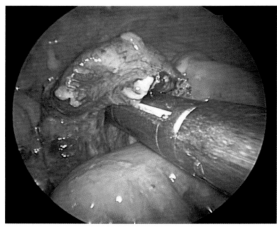

Figure 14-4. After ligation and division of the appendix, the mesoappendix is ligated and divided with the stapler, using a vascular cartridge.

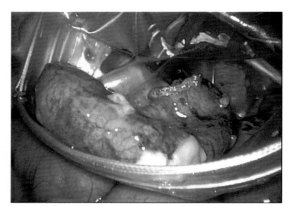

Figure 14-5. Often, the appendix is either too large or too friable to be delivered through the largest cannula. In this situation, an endoscopic retrieval bag is inserted and the appendix is placed in the bag. The bag is then exteriorized after removal of the cannula.

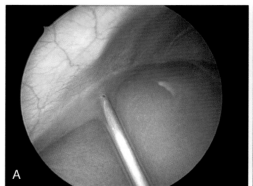
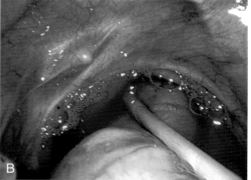

Figure 14-6. When the appendix is perforated and purulent material is throughout the abdominal cavity, the laparoscopic approach is advantageous for evacuation of the purulent material and irrigation. **A,** The purulent material in the suprahepatic area is being evacuated. **B,** The pelvis is being irrigated.

pre-place these stitches before removal of the cannulas. Subcutaneous tissue is closed with an absorbable suture. The skin is then closed with subcuticular running sutures. Butterfly bandage strips or a skin-bonding agent is then used.

PEARLS

1. Sweeping motions are preferred when exposing the appendix.
2. If the appendix is to be grasped, find a healthy or intact portion to avoid rupture and spillage.
3. Use the stapler to divide the appendix to avoid spillage from the appendix.
4. After activating the stapler, orient it with the staples dependent to prevent loose staples from falling when the device is opened.
5. Expand the largest cannula site, if necessary, to remove the endoscopic bag and appendix with the specimen.

PITFALLS

1. Be careful to avoid injuring bowel when exposing the appendix.
2. There is a potential for injury to the ureter when exposing a retroperitoneal or retrocecal appendix.
3. Spillage from the appendix may occur while manipulating it.
4. Be sure to dissect all the way to the base of the appendix before dividing it.
5. The endoscopic bag can break as it is removed from the abdomen. The spillage can lead to intra-abdominal or port site infection.

RESULTS

In the past 10 years, I had 139 cases (82 male patients, 57 female patients) with appendicitis as the primary complaint. Acute appendicitis was suspected in 131 cases, interval appendectomy was planned in five cases, and appendectomy was planned during laparoscopic examination for chronic right lower quadrant pain in three cases. Patient ages ranged from 1 year to 22 years, with a mean age of 11.9 ± 4.5 years. One hundred five cases (75.5%) were planned laparoscopically. Six operations (5.7%) were converted to open cases: two cases involved hostile anatomy, one patient had Meckel's diverticulitis, two patients were toddler-size infants in whom laparoscopic examination revealed that the appendix could be removed through a small right lower quadrant incision, and one case was converted when the dissection coursed into adherent bowel under the umbi-

licus). Thirty-four cases (24.4%) were planned as an open approach.

Of the 131 suspected cases of acute appendicitis, 113 (86.3%) were positive. Twenty (17%) of the positive cases were perforated. Eighteen cases (15.9%) were negative, although a substantial proportion of these patients had symptom relief after appendectomy despite an appendix that appeared normal on histologic examination.

Of three patients who underwent laparoscopic examination and appendectomy for chronic right lower quadrant pain, two had histologically confirmed acute or chronic appendicitis, and one had localized endometriosis that was excised. All had symptomatic relief of their pain.

The following complications were seen in the open group: one rupture of the appendix during removal, necessitating extended antibiotic therapy; one abscess requiring CT-guided drainage; one superficial wound infection; and one readmission for pain (13 days postoperatively) that resolved spontaneously. Of those patients treated laparoscopically for perforated appendicitis, 3 of 13 patients (23%) experienced a postoperative abscess requiring drainage, but none of the seven other patients treated with an open approach experienced this. However, it is important to remember that in this series, the patients treated with open technique were a selected population, generally thin males or small children.

These data indicate the utility and safety of the laparoscopic approach for removal of a diseased appendix in all pediatric age groups. It has become our favored approach for removal of the appendix in children.

SELECTED REFERENCES

1. Gilchrest BF, Lobe TE, Schropp KP, et al: Is there a role for laparoscopic appendectomy in pediatric surgery? J Pediatr Surg 27:209-212, 1992
2. Esposito C: One-trocar appendectomy in pediatric surgery. Surg Endosc 12:177-178, 1998
3. Newman K, Ponsky T, Kittle K, et al: Appendicitis 2000: Variability in practice, outcomes, and resource utilization at thirty pediatric hospitals. J Pediatr Surg 38:371-379, 2003
4. Gollin G, Moores D, Baerg JC: Getting residents in the game: An evaluation of general surgery residents' participation in pediatric laparoscopic surgery. J Pediatr Surg 39:78-80, 2004
5. Oka T, Kurkchubasche AG, Bussey JG, et al: Open and laparoscopic appendectomy are equally safe and acceptable in children. Surg Endosc 18:242-245, 2004
6. Vernon AH, Georgeson KE, Harmon CH: Pediatric laparoscopic appendectomy for acute appendicitis. Surg Endosc 18:75-79, 2004

7. Phillips S, Walton JM, Chin I, et al: Ten-year experience with pediatric laparoscopic appendectomy: Are we getting better? J Pediatr Surg 40:842-845, 2005

8. Aziz O, Athanasiou T, Tekkis PP, et al: Laparoscopic versus open appendectomy in children: A meta-analysis. Ann Surg 243:17-27, 2006

9. Chisolm DJ, Pritchett CV, Nwomeh BC: Factors affecting innovation in pediatric surgery: Hospital type and appendectomies. J Pediatr Surg 41:1809-1813, 2006

10. Tsao KJ, St Peter SD, Valusek PA, et al: Adhesive small bowel obstruction after appendectomy in children: Comparison between the laparoscopic and open approach. J Pediatr Surg 42:939-942, 2007

15
Laparoscopy in the Management of Fecal Incontinence and Constipation

Marc A. Levitt and Alberto Peña

The capacity for voluntary bowel movements may be limited for children born with anorectal anomalies and Hirschsprung's disease, as well as for many patients with spinal anomalies. Some of these patients are distressed with severe constipation, which, if not properly managed, causes overflow pseudoincontinence. Others have true fecal incontinence.

For patients with anorectal malformations with overflow pseudoincontinence, disimpaction, followed by an aggressive laxative regimen, often makes them continent (i.e., capable of having voluntary bowel movements). These children behave like patients with severe idiopathic constipation and encopresis. Surgical resection of a dilated rectosigmoid can dramatically reduce or eliminate daily laxative requirements, improving the quality of life.

In contrast, patients with true fecal incontinence require a management program with a daily enema, which allows them to be kept artificially clean. For these patients, a surgical procedure that allows the daily enema to be administered antegrade is ideal.

The clinician must distinguish between these groups, whose initial presentations are quite similar (i.e., "fecal incontinence"), because the treatments and surgical options differ dramatically.

INDICATIONS FOR WORKUP AND OPERATION

TYPES OF ANORECTAL MALFORMATIONS, SEVERE CONSTIPATION, AND MEGARECTOSIGMOID WITH A GOOD PROGNOSIS

Patients who have undergone an operation for anorectal malformations that had a good prognosis often suffer from varying degrees of hypomotility and dilation of the rectum and sigmoid (megarectosigmoid). These children often underwent a technically correct operation but did not receive adequate postoperative management for constipation. Over time, they develop chronic fecal impaction and overflow pseudoincontinence, and they often present to the clinician with fecal incontinence. Their evaluation requires knowledge of their original anorectal malformation, the quality of their sacrum, and the radiographic anatomy of their rectosigmoid. From this information, it can be predicted whether the patient has the potential for voluntary bowel control, as patients with defects that have a poor prognosis may also suffer from severe constipation. The management of this latter group of patients is markedly different.

Patients belonging to the good-prognosis group are treated as follows. If they are impacted, they are first treated with enemas. Once their colon is radiographically clean, the constipation is treated with large doses of laxatives (not stool softeners), with the laxative amount regulated daily until the proper dosage completely evacuates the colon. If it then becomes evident that the child is capable of having voluntary bowel movements and is actually continent, then the diagnosis is overflow pseudoincontinence. Unfortunately, some of these patients have suffered for years thinking they were incontinent. Medical treatment may then be very difficult because the child has a huge megasigmoid colon and an enormous amount of laxative is required to empty it. In this case, the surgeon can offer an operation to remove the dilated sigmoid (Fig. 15-1A). Sigmoid resection is appropriate, as it is vital in such patients to preserve the distal rectum, which should work very well. The distal rectum acts as a reservoir and may allow a sensation of rectal fullness (i.e., proprioception) (Fig. 15-1B). Moreover, because the anal sphincters and

anal canal failed to develop normally in these patients, the distal rectum may be the key to maintaining adequate propulsion and evacuation with fecal continence.

SEVERE IDIOPATHIC CONSTIPATION AND MEGARECTOSIGMOID

Some patients have never had reconstructive surgery but suffer from severe idiopathic constipation, and the wide spectrum of clinical symptoms in this group ranges from constipation that can be treated with dietary manipulation to severe intestinal pseudo-obstruction needing resection. Only those failing to respond to prolonged medical management come to the attention of a surgeon.

Idiopathic constipation is a common and self-perpetuating condition that, if not treated adequately, allows the patient to proceed through life only partially emptying the colon, leaving larger and larger amounts of stool in the rectosigmoid. This leads to more and more sigmoid colon dilation, which leads to a megasigmoid. Ultimately, the result is encopresis and overflow pseudoincontinence and a most uncomfortable life. This condition is only manageable, not curable, and it requires careful life-long follow-up, with recurrent problems developing if treatment is ignored. Some clinicians recommend colostomies or colonic washouts with the hope that the colonic dilation will improve and laxatives will become more effective. However, once the colostomy is closed or the washouts are discontinued, the symptoms often return rapidly.

In these patients, as in those with severe constipation and anorectal malformations, a study with water-soluble contrast enema is most valuable to confirm the diagnosis of idiopathic constipation. The characteristic image is a megarectosigmoid colon with dilation of the colon

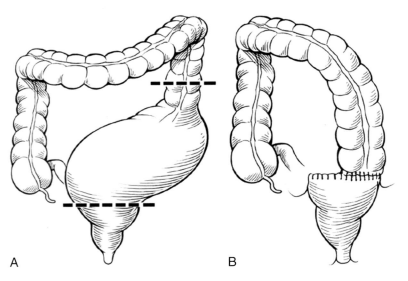

Figure 15-1. **A,** Patients who have undergone an operation for the types of anorectal malformation with a good prognosis often suffer from varying degrees of hypomotility and dilation of the rectum and sigmoid colon. **B,** If medical treatment is not effective because the child has a huge megasigmoid colon and requires an enormous amount of laxative to empty it, the surgeon can offer an operation to resect the dilated sigmoid colon.

A   B

Figure 15-2. **A,** For a patient who has not had reconstructive surgery but suffers from severe constipation, a water-soluble contrast study is most valuable to confirm the diagnosis of idiopathic constipation. The characteristic image is a megarectosigmoid colon with dilation of the colon all the way down to the level of the levator mechanism. (This is in contrast to the transition zone seen in patients with Hirschsprung's disease, where there is usually a dramatic size discrepancy between the normal transverse descending colon and the dilated megarectosigmoid.) **B,** This patient has a normal anal canal and sphincter complex and can be well served with an extensive resection including the entire rectosigmoid colon, very similar to a transanal pull-through for Hirschsprung's disease.

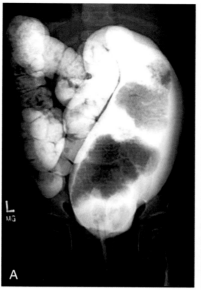
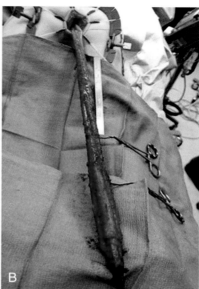

all the way down to the level of the levator mechanism (Fig. 15-2A), in contrast to that seen in patients with Hirschsprung's disease. There is usually a dramatic size discrepancy between a normal transverse and descending colon and the very dilated megarectosigmoid.

After disimpaction and achievement of a laxative dose that successfully empties the colon, resection of the rectosigmoid can be considered if the amount of laxatives required has a negative impact on the patient's bowel habits and quality of life. Because these patients have a normal anal canal and sphincters, a more extensive resection may be considered, such as resection of the entire rectosigmoid colon, much like a Swenson pull-through for Hirschsprung's disease. This operation is performed transanally (Fig. 15-2B), without laparotomy or laparoscopy, and the anal canal and neuromuscular mechanisms are carefully preserved. If the colonic dilation extends proximately to the descending and transverse colon, laparoscopy may help mobilize the splenic and hepatic flexures of the colon.

TRUE FECAL INCONTINENCE IN PATIENTS WITH ANORECTAL MALFORMATIONS, HIRSCHSPRUNG'S DISEASE, OR SPINAL DISORDERS

When a patient has had a previous repair of an anorectal malformation, it must be determined whether the condition is overflow pseudoincontinence or real fecal incontinence with constipation before any surgical option is considered. Failure to make this distinction may lead to an unnecessary operation. A fecally incontinent, constipated child subjected to a colonic

resection without proper indications would change the situation from a tendency to constipation to a tendency toward loose stools, which may be more difficult to manage.

If a patient cannot control the passage of stool even when the constipation is treated adequately, the child has true fecal incontinence. Management with laxatives makes the problem worse by producing liquid stools, which results in more frequent accidents. These patients require a daily enema for bowel management. Moreover, patients with anorectal malformations can often be predicted to have difficulties if the malformation is high and the bony sacrum is deformed radiographically. Other patients, such as those with Hirschsprung's disease who do not have a preserved anal canal, those who have suffered severe perineal trauma, and those with neurologic deficiencies such as spina bifida, may also require a daily enema to remain artificially clean. The enema must be tailored to each patient, and its effectiveness must be monitored with abdominal radiographs.

Most preschool and school-age children enjoy a good quality of life while undergoing the bowel management program. However, as they grow older, they may wish to administer the enemas themselves. For these patients, an operation can be performed to change the route of enema administration. For example, a continent appendicostomy may be created, or a button device is placed in either the cecum or the sigmoid. It should be proven that the child is clean with the regular enema first, as it does not make sense to perform an operation to create another route to administer the enema in a child who has not demonstrated success with a bowel management program.

OPERATIVE TECHNIQUES

SIGMOID RESECTION FOR CONTINENT PATIENTS WITH ANORECTAL MALFORMATIONS AND SEVERE CONSTIPATION, OR WITH MEGARECTOSIGMOID

When sigmoid resection is indicated, the patient is positioned in lithotomy position. The surgeon stands on the patient's right, and the surgical assistant is on the patient's left. Abdominal access is achieved via the umbilicus, and CO_2 is insufflated through this port. The angled telescope attached to the camera is then inserted. Additional ports are placed in the right upper abdomen (5 mm) and the right suprapubic region (12 mm) for the surgeon's right and left hands. A 5-mm port for the surgical assistant is introduced in the left upper quadrant to help hold the sigmoid during the dissection.

The sigmoid colon is mobilized, and the sigmoid mesentery is ligated with an appropriate energy device. Because the sigmoid arcade may have been interrupted during creation of the previous colostomy, the vasculature to the previously pulled-through rectum must be carefully preserved. The sigmoid is mobilized to the peritoneal reflection. The upper rectum is transected with an endovascular stapler, which is inserted and fired through the right lower quadrant port. The proximal bowel is exteriorized through this cannula tract after the incision has been enlarged. The dilated and redundant sigmoid colon is resected just proximal to its most dilated portion, and the anvil of a circular stapler is introduced at the proximal site of the planned anastomosis. The proximal segment, with the anvil in position, is then returned to the abdomen. Interrupted absorbable sutures are placed in the fascia. These sutures are not tied but rather are secured with tourniquets to allow restoration of the pneumoperitoneum and efficient re-entry into the abdomen should the need arise. The anvil is then docked into the pin of the circular endoluminal stapler, which is passed up the rectum, and a circular stapled anastomosis is created. The anastomosis is tested with air and liquid insufflated through the rectum. If there is no leak, the fascial snares are removed and the sutures tied.

Postoperative Care

The patient's diet is advanced rapidly. Laxatives at a smaller dose are reinitiated once a regular diet is started. Occasionally in the postoperative period, gentle irrigations are necessary to relieve colonic distention. These patients must be followed closely because their condition is not being cured by the operation. The remaining rectum is most likely abnormal. Without careful observation and treatment of constipation, the colon can enlarge again. If possible, the dosage of laxatives is tapered over several months, with careful monitoring of the colon with plain abdominal radiographs.

PEARLS AND PITFALLS

1. The sigmoid arcade may have been interrupted during creation of the colostomy, so the blood supply to the previously pulled-through rectum must be preserved. The surgeon cannot ligate the inferior mesenteric artery, because the intervening arcades might have been interrupted when the colostomy was created.
2. With the surgeon on the patient's right side, the operating table should be elevated with left side up to facilitate dissection.
3. The assisting port in the left upper abdomen is very helpful to splay out the sigmoid mesentery.
4. The dissection should begin directly on the bowel wall and continue distally.
5. A window in the mesentery facilitates dissection on the left side of the colon and allows good visualization of the left ureter.
6. There is always a significant size discrepancy for the anastomosis. It is easier for orientation purposes if the anvil is positioned anterior to the transected rectal staple line.

TRANSANAL RECTOSIGMOID RESECTION

For patients who have severe idiopathic constipation, who have not had previous anorectal surgery, and who are unresponsive to enormous laxative dosages intended to empty a dysmotile rectosigmoid colon, a transanal rectosigmoid resection may be considered.

Preoperative bowel preparation is mandatory. The patient is placed in the prone position with the buttocks elevated. A Lone Star retractor (Lone Star Medical Products, Inc., Stafford, TX) is placed in the anus, making sure to preserve 1.5 to 2 cm of the anal canal. Optimal placement is facilitated by inserting the pins circumferentially, then moving them more cephalad. Multiple 5-0 silk sutures are then placed in the mucosa circumferentially, starting 1.5 to 2 cm from the dentate line, and a full-thickness transanal dissection is begun. This is similar to a Swenson procedure for Hirschsprung's disease. As the rectum is mobilized, the bands are dissected and ligated. The surgeon must stay precisely on the rectal wall so as not to injure surrounding structures. Once the dissection proceeds above the level of the rectum, sigmoid vessels are encountered and are ligated. Mobilization is continued until the loop of the sigmoid has been straightened, and the nondilated portion of the upper sigmoid is visualized (Fig. 15-3). At this point, the colon is transected (Fig. 15-4A), and an interrupted, circular, two-layer coloanal anastomosis is performed with long-term absorbable suture (Fig. 15-4B).

Postoperative Care

Because of the low coloanal anastomosis, we allow these patients nothing by mouth and keep them on intravenous hyperalimentation for 7 days before a diet is restarted. Occasionally, transanastomotic irrigations are required to relieve colonic distention. The patients must be watched very closely for several weeks after the resection, and proximal colonic distention must be treated. Laxatives are reinitiated at a lower dose and tapered over weeks, or months if possible.

PEARLS AND PITFALLS

1. Preservation of the anal canal is vital and is facilitated by the Lone Star retractor, with the prongs positioned above the dentate line.

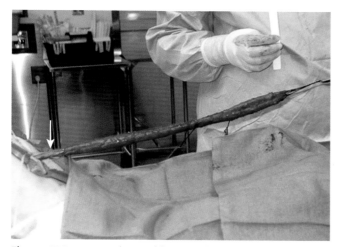

Figure 15-3. For patients with severe idiopathic constipation without previous anorectal surgery, transanal rectosigmoid resection can be performed. Mobilization of the descending colon is continued until the loop of the sigmoid colon has been straightened and the nondilated portion of the upper sigmoid is visualized (*arrow*).

Figure 15-4. Once the nondilated portion of the upper sigmoid is visualized, the colon is transected. **A,** The anterior aspect of the pull-through colon has been incised, and the anterior portion of the coloanal anastomosis is being performed. **B,** The complete coloanal anastomosis is visualized.

2. Dissection must stay very close to the rectal wall.
3. The surgeon should cauterize the sigmoid vessels completely, as they can retract up into the abdomen.
4. Additional silk sutures placed on the sigmoid colon as the dissection progresses help maintain the circumferential tension.
5. When using the cautery, we prefer to burn the most peripheral branches of the vessels as close as possible to the bowel wall, rather than cauterizing the main vascular trunks.

LAPAROSCOPIC APPENDICOSTOMY

For patients who require a daily enema as part of a successful bowel management program, an appendicostomy is the preferred route for antegrade enema administration.

The operation consists of attaching the appendix to the abdominal wall (usually at the umbilicus, sometimes in the left or right lower quadrants) and creating a valve mechanism that allows catheterization of the appendix but avoids retrograde leakage of stool (Fig. 15-5). If the child has previously had an appendectomy, it is possible to create a neoappendicostomy from the cecum.

Umbilical access is obtained and the abdomen is insufflated with CO_2. Care should be taken to open the umbilical skin in a V fashion for the appendix-to-skin Y-V anastomosis. This reduces the incidence of anastomotic stricture. Cannulas are introduced in the left upper quadrant and in the left lower quadrant for the surgeon's right and left hands. The appendix is identified. The right colon is then mobilized off its peritoneal reflection until the cecum easily reaches the umbilicus. The fascia and skin inferior to the umbilicus is then opened for 2 to 3 cm, and the cecum is delivered extracorporeally. Windows in the appendiceal mesentery are created (Fig. 15-6A), and the cecum is plicated around

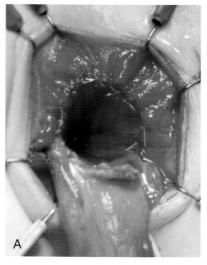
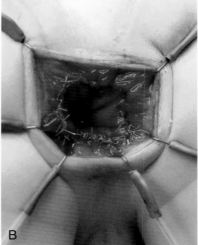

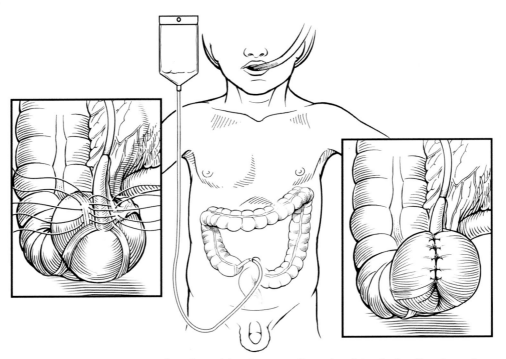

Figure 15-5. Laparoscopic appendicostomy consists of attaching the appendix to the abdominal wall and creating a valve mechanism that allows catheterization of the appendix but avoids retrograde leakage of stool. The appendix is usually exteriorized at the umbilicus, but the right or left lower abdominal wall can be used on occasion.

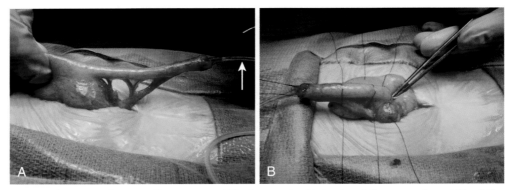

Figure 15-6. To create a laparoscopic appendicostomy, umbilical access is obtained and the cecum is mobilized through instruments inserted through the left upper and left lower abdominal quadrants. Once mobilized, the cecum is then delivered extracorporeally. **A,** Windows in the appendiceal mesentery have been created. A #8 feeding tube (*arrow*) has been inserted through the lumen of the appendix and into the cecum. **B,** The cecum is being plicated around the appendix to create the valve mechanism that will help prevent retrograde flow of stool out the appendicostomy.

the appendix to create a valve mechanism (Fig. 15-6B). The tip of the appendix is opened, and a #8 feeding tube is inserted through its lumen into the cecum. The cecum is fixed to the fascial closure. The tip of the appendix is opened along its posterior aspect and anastomosed to the umbilical skin in a Y-V fashion (Fig. 15-7).

If the appendix was previously removed, a neoappendix can be created from a cecal (or sigmoidal) flap through the same umbilical incision. To create the new appendix, a flap of the medial portion of the cecal wall

is developed (Fig. 15-8). The base of the flap must be oriented so that, when folded over, it can be easily plicated and is in the direction of the planned orifice at the skin level. It is created with one or two of the mesenteric vessels at its base providing the blood supply for the flap. The length of the flap is about 6 to 8 cm, and the width must be sufficient to allow tubularization around a #10 feeding tube without tension. The tube is created with long-term absorbable interrupted sutures, and the defect in the cecum is closed. The neoappendix is then laid down on the colonic wall, which is plicated

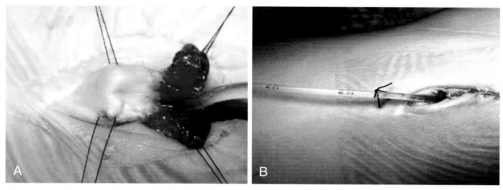

Figure 15-7. A, The cecum has been fixed to the fascial closure, and the tip of the appendix is opened along its posterior aspect. **B,** The two edges of the appendix have been anastomosed to the umbilical skin in a Y-V fashion. The feeding tube is then exteriorized through the umbilical opening.

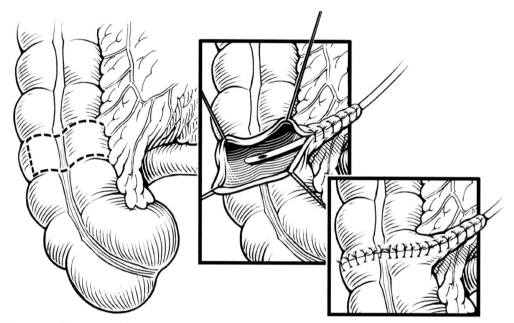

Figure 15-8. If the appendix was previously removed, a neoappendix can be created with a cecal flap through the umbilical approach that was described for a laparoscopic appendicostomy. To create the new appendix, a flap of the medial portion of the cecal wall is developed. The base of the flap must be oriented so that, when folded over, it can easily be plicated and is in the direction of the planned orifice at the skin level. One or two mesenteric vessels are needed at its base to provide the blood supply for the flap. The length of the flap is about 6 to 8 cm, and the width must be sufficient to allow tubularization around a #10 feeding tube without tension.

around it (Fig. 15-9). The sutures of the neoappendix should not lie in contact with the colonic sutures. The appendiceal tip is then anastomosed to the umbilical skin in a Y-V fashion, as described previously.

Postoperative Care
If the patient's native appendix is used, it is catheterized at the conclusion of the operation, and daily irrigations are begun 24 hours after initiation of a regular diet. After 2 weeks, the catheter is removed, and the family and patient are taught to pass it daily.

If a neoappendix is created, the catheter is left in place for 1 month before removing it. At that time, the patient

and family are taught how to pass it. In the interim, small-volume rectal enemas are continued for bowel management.

PEARLS AND PITFALLS

1. With the surgeon on the patient's left, the table is rotated right side up to facilitate the dissection.
2. Grasping of the cecum shows the tension lines along the right retroperitoneum, and the dissection proceeds in this avascular plane.

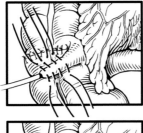
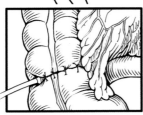
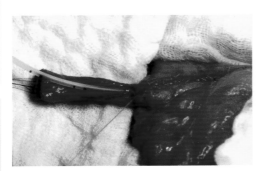

Figure 15-9. The cecum is plicated around the tubularized cecal flap. The sutures of the neoappendix should not lie in contact with the colonic sutures. The tip of the appendix is then anastomosed in the umbilical skin in a Y-V fashion as described in the text.

3. Orientation of the colonic flap must be planned so that once the tube is created, it can be folded back on the colon and is facing in the direction of the planned orifice at the skin level.
4. After each plication suture of the cecum around the appendix, the surgeon should pass the feeding tube to be certain that the tract has not been kinked.
5. The Y-V anastomosis creates a skin-lined tract and avoids a circular anastomosis, which can stricture.

CECOSTOMY OR SIGMOID BUTTON

A button device can also be used for antegrade enema administration. However, this approach is not our preference, as it leaves a foreign body at the site. Moreover, we have found it to be less cosmetically pleasing and more uncomfortable for the patient than the appendicostomy. On the other hand, we have found it ideal for certain patients, particularly those with a thick abdominal wall. The different types of device are available, and the device can be placed in the cecum or sigmoid using a laparoscopic approach. This technique is almost identical to that described for laparoscopic gastrostomy (see Chapter 6). The cecum or sigmoid is identified and mobilized so that it easily reaches the anterior abdominal wall. This often requires no mobilization at all. Two U-stitches are placed through the abdominal wall and into the colon, and a stab incision is made between them. A guidewire is passed through a needle into the cecum or sigmoid. Vascular dilators are then passed over the wire, and the button device is inserted over the wire. The crosspiece is secured to the skin and the U-stitches are tied over the crosspiece.

Postoperative Care

Patients require simple local care of the button device, and enemas can be initiated within 24 to 48 hours. The U-stitches are left in place for 7 days. The button device is irrigated with 10 mL of water for 2 weeks postopera-

tively, after which time full colonic irrigations are performed.

PEARLS AND PITFALLS

1. Local care around the button helps to prevent infectious problems and skin irritation.
2. Sigmoid buttons allow complete left-colonic evacuations, and they work faster with less cramping than cecal buttons.

RESULTS

Over a 15-year period, we have followed 237 patients suffering from idiopathic constipation. Seventeen of them elected to have an operation. We also treated 315 patients suffering from constipation and anorectal malformations, and 53 of these underwent a sigmoid resection. For nine of these cases, the laparoscopic approach was used. The degree of improvement in these patients varied. After sigmoid resection, 10% of patients did not require any more laxatives, had bowel movements every day, and did not exhibit any soiling. Thirty percent of patients decreased the laxative requirement by 80%. The remaining 60% of patients decreased the laxative requirement by 40%.

The transanal rectosigmoid resection for idiopathic constipation is a relatively new concept. Thus far, we have performed this operation on three patients. Excellent results were achieved in two: the daily laxative requirement was dramatically reduced in one and eliminated in the other. The third suffers from severe dysmotility and requires a daily irrigation to empty his colon. He is being considered for further colonic resection.

We have performed 110 appendicostomies and 30 neoappendicostomies. All patients had achieved success with a bowel management program before the operation, and the operations were 100% successful. All patients receive a daily enema, and they are clean and wear normal underwear. The incidence of stoma stricture is 4%, and leakage is 5%. In the last 27 patients, the Y-V anastomosis was used rather than a circular anastomosis between the skin and umbilicus. With this technique, we have not had a stricture and the leakage rate was unchanged.

Our experience with buttons for antegrade enemas is limited, and we defer to results in the published data in the references.

SELECTED REFERENCES

1. Peña A, El-Behery M: Megasigmoid: A source of pseudoincontinence in children with repaired anorectal malformations. J Pediatr Surg 28:1-5, 1993
2. Chait PG, Shandling B, Richards HF: The cecostomy button. J Pediatr Surg 32:849-851, 1997
3. Levitt MA, Soffer SZ, Peña A: The continent appendicostomy in the bowel management of fecally incontinent children. J Pediatr Surg 32:1630-1633, 1997
4. Peña A, Guardino K, Tovilla JM, et al: Bowel management for fecal incontinence in patients with anorectal malformations. J Pediatr Surg 33:133-137, 1998
5. Wheatley JM, Hutson JM, Chow CW, et al: Slow-transit constipation in childhood. J Pediatr Surg 34:829-833, 1999
6. Marshall J, Hutson JM, Anticich N, et al: Antegrade continence enemas in the treatment of slow-transit constipation. J Pediatr Surg 36:1227-1230, 2001
7. Peña A, Levitt MA: Colonic inertia disorders in pediatrics. Curr Probl Surg 39:666-730, 2002
8. Chait PG, Shlomovitz E, Connolly BL, et al: Percutaneous cecostomy: Updates in technique and patient care. Radiology 227:246-250, 2003
9. Levitt MA, Carney DE, Powers CJ, et al: Laparoscopically assisted colon resection for severe idiopathic constipation with megarectosigmoid. Pediatr Endosurg Innov Tech 7:285-289, 2003
10. Malone PS: The antegrade continence enema procedure. Br J Urol 93:248-249, 2004
11. Yagmurlu A, Harmon CM, Georgeson KE: Laparoscopic cecostomy button placement for the management of fecal incontinence in children with Hirschsprung's disease and anorectal anomalies. Surg Endosc 20:624-627, 2006

16

Laparoscopic Segmental Colectomy

Steven S. Rothenberg

The efficacy of laparoscopic colon resection has been demonstrated in a number of conditions, including Hirschsprung's disease and inflammatory bowel disease. These procedures can be quite extensive and usually include at least a proctocolectomy. However, for a number of conditions, it may be sufficient to perform a lesser or more limited colon resection, which can give the same benefits that are observed with the more extensive procedures. This is true whether all of the procedure is performed intracorporeally or whether a portion, such as the anastomosis, is performed extracorporeally.

INDICATIONS FOR WORKUP AND OPERATION

The indications for segmental colon resection are a bit more varied and more infrequent than those for colon pull-through or total colectomy. They include strictures secondary to necrotizing enterocolitis (NEC), colon duplications, segmental inflammatory bowel disease, and chronic constipation. The workup depends on the disease process. Usually, at the least, a barium enema is required. This can usually identify the area of stricture or obstruction. Occasionally, colonoscopy is desirable to help define the type and extent of the lesion. A computed tomographic scan may also be helpful in cases of colonic duplication. In patients with chronic constipation, a barium enema often shows a dilated and tortuous sigmoid colon. Before resection, the patient should have failed an extensive bowel management program.

OPERATIVE TECHNIQUE

Before surgery, the patient can be given a mechanical bowel preparation if there is not a complete or near-complete obstruction. A Golytely prep (Braintree Laboratories, Braintree, MA) is usually adequate and may be supplemented by saline enemas. Irrigations can also be performed in the operating room after the patient is placed under general anesthesia. A patient who is nearly obstructed should be restricted to clear liquids or receive nothing by mouth for 2 to 3 days before the operation, especially if a primary anastomosis is planned.

The patient's position depends on the site of the lesion. In general, the patient is placed supine on the operating table. If the area of resection includes the transverse colon, larger patients should be placed in a modified decubitus position with the legs in stirrups and angled down 60 degrees. Such positioning allows the surgeon to stand between the legs, which is the most ergonomic position for mobilizing the transverse colon. The viewing monitors are placed directly in front of the surgeon, in line with the area of pathology. For the sake of illustrating the operative technique, a segmental sigmoid resection will be described (Fig. 16-1).

A routine skin preparation is performed and the patient is sterilely draped. The abdomen is then insufflated through a 5-mm umbilical ring incision using

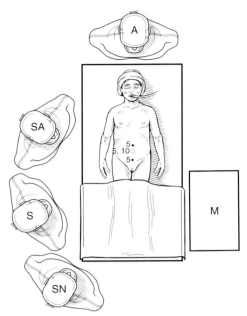

Figure 16-1. In general, patients are positioned supine on the operating table for colonic procedures involving either the right, left, or sigmoid colon. For operations involving the transverse colon or rectum, placing the legs in stirrups and angled down 60 degrees is advantageous. This allows easy access to the rectum for insertion of a curved intraluminal stapling device, if needed. Also, the surgeon can stand between the patient's legs to access the transverse colon. In this diagram, a sigmoid resection will be performed. Therefore, the surgeon (S) and surgical assistant (SA) are positioned to the patient's right side, with the monitor (M) over the patient's lower left side. This allows an in-line view of the target organ. The scrub nurse (SN) is to the right of the surgeon. Initially, a 5-, 10-, or 12-mm port is inserted through the umbilicus. A 12-mm port is used if an intracorporeal anastomosis is planned. This large incision allows removal of the specimen through this site as well. Two other ports are then introduced, one above and one below the umbilicus, to create the appropriate 90-degree approach for colon mobilization and anastomosis. These two ports are usually 5 mm in size. A, anesthesiologist.

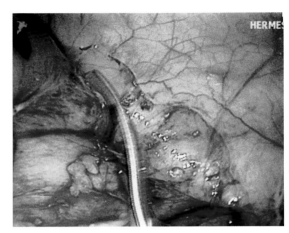

Figure 16-2. The first step for sigmoid resection is mobilization of the involved segment. In this view, scissors are being used to sharply divide the lateral peritoneal attachments to the descending colon.

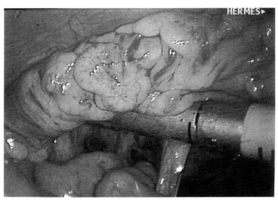

Figure 16-3. After division of the colon proximal to the site of the pathologic lesion with one or two tissue loads, the mesentery can be divided with a number of instruments, such as monopolar cautery, the ultrasonic scalpel, the Ligasure, or the endoscopic stapler that is shown here.

either a Veress needle or the open technique, depending on surgeon preference. A 10- or 12-mm port is inserted in the umbilicus if the plan is to perform the resection and anastomosis intracorporeally. This large incision and cannula allow removal of the specimen through the umbilicus.

At least two other ports are needed. They are inserted above and below the umbilical port to create the appropriate 90-degree approach for colon mobilization and anastomosis (Fig. 16-1). The first step is mobilization of the involved segment. The lateral peritoneal attachments can be mobilized by sharp dissection, as this is an avascular plane (Fig. 16-2). Once an adequate segment is laterally mobilized to allow resection and anastomosis, the bowel is divided proximally and distally. The method for bowel division depends on the size of the patient. In larger patients, an endoscopic stapler is introduced

through the 12-mm umbilical port. The colon is divided proximal to the site of pathology with one or two tissue loads. The mesentery is then divided using either monopolar cautery, the ultrasonic scalpel, Ligasure (Covidien, Mansfield, MA), or another sealing technology. The endoscopic stapler can also be used to divide the mesentery (Fig. 16-3). Dissection is maintained near the bowel wall, as these vessels tend to be smaller than those found at the root of the mesentery. Moreover, this approach decreases the risk of injury to adjacent structures such as the ureters. Usually, the mesenteric division is facilitated by working from the proximal end of the divided bowel and progressing distally. Once the distal end of the diseased colon is reached, the bowel is again divided. A side-to-side anastomosis can then be performed using the endoscopic stapler (Fig. 16-4). Details are described in Chapter 12.

In smaller patients, such as those with strictures secondary to necrotizing enterocolitis, the bowel is divided and an end-to-end anastomosis performed. When performing the anastomosis, it is important to limit intraperitoneal contamination by creating a small enterotomy first and then using a laparoscopic suction device to evacuate the bowel contents. The anastomosis can then be done with running or interrupted sutures. Stay sutures are placed at the apex and the lower part of the two colon ends to be anastomosed to align and stabilize the bowel segments (Fig. 16-5A). These stay sutures can be used to tie to at the end of the suture line. A running suture line is usually preferable. The anastomosis is started on the back wall with a continuous suture using 3-0 Vicryl or PDS (Ethicon, Inc., Somerville, NJ). The anterior wall is then anastomosed using a continuous suture (Fig. 16-5B). If needed, the assistant can use a small clamp placed through a fourth port in the left upper quadrant to follow the suture line and facilitate suturing. After completion of the anastomosis, the mesenteric defect should be closed with a few interrupted sutures, and the resected bowel is placed into an endoscopic bag that is exteriorized through a slightly extended umbilical incision.

If the surgeon is not comfortable with performing an intracorporeal anastomosis, the bowel can be mobilized in the same fashion as described but brought out through a small muscle-sparing lower abdominal incision (Fig. 16-6). The bowel is then divided and the anastomosis is performed extracorporeally.

POSTOPERATIVE CARE

A nasogastric tube is usually left for 24 hours, and broad-spectrum antibiotics are continued for 2 days. Oral intake is initiated after the patient has passed flatus

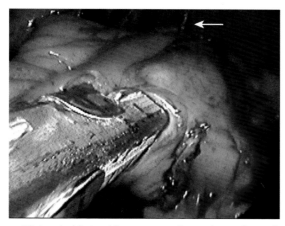

Figure 16-4. A side-to-side anastomosis can be performed with the endoscopic stapler. In this view, the two ends to be anastomosed have been positioned side by side. Each arm of the stapler has been introduced through an enterotomy in each limb. The stay suture (*arrow*) at the top of the photograph was placed to align the two segments of bowel.

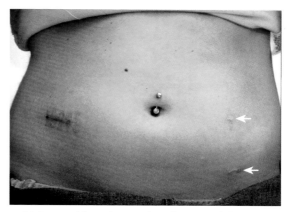

Figure 16-6. In this patient undergoing a partial right colectomy, an extracorporeal anastomosis was performed through a small right lower quadrant incision. The belly-button ring was removed and the umbilicus utilized for one of the port sites. The other two port sites are marked with *arrows*.

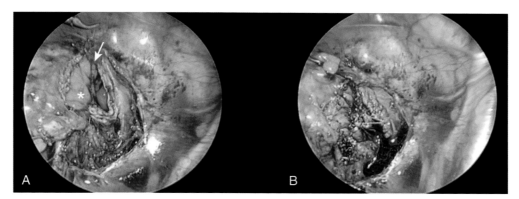

Figure 16-5. In this patient, an intracorporeal anastomosis was performed. **A,** The two ends of the bowel to be anastomosed are aligned. A portion of the posterior suture line has been completed (*arrow*). The mucosa of the proximal segment of colon is marked with an *asterisk*. The distal lumen is well visualized. **B,** The anterior suture line has been completed.

or stool, which usually occurs within 48 hours. A number of patients are actually ready for oral intake after 24 hours.

PEARLS

1. Align the bowel ends so that suturing is performed with the optimal angle (90 degrees) between the left- and right-hand operating ports. Always sew toward yourself.
2. If the proximal bowel is grossly dilated, an angiocatheter can be inserted through the abdominal wall to decompress the bowel before its mobilization.
3. Make a small enterotomy proximally and insert a suction device (which is introduced through the assistant's port) to minimize or avoid peritoneal contamination.
4. Know the extent of the strictured or diseased bowel as much as possible with adequate preoperative imaging (contrast) studies. This avoids the guesswork that prolongs operating time.

PITFALLS

1. If the anastomosis is performed extracorporeally, the bowel may become congested, making it difficult to reduce it back through the lower abdominal incision.
2. Pulling a running suture line too tight can result in an unrecognized stricture. The bowel anastomosis needs to be secure but not stenosed. If you are not sure, then run one part of the anastomosis and interrupt the other side.
3. Inadequate mobilization of the bowel can result in too much tension on the anastomosis, making it technically much more difficult. This can be hard to judge intracorporeally. The two colonic ends should lie next to each other without being held.
4. A low anterior anastomosis can be difficult to sew laparoscopically. Consider using a curved intraluminal stapler inserted through the anus.

RESULTS

Over the past 10 years, 21 patients have undergone laparoscopic segmental colon resection with primary anastomosis. This group included 13 patients with intestinal strictures secondary to NEC, six patients with chronic constipation and a redundant sigmoid colon, one patient with a stricture at a previous colon anastomosis, and one patient with a mesenteric cyst. The patients' ages ranged from 2 months to 14 years, and their weight from 3 to 60 kg. All underwent laparoscopic mobilization and resection. Five patients with NEC stricture had an extracorporeal anastomosis performed and the rest had an intracorporeal anastomosis. All NEC patients had an end-to-end, hand-sewn anastomosis. Among those requiring sigmoid resection, an end-to-end anastomosis was performed in five, the anastomosis was hand sewn in two, and a curved intraluminal stapler inserted through the anus was used in three. One patient had an intracorporeal stapled anastomosis. The patient with the anastomotic stricture had a hand-sewn anastomosis. In this series, the average operative time was 110 minutes. A nasogastric tube was left for 24 hours in all cases, and all patients were started on oral feedings by the second postoperative day. The postoperative hospitalization ranged from 3 to 7 days.

SELECTED REFERENCES

1. Ramos JM, Beart RW Jr, Goes R, et al: Role of laparoscopy in colorectal surgery: A prospective evaluation of 200 cases. Dis Colon Rectum 38:494-501, 1995
2. Rothenberg SS: Experience with advanced endosurgical procedures in neonates and infants under 5 kg. Pediatr Endosurg Innov Tech 2:107-110, 1997
3. Carvalho JL, Campos M, Soares-Oliveira M, et al: Laparoscopic colonic mapping of dysganglionosis. Pediatr Surg Int 17:493-495, 2001
4. Rothenberg SS: Laparoscopic segmental intestinal resection. Sem Pediatr Surg 11:211-216, 2002
5. Simon T, Orangio G, Ambroze W, et al: Laparoscopic-assisted bowel resection in pediatric/adolescent inflammatory bowel disease: Laparoscopic bowel resection in children. Dis Colon Rectum 46:1325-1331, 2003

17

Laparoscopic Total Colectomy with Pouch Reconstruction

Robert Cina and Keith E. Georgeson

Many children with familial polyposis and ulcerative colitis can be medically managed into adulthood. On the other hand, some suffer from refractory disease, experience adverse disease sequelae (growth retardation and delayed puberty), or suffer treatment-related complications. For these patients, restorative proctocolectomy with ileal pouch–anal anastomosis provides an effective surgical alternative to continued ineffective medical management.

PREOPERATIVE PREPARATION

A mechanical bowel preparation is administered the day before surgery. The addition of an enteral antibiotic preparation is employed by some, although this practice has become controversial in recent years. Broad-spectrum antibiotics should be administered 30 minutes before the incision and the dose repeated during the procedure as appropriate. The patient is placed in a modified lithotomy position using stirrups. All pressure points should be well padded to avoid pressure injuries. Excessive flexion at the hips and knees should also be avoided, because this may provide a physical barrier to the mobility of the laparoscopic instruments. The arms are tucked at the patient's side. A urinary catheter is inserted. The surgeon and camera holder stand opposite the area being resected during the procedure, and the assistant initially stands at the foot of the bed between the legs (Fig. 17-1).

OPERATIVE TECHNIQUE

Five or six 5-mm ports are required to access and mobilize the colon laparoscopically (Fig. 17-2). Access to the abdomen is obtained through the umbilicus. A suprapubic midline port and right and left lower quadrant midclavicular ports are inserted. A fifth port is situated in the right upper quadrant in the midclavicular line to assist in accessing the splenic flexure of the colon. Sometimes a sixth port (5 mm) in the left upper quadrant in the midclavicular line is used for better access to the hepatic flexure of the colon. Colon mobilization is initiated at the rectosigmoid mesocolon just proximal to the rectosigmoid junction. The division of the mesocolon is optimally achieved with the use of an ultrasonic scalpel. Dissection with the ultrasonic scalpel is kept close to the wall of the colon, which promotes the division of smaller vessels as opposed to the larger vessels near the mesenteric root (Fig. 17-3). Keeping the dissection close to the colon adds a level of safety to the operation, as the mesentery of children with ulcerative colitis is often thick as a result of their chronic inflammatory state and the use of steroids. Alternatively, dissection close to the root of the mesocolon can be performed using vascular clips or a stapler to control the larger vessels.

After a window has been developed in the rectosigmoid mesocolon, dissection is carried proximally from this point. Care must be taken to avoid injury to the left ureter, especially when taking down the lateral

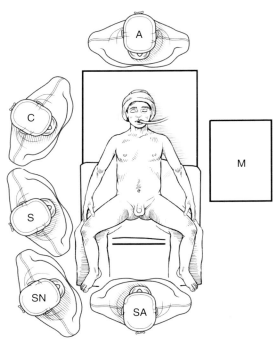

Figure 17-1.   Personnel positioning for a laparoscopic total colectomy at the initial step in the operation, which is mobilization of the upper rectum, sigmoid, and left colon. The surgeon (S) and camera holder (C) stand opposite the colon segment that is being mobilized. The telescope and camera are initially inserted through the umbilical cannula but are rotated among the ports depending on where the colon mobilization is occurring. A, anesthesiologist; M, monitor; SA, surgical assistant; SN, scrub nurse.

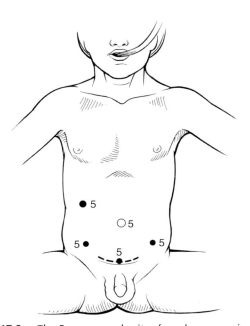

Figure 17-2.   The 5-mm cannula sites for a laparoscopic-assisted proctocolectomy with J-pouch pull-through. A left upper quadrant port is sometimes added for help with the dissection of the hepatic flexure of the colon. The rectal dissection and formation of the J-pouch are performed through the small suprapubic incision.

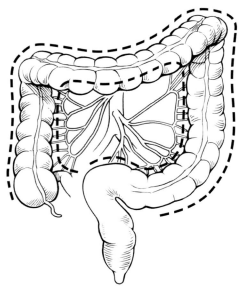

Figure 17-3.   The lateral peritoneal attachments and mesentery of the colon are divided to fully mobilize the colon. A variety of instruments can be used to mobilize the colon, including scissors, the ultrasonic scalpel, Ligasure, and stapler for a thickened mesentery.

peritoneal attachments of the colon to the abdominal wall. This lateral fusion fascia is divided with either scissors or hook cautery. These instruments perform this task faster than the ultrasonic scalpel. There is usually minimal bleeding from the fusion fascia. The mesenteric dissection becomes more difficult as the splenic flexure is approached. Although the mesocolon at this level can be divided by either a medial or a lateral approach, retraction of the colon medially with lateral division of the mesocolon is often safer. As the dissection becomes more difficult and confusing, the gastrocolic ligament should be divided beginning on the right side of the patient, just to the left of the falciform ligament. Care must be taken to avoid dividing both the gastrocolic ligament and the transverse colon mesentery simultaneously, as these two structures are frequently closely adherent. The gastrocolic ligament is divided to the level of the ileocolic ligament, which is also severed. The mesocolon around the splenic flexure is divided by alternating the proximal and distal approaches. The mesocolon can be visualized by elevating the colon toward the anterior abdominal wall or by pulling the colon centrally and dividing the mesocolon lateral to the colon. After the splenic flexure of the colon has been separated from the mesocolon, the operating surgeon changes position from the right side of the operating table to a point between the patient's legs. The operation continues with mobilization of the transverse mesocolon. This maneuver is aided by placing the patient in a reverse Trendelenburg position, allowing gravity to pull the small bowel and omentum into the pelvis. Some surgeons advocate preserving the greater omentum, but we prefer to resect the omentum with the colon.

The gastrocolic and hepatocolic ligaments are divided to the hepatic flexure. It is important to identify and avoid injury to the duodenum during the dissection of the right transverse mesocolon. Mobilization of the hepatic flexure can be difficult. Dissecting the cecum and ascending colon first can make this process easier.

The cecum and terminal ileum are mobilized by dividing the retroperitoneal attachments to the appendix and cecum. The right fusion fascia is also incised sharply. Tilting the table to the patient's left aids in the dissection of the hepatic flexure and ascending colon. The right mesocolon is divided as close to the colon as possible to save the right colic artery and marginal artery branches, which sometimes serve as the main blood supply to the terminal ileum and the J-pouch.

After complete devascularization of the colon and division of all of its abdominal attachments, a suprapubic transverse incision is made. Upon entering the peritoneal cavity, the distal colon is divided with a gastrointestinal (GI) stapling device. In a similar fashion, the terminal ileum is divided with the GI stapler and the specimen is removed. Construction of the J-pouch follows. A point approximately 10 to 20 cm proximal to the ileocecal valve is chosen for construction of the J-pouch. It is important to assess the amount of pouch mobility. The apex of the future J-pouch should reach the base of the penis in males and the clitoris in females. Several techniques can be used to increase pouch mobility. Transverse incisions in the anterior and posterior small-bowel mesentery overlying the superior mesenteric artery and vein usually allow several centimeters of additional length (Fig. 17-4). Further length can be obtained by dividing the restraining superior mesenteric artery vessels, provided that an assessment of the collateral blood supply is made first. This assessment is performed by placing a small bulldog clamp on the restraining vessels and observing whether ischemic changes develop anywhere in the pouch.

The ileum is then folded on itself and secured with stay sutures. Each limb should be approximately 6 to 8 cm in length. A small incision is made in the apex of the folded ileum, through which a GI stapler is inserted with one arm in each limb of the folded ileum (Fig. 17-5). The stapler is locked and fired, creating the J-pouch. The enterostomy at the apex of the J-pouch is closed with a purse-string polypropylene suture. Next, the mesentery of the distal sigmoid colon and proximal rectum is divided down to the level of the peritoneal reflection. Dissection of the rectum is continued very close to the rectal wall. Hemostasis with electrocautery or the ultrasonic scalpel is helpful to minimize bleeding in the pelvis. The dissection around the rectum is continued circumferentially until the entire rectum is separated from the pelvic structures to within 1 to 2 cm of the dentate line. Some

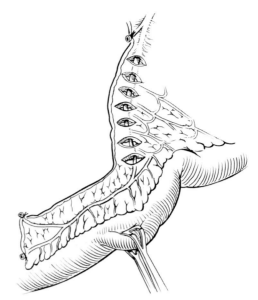

Figure 17-4. Lengthening of the vascular pedicle to the J-pouch can be accomplished by making multiple crosshatches over the mesenteric vessels. Care must be taken not to injure the vessels. This crosshatching can be done on both the anterior and the posterior surfaces of the small-bowel mesentery. The mesenteric vessels can be divided if there is adequate collateral circulation, but only if an adequate pedicle length cannot be obtained any other way.

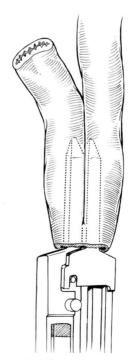

Figure 17-5. The terminal ileum is folded back on itself. A 75- to 100-mm stapler is applied on each side of the J-pouch spur and fired, avoiding the mesenteric vessels.

of this dissection is performed bluntly, but much of it is performed using a right-angle clamp and electrocautery. Retracting the rectum upward facilitates this low rectal dissection.

The patient's legs are flexed in the stirrups to allow easier access to the anus. A long clamp is passed through the anus into the mobilized rectum and rectosigmoid colon. The stapled proximal end of the rectosigmoid colon is grasped, and the rectal sleeve is inverted (Fig. 17-6A). The surgeon should then note whether the dissection of the rectum has been adequate. If the rectum cannot be inverted within 1 to 2 cm of the dentate line, further dissection should be performed transabdominally. The inverted rectum is then stapled externally

between the buttock cheeks as close to the anus as possible (see Fig. 17-6B). The anvil of the circular endoluminal stapler is inserted inside the J-pouch and the purse-string suture closed snugly around it. The blunt portion of the circular endoluminal stapler is passed through the anus. The spike is deployed through one side of the anorectal staple line (Fig. 17-7A) and the anvil in the J-pouch is securely attached to the spike. The stapler is then fired and disengaged from the rectum (see Fig. 17-7B). Two complete colon rings should be identified on the stapler. The anastomosis can also be evaluated by careful digital examination.

The operative team returns to the abdominal field after changing their gloves and gowns. The small bowel

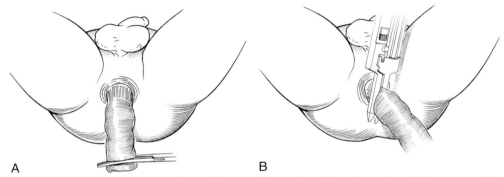

Figure 17-6. **A,** The rectum is being inverted out through the anus by passing a long clamp through the anus and grasping the staple line at the rectosigmoid junction. **B,** The rectum is transected through the transitional mucosa less than 2 cm above the dentate line.

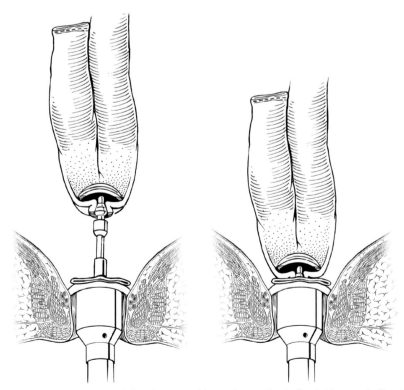

Figure 17-7. **A,** The spike is docked with the anvil (in the J-pouch). **B,** The stapler is fired. The staple line is carefully palpated transanally.

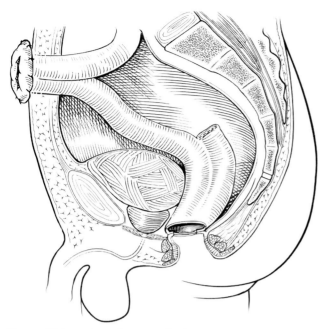

Figure 17-8. A loop ileostomy is almost always used to protect the J-pouch and the anorectal anastomosis. This ileostomy can be closed 6 to 8 weeks after formation of the J-pouch.

and its pedicle are examined carefully to ensure an adequate blood supply. The mesenteric defect is closed using nonabsorbable suture. This closure should be very carefully performed so as to avoid encroachment on the nourishing blood vessels contained in the vascular pedicle. Failure to completely obliterate the defect behind the small-bowel pedicle can result in an internal hernia with future bowel obstruction. The small bowel and its pedicle should also be checked to ensure that no twists in the mesenteric pedicle have occurred. The pedicle should be relatively tension free.

After completion of the anorectal anastomosis and closure of the posterior mesenteric defect, a protective loop ileostomy is created 20 to 30 cm proximal to the J-pouch (Fig. 17-8). A loop ileostomy is usually easier to construct and subsequently close than an end ileostomy. At times, the abdominal wall is so thick or the mesentery is so short that an end ileostomy is the only possible stoma that can be formed. In this instance, the distal ileum should be tacked to the proximal ileum, close to its exit through the abdominal wall to facilitate reestablishment of continuity at the time of ileostomy closure. Additionally, the ileostomy in children should be attached to the anterior fascia of the abdominal wall to reduce the incidence of peristomal herniation. The suprapubic incision is irrigated and closed using standard technique, as are the laparoscopic incisions.

POSTOPERATIVE CARE

Postoperatively, broad-spectrum antibiotics are continued for 24 hours. Bowel function usually returns on the second to fourth day. Patients are usually ready for discharge by the fifth or sixth postoperative day.

PEARLS

1. Dissection of the mesentery close to the colon with the ultrasonic scalpel minimizes bleeding and avoids injury to important retroperitoneal structures.
2. Swinging the colon medially and dividing the mesocolon lateral to the colon improves the speed and safety of the dissection.
3. A small suprapubic incision is faster and safer for the rectal dissection and formation of the J-pouch than the laparoscopic approach.

PITFALLS

1. Placement of the lateral ports too far laterally makes them less effective when the patient is tilted toward the side of the laterally placed cannula.
2. A long J-pouch (greater than 10 cm) can lead to dysfunctional evacuation of the pouch.
3. Careless closure of the potential hernia space behind the small bowel mesentery can lead to internal herniation and a subsequent bowel obstruction.

RESULTS

Large series of patient outcomes have been reported for both open and laparoscopic proctocolectomy with J-pouch formation in adults. Daytime continence is reported in about 80% of patients, with 70% of patients reporting nighttime continence. Severe incontinence is seen in only about 5% of patients. We have performed over 30 laparoscopic-assisted proctocolectomies with even better daytime and nighttime continence outcomes. Other postoperative complications include pouchitis in about 40% of patients, which almost always responds to metronidazole, bowel obstruction in 10%, and anorectal stenosis in less than 5% of patients. Proctocolectomy with J-pouch construction seems to be well tolerated by adolescent patients.

SELECTED REFERENCES

1. Marcello PW, Milson JW, Wong SK, et al: Laparoscopic restorative proctocolectomy. Dis Colon Rectum 43:604-608, 2000
2. Georgeson KE: Laparoscopic-assisted total colectomy with pouch reconstruction. Semin Pediatr Surg 11:223-226, 2002
3. Rintala RJ, Lindahl HG: Proctocolectomy and J-pouch ileoanal anastomosis in children. J Pediatr Surg 37:66-70, 2002

4. Wexner SD, Johansen OB, Nogueras JJ, et al: Laparoscopic total abdominal colectomy: A prospective trial. Dis Colon Rectum 35:651-655, 2002
5. Baixauli J, Delaney CP, Wu JS, et al: Functional outcome and quality of life after repeat ileal pouch-anal anastomosis for complications of ileoanal surgery. Dis Colon Rectum 47:2-11, 2004
6. Shen B, Fazio VW, Remzi FH, et al: Comprehensive evaluation of inflammatory and noninflammatory sequelae of ileal pouch-anal anastomoses. Am J Gastroenterol 100:93-101, 2005
7. Remzi FH, Fazio VW, Gorgun E, et al: The outcome after restorative proctocolectomy with or without defunctioning ileostomy. Dis Colon Rectum 49:470-477, 2006

18
Laparoscopic-Assisted Pull-Through for Hirschsprung's Disease

Michael J. Morowitz and Keith E. Georgeson

Surgical correction of Hirschsprung's disease can be safely achieved in most patients with a primary, one-stage procedure. A simple laparoscopic approach for correcting Hirschsprung's disease is the laparoscopic-assisted endorectal pull-through adapted from Soave and Boley. Since this procedure was first reported in 1995, experience has demonstrated that it can also be successfully performed as a transanal one-stage endorectal pull-through without laparoscopy. However, the laparoscopic-assisted approach offers significant advantages. First, obtaining leveling biopsies with laparoscopic guidance provides the surgeon with valuable confirmation of the specific location of the pathologic transition zone. Second, laparoscopic dissection of the proximal rectum and mesorectum allows an easier transanal dissection resulting in less retraction of the sphincters. Minimizing the extent of the transanal dissection and retraction is desirable for better long-term continence. Additionally, proximal tethering of the neorectum is also lessened by dividing the fusion fascia and developing a mesenteric pedicle when using the laparoscopic technique. This chapter describes the perioperative considerations and operative technique for performing the one-stage laparoscopic-assisted pull-through.

INDICATIONS FOR WORKUP AND OPERATION

Biopsy of the rectal wall provides the most accurate means of diagnosing Hirschsprung's disease, which should be considered in any child with a history of severe constipation since birth. Histologic findings supporting the diagnosis include the absence of ganglion cells, the presence of hypertrophied nerve trunks, and increased acetylcholinesterase staining in the muscularis mucosa. In most patients, primary laparoscopic-assisted endorectal pull-through may be performed soon after firmly establishing the diagnosis. A contrast enema delineating the colonic transition zone aids in planning the operation. In newborns, retained contrast seen on a follow-up film 1 day after the contrast enema often demonstrates the apparent transition zone. Relative contraindications to a primary one-stage approach include severe enterocolitis, major comorbidities, and the inability to determine the site of normal ganglion cells above the transition zone. Also, massive diffuse colonic dilation caused by chronic obstruction is a contraindication to primary pull-through. For patients with transition zones proximal to the mid-transverse colon, a single or multistage laparoscopic Duhamel procedure is probably more appropriate than the endorectal pull-through.

All patients with Hirschsprung's disease receive preoperative parenteral antibiotics. Because bowel distention interferes with laparoscopic visualization of the colon and its mesentery, the gastrointestinal tract should be decompressed. Digital manipulation every 3 hours for 2 to 3 days before surgery may provide adequate decompression, but sometimes rectal irrigation with the tip of the rectal tube above the transition zone is necessary. In older children with chronic disease, the administration of an oral cathartic is recommended.

OPERATIVE TECHNIQUE

After induction of general endotracheal anesthesia, infants and small children are positioned transversely across the operating table (Fig. 18-1A). If necessary, placing arm boards parallel to the main axis of the table will lengthen the surface available for patient positioning. Larger children should be positioned in the lithotomy position along the long axis of the table, with the legs in stirrups. Broad-spectrum antibiotics are administered, and an orogastric tube is inserted to decompress the stomach. Preparation of the patient includes wide cleansing of the trunk from the nipples to below the level of the buttocks. For small children in the supine position, the buttocks and legs are cleansed circumferentially to the tips of the toes, and sterile stockings are placed on both legs (see Fig. 18-1B). The surgeon and assistant stand above the infant's head with the monitor positioned beyond the infant's feet (Fig. 18-2A).

A 5-mm port is inserted through the umbilicus and carbon dioxide pneumoperitoneum is established. Two additional 4-mm working ports are positioned in the right upper and lower quadrants (Fig. 18-2B). For patients with a transition zone proximal to the sigmoid colon, a fourth working port in the left upper abdomen along the midclavicular line can be used for retraction.

The operation begins by defining the location of the colonic transition zone and thus determining which segment of colon can be safely pulled through to serve as a functional neorectum (Fig. 18-3). Seromuscular biopsy specimens are obtained along the length of the colon with laparoscopic Metzenbaum scissors and fine-tipped grasping forceps such as the Maryland dissector. Blunt-tipped graspers are more likely to yield a full-thickness biopsy and should be avoided during this step of the procedure. To initiate the biopsy, the wall of the colon is elevated with the fine-tipped forceps, and shears are used to incise the seromuscular wall. The cut end is grasped and then undermined with the shears to complete the biopsy (Fig. 18-4A). Biopsy sites should be closed laparoscopically with sutures if the mucosa has been violated. An alternative approach is to deliver the colon through the umbilical incision (after removing the cannula) and perform an extracorporeal biopsy (Fig. 18-4B). This technique works well for biopsy of the sigmoid colon, as it is quite mobile.

Usually three or four biopsy specimens are evaluated by rapid frozen section analysis to determine the level of normally ganglionated colon. If this initial pathologic review indicates a transition zone proximal to the mid-transverse colon, it is prudent to halt the procedure at this point and wait for permanent section confirmation of aganglionosis (Fig. 18-5). In this relatively uncommon scenario, the appropriate surgical procedure may then be completed 1 or 2 days later after permanent histologic evaluation of the biopsy sites.

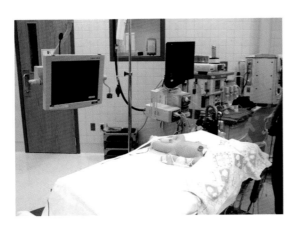
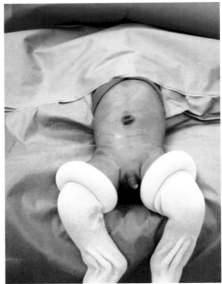

Figure 18-1. After induction of general endotracheal anesthesia, infants and small children are positioned transversely across the operating table (*left*). The monitor is placed at the infant's feet for viewing by the surgeon, who will be positioned above the infant. On the *right*, the buttocks and legs have been cleansed circumferentially to the tips of the toes, and sterile stockings have been placed on both legs. The infant's lower back is also sterilely prepped and draped.

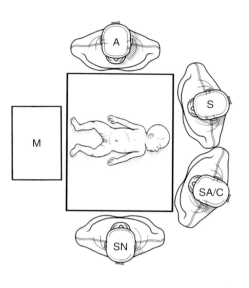

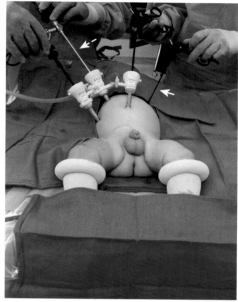

Figure 18-2.   The surgeon (S) and surgical assistant/camera holder (SA/C) stand above the patient's head with the monitor (M) positioned beyond the infant's feet. The scrub nurse (SN) can be positioned according to the surgeon's preference, although being positioned at the foot of the operating table appears to be ideal. A, anesthesiologist. The photograph shows port placement for this operation. Usually three or four ports are required. The umbilical port is inserted using an open technique and the other ports are introduced under direct visualization. The telescope (*dotted arrow*) is placed through the 5-mm port in the right upper abdomen. The surgeon's two primary working ports are the umbilical port for the left hand and the right lower abdominal port for the right hand. A retracting instrument (*solid arrow*) is often helpful and can be inserted through a stab incision in the infant's left upper abdomen. A urinary catheter has been introduced to help decompress the bladder.

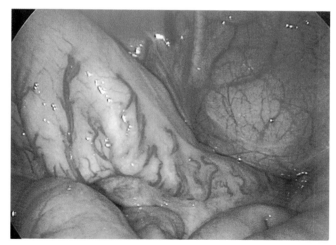

Figure 18-3.   In this view, taken in an 18-month-old with chronic constipation, a well-visualized transition zone between the ganglionic sigmoid colon and aganglionic rectum is seen. Biopsy specimens should be obtained for frozen section analysis before initiating any colonic dissection and mobilization.

In most cases, the frozen section biopsy indicates the presence of normal ganglion cells in the distal sigmoid colon or upper rectum, thus confirming a relatively short, left-sided aganglionic segment. It is important for the surgeon to wait for the biopsy results before proceeding with laparoscopic mobilization of the rectum and colon. The distal sigmoid colon is distracted toward the anterior abdominal wall with a grasper in the surgeon's left hand. A hook cautery is used to create a defect in the mesocolon close to the colon wall (Fig. 18-6A). Staying as close as possible to the wall of the colon spares the superior rectal artery and minimizes intraoperative bleeding (Fig. 18-6B). Mesenteric vessels are divided with cautery from the level of the transition zone proximally to the level of the peritoneal reflection distally (Fig. 18-6C). It is especially important to understand the location of the ureters during this dissection (Fig. 18-7).

When the transition zone is demonstrated to be proximal to the mid-sigmoid colon, a pedicled colon flap must be developed for endorectal pull-through. In this situation, the flap will derive its vascular supply from the marginal artery. To this end, the mesocolon adjacent to the healthy ganglionated bowel should be divided further from the colon wall in a position medial to the marginal artery. To mobilize the descending colon and splenic flexure, it is usually necessary to ligate and divide the proximal inferior mesenteric artery (Fig. 18-8). By dividing the arterial supply at this point, the marginal artery is left intact to supply the splenic flexure and descending colon. This preserves an intact vascular supply to the colon pedicle.

The final steps of the abdominal portion of the procedure are selecting a site along the colon for the

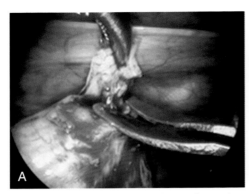 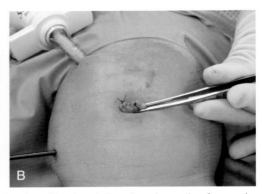

Figure 18-4.   **A,** An intracorporeal biopsy is being performed on the sigmoid colon. A fine-tipped grasping forceps has been used to grasp the biopsy site, and Metzenbaum scissors are used to take the biopsy. **B,** This biopsy was performed through the umbilical incision. One port and another instrument have been introduced through the infant's abdominal wall. A site on the colon for the biopsy was visualized and delivered just under the umbilical cannula. The umbilical cannula was removed and this portion of the colon was grasped and exteriorized. An extracorporeal biopsy was obtained and the biopsy site was closed. This is an alternative means for obtaining the biopsy.

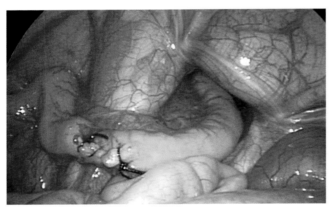

Figure 18-5.   The biopsy specimen taken from this site in the upper rectum did not show ganglion cells. This view shows no evidence of a transition zone. After several biopsies, which all returned aganglionic colon, the operation was halted and the surgeon waited for permanent sections. Permanent sections revealed the infant had total colonic aganglionosis, and an ileostomy was created 2 days later.

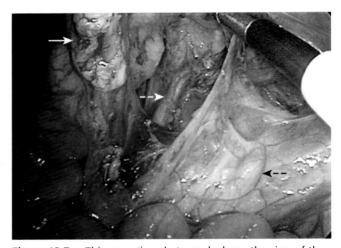

Figure 18-7.   This operative photograph shows the view of the pelvis after most of the mesocolonic dissection. The sigmoid colon (*solid arrow*) has been retracted toward the anterior abdominal wall. It is important to know the location of each ureter during this dissection. The left ureter is identified with a *white dotted arrow* and the right with a *black dotted arrow*.

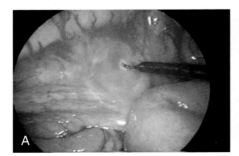 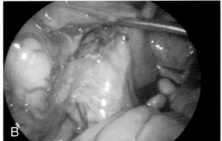 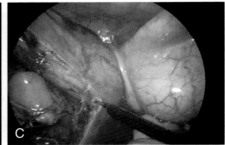

Figure 18-6.   **A,** The sigmoid colon is being distracted toward the anterior abdominal wall with a grasper in the surgeon's left hand. The hook cautery is being used to create a defect in the mesocolon close to the colonic wall to initiate the colonic mobilization. **B,** The hole in the mesocolon has been extended toward the colon. **C,** The mesocolonic dissection is carried down near the peritoneal reflection.

intended coloanal anastomosis and ensuring that this segment of the colon is sufficiently mobile to reach the pelvis. Some authors have argued that the segment of ganglionated colon just proximal to the transition zone is functionally abnormal. Therefore, when possible, 5 to 10 cm of ganglionated colon proximal to the transition zone should be removed, so that the coloanal anastomosis will involve nearly normal colon wall. The

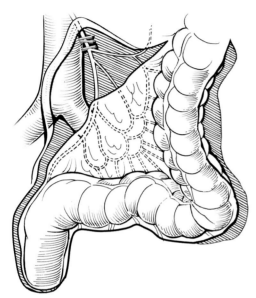

Figure 18-8. When the transition zone is seen proximal to the mid-sigmoid colon, a pedicled colon flap must be developed for the endorectal pull-through. In this situation, the pull-through colon will derive its vascular supply from the marginal artery. Therefore, to mobilize the descending colon and splenic flexure, it is necessary to ligate and divide either the inferior mesenteric artery just distal to its origin from the aorta (as seen in this drawing) or the left colic artery just after it arises from the inferior mesenteric artery. By ligating these vessels at these sites, the arterial supply through the marginal artery is not compromised.

desired site of the intended anastomosis is grasped and pushed far down into the pelvis. If there is insufficient laxity of the mobilized colon, laparoscopic mobilization should continue. In cases of long aganglionic segments, it may be necessary to divide the lateral peritoneal attachments or, rarely, the gastrocolic ligament to adequately mobilize the colon (Fig. 18-9). The ability to mobilize the colon to ensure a tension-free anastomosis is a significant advantage of the laparoscopic-assisted approach.

After dissection and mobilization of the ganglionated colon, attention is turned to the perineum. Children in the supine position are repositioned by flexing their legs and securing their feet over their head.

The perineal dissection begins with placement of circumferential 2-0 silk traction sutures from the dentate line to the perineum approximately 2 to 3 cm outward from the anus (Fig. 18-10A). The Lone Star retractor

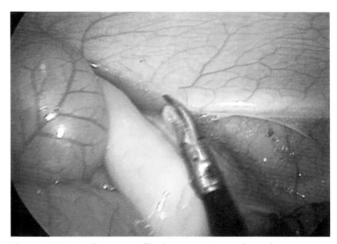

Figure 18-9. When aganglionic segments are long, it may be necessary to divide the lateral peritoneal attachments to mobilize the descending colon. This photograph shows the peritoneal attachments to the upper descending colon and splenic flexure being divided sharply with scissors.

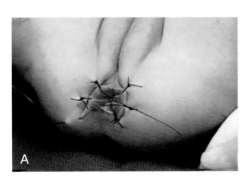
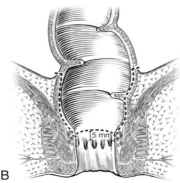
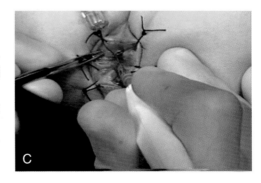

Figure 18-10. **A,** The perineal dissection begins with the placement of circumferential 2-0 silk traction sutures from the dentate line to the perineum approximately 2 to 3 cm outward from the anus. **B** and **C,** A needle-tipped electrocautery is used to circumferentially incise the rectal mucosa approximately 5 mm proximal to the anal columns. Fine silk traction sutures are then placed in the rectal mucosa to help retract the mucosa during circumferential dissection.

(Lone Star Medical Products, Inc., Stafford, TX) can also be helpful for further exposing the anus. Great care must be taken throughout the transanal dissection to avoid over-retraction of the anal sphincters. Hyper-retraction of the internal sphincter can lead to fecal soiling later in life. A needle-tipped electrocautery is used to circumferentially incise the mucosa 5 mm proximal to the dentate line (Fig. 18-10B,C). Fine silk traction sutures are then placed in the proximal rectal mucosa. The plane between the submucosa and the circular smooth muscle should be developed and extended laterally in either direction. The surgeon should identify the white muscle fibers of the circular smooth muscle and remain just inside this plane (Fig. 18-11). Bleeding is controlled with the judicious use of electrocautery. Gentle and steady traction applied to the sutures in the mucosa allows the circumferential plane to be deepened with fine scissors or the cautery. Sutures are added as needed to maintain tension along the length of the submucosal plane. Once the mucosa begins to separate crisply and easily, blunt dissection with a cotton swab or suction tip is sufficient to continue the dissection proximally until the smooth muscle cuff of rectum prolapses. The cessation of bleeding from the endorectal dissection

indicates that the devascularized rectosigmoid has been reached. At this point, the submucosal dissection has proceeded far enough, and the muscular wall of the rectum is divided circumferentially. Spontaneous evacuation of residual CO_2 upon transecting the colon wall confirms entry into the peritoneal cavity.

Next, the muscular cuff is split posteriorly in the midline to provide space for a neorectal reservoir. This cuff division is extended distally to the level of the intended anastomosis, approximately 1 to 2 cm above the dentate line (Fig. 18-12). After proximal division of the cuff, it is pushed back into the pelvis.

With the muscular cuff of rectum divided and returned to its normal anatomic position, the ganglionated colon is grasped and drawn through the anal canal until the appropriate biopsy site is seen (Fig. 18-13). Additional mesocolon can be divided transanally, if necessary. As mentioned previously, the colon should then be transected approximately 5 to 10 cm above the transition zone when possible. A longitudinal to transverse neorectoplasty can be used to create a mini-reservoir in patients with a long aganglionic segment (Fig. 18-14). A secure anastomosis is then fashioned between the neorectum and the anus with interrupted absorbable

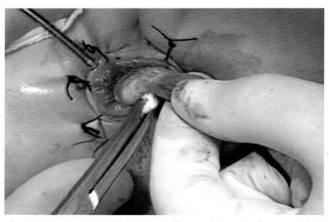

Figure 18-11. The white muscle fibers of the circular smooth muscle can be easily identified during this endorectal dissection. A Kitner can be a useful instrument to push the circular smooth muscle away from the submucosa.

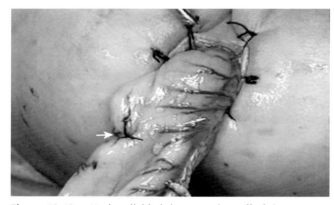

Figure 18-13. Having divided the muscular cuff of the rectum, the ganglionated colon is grasped and exteriorized through the anal canal. Note the biopsy site (*arrow*).

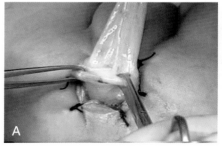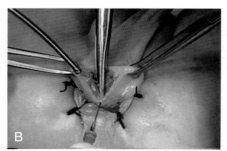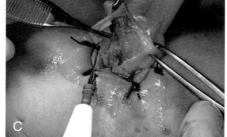

Figure 18-12. After endorectal mobilization, the muscular cuff is grasped with two Allis clamps (**A**) and then is incised with the cautery (**B**) distally toward the dentate line. The cuff is then circumferentially excised (**C**).

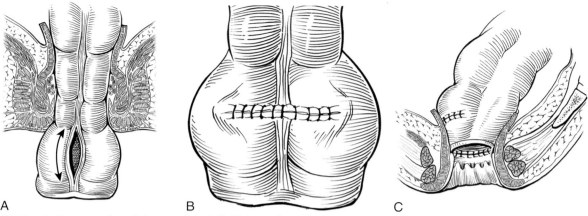

Figure 18-14.   A, To create the mini-reservoir, a full-thickness linear incision is made through the anterior wall of the ganglionic colon beginning 1.5 cm above the transected bowel and continuing for 3 cm proximally. **B,** The linear incision is then closed transversely in a Heineke-Mikulicz fashion. **C,** The coloanal anastomosis and the reservoir closure are seen.

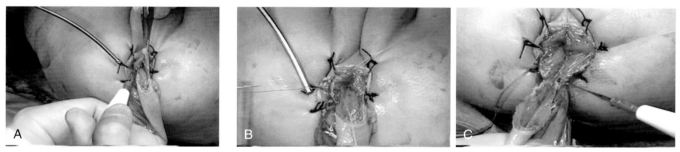

Figure 18-15.   After the mini-reservoir is created, the anastomosis is performed. **A, The pull-through colon is being transected with the cautery. **B,** Approximately half of the circumference of the pull-through bowel is incised, and quadrant sutures are placed at 12 o'clock, 9 o'clock, and 3 o'clock. **C,** After placing the 3-o'clock suture, the pull-through colon is completely transected and made ready for the anal anastomosis.

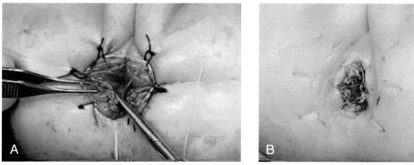

Figure 18-16.   A, The anastomosis is being performed with interrupted 4-0 absorbable sutures. **B,** The everting stay sutures have been cut.

sutures just proximal to the dentate line (Figs. 18-15 and 18-16). Removal of the outer traction sutures returns the anus to its native position. Finally, attention is redirected to the abdomen and the pneumoperitoneum is reestablished. The segment of colon that was drawn into the pelvis is inspected for twists or potential sites of internal herniation. Any tethering of the neorectum should be released by dividing the fusion fascia or lengthening the mesocolic pedicle. Port site incisions are closed with absorbable suture and sterile dressings are applied.

POSTOPERATIVE CARE

Patients may be safely fed on the first postoperative day. Typically, bowel function returns at this point. Discharge from the hospital may be anticipated by postoperative day 3.

PEARLS

1. Before obtaining seromuscular colon biopsies laparoscopically, orient the colon at a right angle from the camera to provide good visualization as the biopsy is taken.
2. When possible, obtain biopsies along the teniae coli, which are the thickest areas of the colon wall and the least likely area to yield a full-thickness biopsy.
3. Place the right lower quadrant port about 1 cm medial to the anterior axillary line. Placing the port too far laterally can result in manual difficulty and awkwardness when exchanging instruments.
4. Divide the mesocolon and the rectal attachments down to the peritoneal reflection to make the transanal dissection easier to perform with minimal anal retraction.
5. Be sure to split the rectal cuff posteriorly to avoid a contracted rectal reservoir.

PITFALLS

1. Beware of injury to the liver when placing the right upper abdominal port. This is particularly important for neonates, in whom the liver tends to extend relatively far below the costal margin.
2. Avoid retraction of the sphincters during transanal dissection. Hyperstretching of the internal sphincter can lead to fecal soiling later in life.
3. Tethering of the neorectum will widen the anorectal angle, which can make eventual continence less satisfactory.

RESULTS

Since the 1980s, the approach to surgical correction of Hirschsprung's disease has shifted from a staged procedure to a one-stage pull-through. The primary laparoscopic-assisted endorectal pull-through is a one-stage, minimally invasive procedure that was first reported in 1995 (Georgeson et al. 1995). The largest series published thus far was a 1999 report of 80 infants treated with this approach (Georgeson et al. 1999). In this report, nearly all patients were younger than 6 months, and only two of the patients required conversion to an open procedure. The average time to discharge was 3.7 days. Long-term follow-up of these patients has not yet been reported, but early experience has suggested that functional results are similar to those seen with open approaches.

SELECTED REFERENCES

1. Carassone M, Morrison-Lacombe G, Le Tourneau JN: Primary corrective operation without decompression in infants less than three months of age with Hirschsprung's disease. J Pediatr Surg 17:241-243, 1982
2. Georgeson KE, Fuenfer MM, Hardin WD: Primary laparoscopic pull-through for Hirschsprung's disease in infants and children. J Pediatr Surg 30:1-7, 1995
3. So HB, Becker JM, Schwartz DL, et al: Eighteen years' experience with neonatal Hirschsprung's disease treated by endorectal pull-through without colostomy. J Pediatr Surg 33:673-675, 1998
4. Georgeson KE, Cohen RD, Hebra A, et al: Primary laparoscopic-assisted endorectal colon pull-through for Hirschsprung's disease. Ann Surg 229:678-683, 1999
5. Georgeson KE: Laparoscopic-assisted pull-through for Hirschsprung's disease. Semin Pediatr Surg 11:205-210, 2002
6. Teitelbaum DH, Wulkan ML, Georgeson KE, et al: Hirschsprung's disease. In Ziegler MM, et al (eds): Operative Pediatric Surgery. New York, McGraw-Hill, 2003, pp 617-646

19
Laparoscopic Duhamel Procedure

David C. van der Zee

Treatment of Hirschsprung's disease consists principally of resection of the aganglionic bowel with preservation of the anal sphincter complex. Several techniques have emerged over the past 50 years. The proposed advantage of the Duhamel side-to-side anastomosis is the avoidance of dissection of the anterior and lateral part of the distal rectum, preserving the nerve fibers to the adjacent bladder. In the open approach, the Duhamel procedure is a fairly straightforward operation and is known for its good results. Laparoscopically, the procedure is more difficult because it requires the intracorporeal suturing of the rectal stump. To date, results seem to be promising. This chapter describes our laparoscopic Duhamel technique and documents our results.

INDICATIONS AND PREOPERATIVE WORKUP

Indications for the laparoscopic Duhamel procedure do not differ from those for the open operation. The diagnosis of Hirschsprung's disease is determined by rectal suction biopsies. In unclear cases, full-thickness rectal biopsies may be needed, although the site of the biopsy may interfere with the future location of the side-to-side anastomosis. Alternatively, anorectal manometry may give additional information that is helpful in making the diagnosis of Hirschsprung's disease. Generally, when a child is referred with suspected Hirschsprung's disease, rectal washouts, 10 to 20 mL/kg each time, are initiated until clear fluid is returned and the abdominal distention has reduced. Parents are then taught to perform the daily rectal washouts at home until the child is admitted for the Duhamel procedure. Children are admitted 2 days before the operation for intravenous hydration and for an antegrade bowel preparation the day before surgery through a nasogastric tube.

OPERATIVE TECHNIQUE

The infant or child is placed supine on the operating table. Infants are placed transversely at the lower end of a short operating table to allow the surgeon to stand comfortably at the cranial side of the child. Armrests covered with gel pads on one or both sides of the table allow somewhat older children to be positioned likewise. Endotracheal anesthesia is supported by epidural regional anesthesia. Before the procedure, the cleanliness of the rectosigmoid colon is checked by a rectal washout on the operating table. The patient is prepped from the costal margin down to the lower legs. The legs are covered with separate drapes so they can be moved during the perineal phase of the procedure. The children receive intravenous antibiotics for 24 hours. A urinary catheter is inserted after the patient has been draped.

The first 5.5-mm port is placed in the subumbilical fold by an "open" technique and secured to the fascia with 2-0 Vicryl (Ethicon, Inc., Somerville, NJ) suture. (By simply tying this suture at the end of the procedure, the subumbilical defect is closed.) A 3.5- or 5.5-mm port is placed in the right lower abdomen under direct vision for instrumentation. A second port is placed in

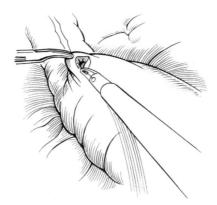 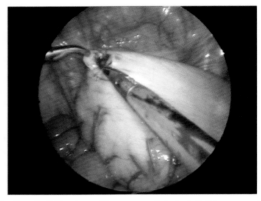

Figure 19-1. Biopsies of the colon are important to determine the level of the transition zone. It is helpful to grasp the biopsy site with a fine-tip grasper (such as a Maryland dissecting instrument) and then to incise the serosa and muscularis sharply with scissors, as shown.

the right upper quadrant, also for instrumentation. A third port is placed in the left lower abdomen for insertion of a grasping forceps to hold up and manipulate the bowel. The surgeon and surgical assistant/camera holder stand above the head of the patient. These port and personnel positions are similar to those described in Chapter 18.

The procedure is started by taking biopsies of the colon for frozen section analysis of ganglion cells (Fig. 19-1). The first biopsy is taken at the "transition zone," a second one more proximal in "normal-feeling" tissue. Care is taken to avoid mucosal entry. Vicryl sutures are used to close the biopsy sites. It is advantageous to leave the most proximal suture a little long, to mark the site for the coloanal anastomosis.

Using monopolar cautery, dissection of the aganglionic colon is started on the medial side close to the bowel wall at the level of the rectum by incising the peritoneal attachment and cauterizing the small vessels. When a sufficient mesenteric window has been made, dissection is moved to the patient's left side, first cauterizing the vessels close to the bowel wall and then opening the peritoneum on the lateral side of the distal colon. In older children, an ultrasonic scalpel may be used to dissect further down the pelvis. At all times, notice should be taken of both ureters and, in boys, the ducti deferentes, which may run close to the dissection. At the peritoneal reflection in the pelvis, the peritoneum is opened anteriorly to allow more traction on the distal rectum, although, to preserve nerve fibers running to the bladder, it is not extensively dissected inferiorly. Dissection is continued dorsally and laterally to the median hemorrhoidal vessels. The retrorectal space is then opened and spread to facilitate the pull-through of the mobilized bowel (Fig. 19-2). When the retrorectal space has been sufficiently enlarged, the grasping forceps can be palpated from the perineum at the level of the dentate line.

Dissection is then turned upward in the direction of the most proximal positive biopsy, again staying close

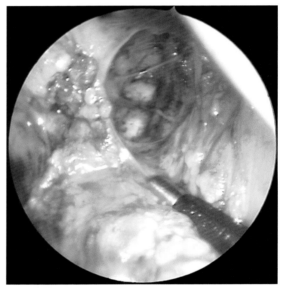

Figure 19-2. This laparoscopic view shows that the retrorectal space has been opened and made ready for the Duhamel pull-through.

to the bowel wall. When the mobilization needs to extend higher to the splenic flexure and beyond, the middle colic vessels should be ligated near the aorta. If the aganglionosis extends to the hepatic flexure, the surgeon should consider using the ileocolic artery for the vascular supply to the pull-through colon.

After the colon has been mobilized, a 2-0 Vicryl ligature is placed around the rectum, approximately 3 cm proximal to the peritoneal reflection. A suction device is introduced transanally and the rectum further cleansed. The rectum is elevated with a grasping forceps that has been inserted through the port in the lower left abdomen. While elevating the rectum, the rectum is sharply transected approximately 2 cm above the peritoneal reflection (Fig. 19-3). In dividing the rectum, first the anterior wall is incised, after which the grasping forceps is used to grasp the anterior wall of the rectum

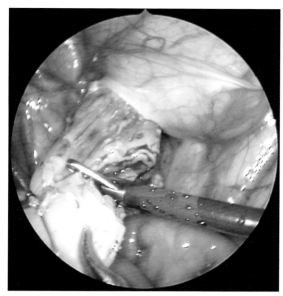

Figure 19-3. While elevating the aganglionic rectum, the rectum is sharply transected approximately 2 cm above the peritoneal reflection. The anterior wall is usually incised first, followed by incision of the posterior aspect of the rectal wall.

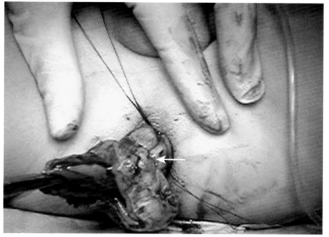

Figure 19-4. This external view shows the mobilized colon being exteriorized through the anal incision to the point where the most proximal biopsy was taken (*arrow*). It is important to ensure that the pulled-through colon is not twisted and lies with its antimesenteric surface facing anteriorly.

to avoid retraction of the stump. Once the anterior wall of the rectal wall is grasped, the posterior aspect of the rectal wall is incised. A grasping forceps is then introduced through the right midabdominal cannula and positioned in the retrorectal space just proximal to the dentate line.

The legs of the patients are lifted and two small retracting hooks are carefully introduced into the anus. By pushing down on the grasping forceps that was positioned in the retrorectal space, the correct location for the incision in the posterior wall of the rectum just above the dentate line can be determined. An incision in the posterior aspect of the rectum is made 0.5 cm above the dentate line using a knife or diathermia tip right over the grasping forceps. The grasping forceps can then be exteriorized through this incision in the posterior anus. Two 4-0 Vicryl sutures are placed full thickness through the anterior proximal side of the incision for the future coloanal anastomosis. This incision in the native rectum is then extended laterally to each corner, parallel to the dentate line, where two additional corner sutures are placed. Finally, a suture is placed on the anterior edge of this incision in the posterior native rectum in the midline. The protruding grasping forceps is then secured with an artery clamp and both are returned to the abdominal cavity. After readjusting the camera, the clamp can be seen on the inside, and the transected pull-through rectum or colon can be secured into the artery clamp.

With the grasping forceps that was inserted through the lower left abdominal port, the anterior wall of the rectal stump can be secured and lifted up to avoid the stump being drawn deep into the pelvis. Under direct vision and with the guidance of the grasping forceps through the right midabdominal port, the artery clamp containing the mobilized colon can be exteriorized to the point where the most proximal biopsy was taken (Fig. 19-4). Care is taken so that the pulled-through colon is not twisted and lies with its antimesenteric surface facing anteriorly. The adequacy of the blood supply to the pull-through colon is checked, especially in the more extended resections. Also, the small bowel should be withdrawn from under the pulled-through bowel.

Once the ganglionic bowel has been pulled through the incision in the native rectum, the anterior surface of the pull-through colon just proximal to the biopsy site is incised and anastomosed using the two sutures previously placed on the ventral side of the posterior incision in the native rectum. The sutures are left long for traction when using the endoscopic stapler device later. The incision in the pulled-through bowel is extended laterally. The lateral corners of the ganglionic pull-through are anastomosed to the corners of the native rectum, and these sutures are also left long for traction. The pulled-through colon is then transected completely and the posterior suture line is created. (This coloanal anastomosis is the same as in the open Duhamel technique.) Alternatively, an eversion technique can be used with external resection of the aganglionic bowel, followed by the coloanal anastomosis.

By pulling on the previously mentioned two ventrally placed sutures, which now have secured the pull-through colon and native rectum, the lumens of the rectum and the pulled-through colon can be seen. A 45-mm EndoGIA (Ethicon Endosurgery, Cincinnati, OH) stapler can be introduced, with one leg in each opening, between these two sutures (Fig. 19-5). From inside the abdomen, the correct position of the EndoGIA can

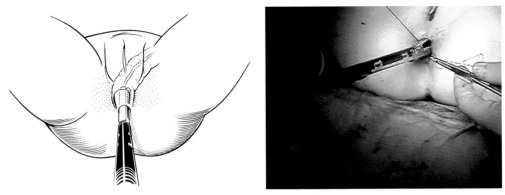

Figure 19-5. A 45-mm endoscopic stapler is introduced in both the native aganglionic rectum and the ganglionic pull-through colon to create a common cavity between the lumens of each limb.

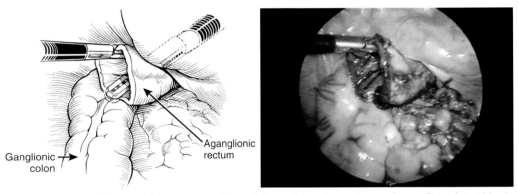

Figure 19-6. From inside the abdomen, the correct position of the endoscopic stapler can be confirmed. In this view, the endoscopic stapler and the aganglionic rectal segment are visualized.

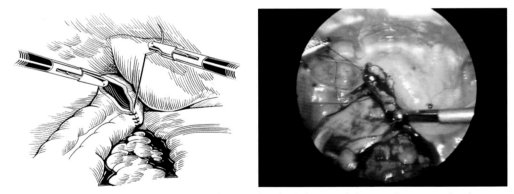

Figure 19-7. The final step in the Duhamel procedure is intra-abdominal closure of the rectal stump, using intracorporeal suturing. Closure of the anterior wall of the newly created common rectal cavity is seen in the drawing and operative photograph.

be confirmed (Fig. 19-6). By pushing the handle once, the correct position of the stapler for firing can be checked a final time. If the surgeon is not satisfied with the position of the stapler, the device can easily be opened again. Once the surgeon is satisfied with the stapler position, the stapler is fired, thus creating the side-to-side anastomosis. After checking that the device was fired completely, the handle on the side of the stapler is pulled back and the device is withdrawn care-

fully. Often, a second loading is necessary to complete the anastomosis.

The final part of the operation is intra-abdominal closure of the rectal stump using intracorporeal suturing techniques (Fig. 19-7). If the side-to-side colorectal anastomosis has been extended sufficiently far enough cephalad, the rectal stump can be closed without leaving a blind sac. A 4-0 Vicryl running suture is used, starting from the superior part of the rectal stump and coming down to the side-to-side anastomosis. If necessary, a second suture can be used running upward, and the two sutures can be tied, completing the closure.

If deemed necessary, a transrectal transanastomotic siliconized drain can be introduced under direct vision and left for colonic decompression for a few days after the operation. Under direct vision, the ports are removed and the fascial defects are all closed using 4-0 Vicryl. The skin is approximated with sterile strips.

POSTOPERATIVE CARE

Antibiotics are continued for the first 24 hours. Pain medication is prescribed in consultation with the anesthesiologist. If the child has received an epidural catheter, the urinary catheter will remain until the epidural catheter has been removed; otherwise, it may be removed at the end of the procedure. The child receives nothing by mouth until the next day or until flatus or stool has been passed. A transanastomotic drain, usually kept in place for 1 to 2 days, is rinsed twice daily with 10 to 20 mL of saline. The child usually goes home by postoperative day 4 or 5, with a normal diet and without any medication.

The children are seen in follow-up at 2, 6, and 12 weeks postoperatively, according to the protocol of the Dutch Society of Pediatric Surgery, or sooner in case of problems.

PEARLS

1. By performing rectal washouts, rectal decompression can, in most instances, be accomplished and the creation of a colostomy at the end of the operation is unnecessary.
2. By placing the infant transversely at the lower end of a short table, the surgeon and assistant can stand comfortably at the head of the patient and work over the baby's head and neck.
3. Postoperative rectal retention, which develops if the child keeps the buttocks tightly together, can be avoided by placing a transanastomotic tube for the first few postoperative days.
4. Nationwide consensus on the treatment and follow-up of patients with Hirschsprung's disease will contribute to the improvement of quality care.

PITFALLS

1. Suturing of the biopsy sites avoids unnecessary spill of bowel contents in case of mucosal perforation.
2. It is better to temporarily terminate the planned operation when the frozen section biopsy is inconclusive.

3. Excessive coagulation causes thermal damage to surrounding tissues such as the bowel and may lead to intestinal perforation.
4. Do not twist the pulled-through bowel.
5. Make the side-to-side anastomosis long enough, and do not leave a blind rectal stump.

RESULTS

Over the past 10 years, we have managed 55 patients with a laparoscopic Duhamel procedure. Sixteen children had additional abnormalities, of which Down syndrome was the most frequent (Van der Zee and Bax 2000). The male-to-female ratio was 4 : 1. Ten patients had long-segment Hirschsprung's disease. Six of seven children receiving a diverting colostomy had extended Hirschsprung's. One child was given a colostomy because of severe enterocolitis on admission. In all cases, the colostomy was closed during the Duhamel procedure.

A postoperative fever occurred in eight children. In four children, there was local leakage of the rectal stump, which was managed conservatively. One child had leakage at a biopsy site. Two children developed an abscess. In two cases, a re-do Duhamel was necessary because of transitional-zone Hirschsprung's disease. Three children required reoperation for obstruction. At follow-up, 19 patients are experiencing episodes of constipation, for which medication is necessary. Five children display soiling. The other 31 patients are continent.

SELECTED REFERENCES

1. Bax NMA, van der Zee DC: Laparoscopic removal of the aganglionic bowel according to Duhamel-Martin in five consecutive infants. Pediatr Surg Int 10:226-228, 1994
2. Van der Zee DC, Bax NMA: Duhamel-Martin procedures in neonates and infants for Hirschsprung's disease: One-stage operation. J Pediatr Surg 31:901-902, 1996
3. Bufo AJ, Chen MK, Shah R, et al: Analysis of the costs of surgery for Hirschsprung's disease: One-stage laparoscopic pull-through versus two-stage Duhamel procedure. Clin Pediatr (Phila) 38:593-596, 1999
4. Van der Zee DC, Bax NMA: One-stage Duhamel-Martin procedure for Hirschsprung's disease: A 5-year follow-up. J Pediatr Surg 35:1434-1437, 2000
5. Boemers TM, Bax NM, van Gool JD: The effect of rectosigmoidectomy and Duhamel-type pull-through procedure on lower urinary tract function in children with Hirschsprung's disease. J Pediatr Surg 36:453-456, 2001
6. Bonnard A, de Lagausie P, Leclair MD, et al: Definitive treatment of extended Hirschsprung's disease or total colonic form. Surg Endosc 15:1301-1304, 2001
7. Georgeson KE, Robertson DJ: Laparoscopic-assisted approaches for the definitive surgery for Hirschsprung's disease. Semin Pediatr Surg 13:256-262, 2004

20
Laparoscopic-Assisted Anorectal Pull-Through

Keith E. Georgeson

Posterior sagittal anorectoplasty (PSARP) is the current standard for the surgical management of patients with complex anorectal malformations. However, a number of surgeons have reported that outcomes may not be better after PSARP than they are after other operations for anorectal malformations. The goals of the laparoscopic-assisted pull-through for anorectal malformations include avoiding the division and weakening of the external sphincters and diminishing perirectal scarring, while allowing precise placement of the rectum through the external sphincters. Moreover, this approach allows the development of a primary corrective procedure in the newborn that avoids the morbidity of a colostomy.

INDICATIONS FOR WORKUP AND OPERATION

Any infant with an anorectal malformation that does not involve a fistula to the perineum or vestibule is a potential candidate for a laparoscopic-assisted anorectal pull-through. The infant's preoperative evaluation should be similar to that of patients being prepared for PSARP. A distal colostogram is helpful for determining the presence and level of a rectourethral fistula. A careful physical examination and radiographs of the pelvis and sacrum are useful for assessing the patient's potential for continence.

OPERATIVE TECHNIQUE

A proximal sigmoid colostomy should be performed in the newborn patient with an intermediate or high anorectal malformation. The colostomy is placed in the proximal sigmoid colon. The proximal sigmoid colon is divided so that a 1-cm lip of proximal colon can be pulled through the lower left quadrant colostomy site. The sigmoid colon should be divided so that the lateral ligaments to the descending colon tether the colostomy to prevent prolapse of the proximal limb. The distal colon is also prone to prolapse. This prolapse can be prevented by pulling out a small portion of colon 2 cm distal to the staple line dividing the sigmoid colon. The distal colon fistula should be sited so that there is enough length of colon to allow the pull-through to be performed without tension. The distal mucous fistula does not need to be placed laterally, as visualization into the pelvis is adequate as long as the distal fistula is slightly to the left or midline. The opening to the mucous fistula should be no greater than 10 mm. The mucosa of the distal fistula is secured flush with the skin, with no lip.

Several months after creation of the colostomy, the patient is positioned transversely at the end of the operating table. A urinary catheter should always be inserted into the urethra before beginning the laparoscopic dissection. In some patients, this may require cystoscopy with the passage of the catheter over a guidewire. A circumferential prepping is performed from the nipples to the toes. The surgeon and the surgical assistant/camera holder stand above the infant with a single monitor beyond the infant's legs (Fig. 20-1A). A 5-mm

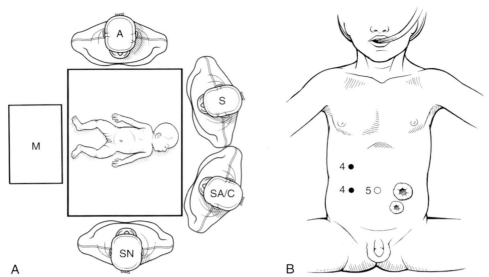

Figure 20-1. **A,** The positions of the operating personnel for the laparoscopic-assisted pull-through. The infant is positioned transversely across the operating table with the surgeon (S) and surgical assistant/camera holder (SA/C) positioned above the infant's head. A, anesthesiologist; M, monitor; SN, scrub nurse. **B,** The cannula sites are shown. The telescope and camera are inserted through the 4-mm right upper abdominal port. The other two ports are the surgeon's working ports.

port is inserted through the umbilicus using an open technique. A pneumoperitoneum with a pressure of 12 mm Hg is established. A 4-mm port is introduced in the anterior axillary line just below the inferior margin of the liver for the telescope attached to the camera. A second 4-mm port is placed in the anterior axillary line in the right lower quadrant (RLQ) (Fig. 20-1B). Instruments are inserted through the umbilical and RLQ ports.

The pelvic dissection is begun at the peritoneal reflection adjacent to the rectum. The hook cautery is useful for this dissection. The dissection is kept adjacent to the muscle wall of the rectum all the way down to the rectourethral fistula or to the blind end of the rectum. Hitching the posterior bladder wall with a U-stitch placed through the abdominal wall improves visualization in the deep pelvis. Traction is applied to the upper rectal wall with a grasper in the surgeon's left hand (through the umbilical port), and the hook cautery (through the RLQ port) is used to dissect through the perirectal plane. By staying close to the rectal wall, injury to adjacent structures in the pelvis is avoided. As the dissection approaches the rectourethral fistula, the rectal circumference can be noted to diminish and taper (Fig. 20-2). If the operating surgeon cannot tell where the junction of the fistula and urethra is located, the fistulous tract can be opened and the indwelling urethral catheter visualized. The rectourethral fistula should be divided about 4 mm proximal to its junction with the urethra. A pre-tied loop ligature is inserted through the 5-mm cannula in the umbilicus and positioned over a Maryland clamp that was inserted through the 4-mm port in the RLQ. The Maryland grasper is then used to grasp the 4-mm cuff of the distal rectourethral fistula

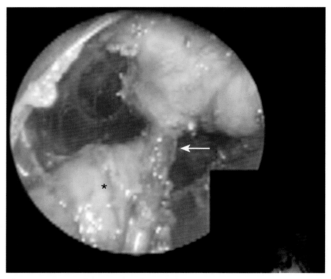

Figure 20-2. The rectum (*asterisk*) is seen tapering in size to the rectourethral fistula (*arrow*) in the pelvis.

(Fig. 20-3A). The loop ligature is tightened snugly around the fistulous stump (see Fig. 20-3B). In a similar fashion, the proximal fistulous opening of the rectum is ligated. In many patients with anorectal malformations, the levator ani muscles can be easily visualized from above through the telescope (Fig. 20-4). In other patients, the levator ani muscles are poorly developed and are difficult to identify.

The transperineal dissection is the next step in this procedure. The infant's knees are flexed and the feet are secured over the head, exposing the posterior perineum. The contractions of the external sphincters are mapped using a cutaneous electrical stimulator on the perineum.

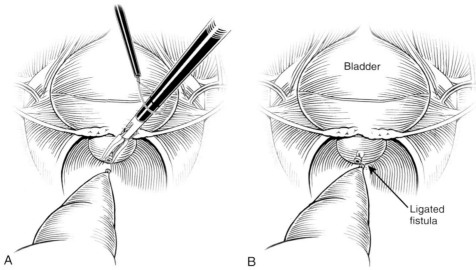

Figure 20-3. After circumferential dissection of the rectum, the fistula has been divided and the rectal end ligated with a pre-tied ligature. **A,** The fistula on the urethral side is grasped with a Maryland clamp preloaded with a pre-tied loop ligature. **B,** The ligature is tightened around the urethral side of the fistula.

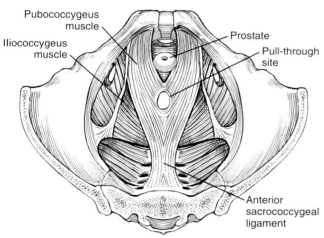

Figure 20-4. This diagram depicts the pelvic anatomy as seen by the surgeon in infants with a well-developed muscle complex.

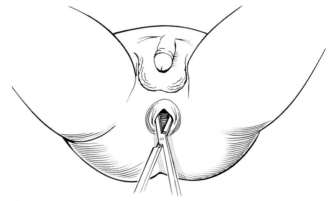

Figure 20-5. Transperineal blunt dissection of the intersphincteric plane is performed through a 1-cm vertical incision using a clamp in the anal incision.

The area inside the point of maximal contraction is marked appropriately with sutures. A 1-cm vertical incision is made in the midline over the point of maximal muscle contraction. A plane is identified by gently dissecting inside the muscle complex. This plane inside the muscle complex is easily dissected for about 2 cm (Fig. 20-5). When blunt dissection is no longer productive, a Veress needle with an expandable sleeve (Step, Covidien, Mansfield, MA) is passed through the plane inside the muscle complex using laparoscopic surveillance from inside the peritoneal cavity. The operating surgeon must remember that, as the Veress needle passes toward the scope, the right and left orientation is reversed on the television monitor. This reversal of right and left can be disorienting to the operator, but this can be overcome by short probes of the needle to identify the precise position of the penetrating needle. Alternatively, if possible, the monitor can be turned upside down to correct this confusing view.

The Veress needle and expandable sheath should be passed directly behind the urethra about 4 mm away from the urethra. It is not necessary to crowd the urethra anteriorly, as the muscle complex is not tightly adjacent to the posterior wall of the urethra. A space between the urethra and the anterior aspect of the encircling levator ani muscles can be clearly seen through the telescope in patients with a well-developed levator muscle complex. The Veress needle and encircling expandable sheath are pushed through the levator fascia directly behind the urethra.

Once the Veress needle has been inserted in the appropriate position, the needle is removed, leaving the

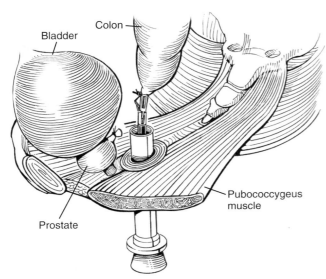

Bladder

Colon

Pubococcygeus muscle

Prostate

Figure 20-6. This schematic diagram shows the 12-mm cannula that has been passed from the perineum between the two bellies of the pubococcygeus muscle into the abdomen. A grasper is advanced through the port to secure the distal end of the dissected rectum. The rectum is then pulled down through the perineum after withdrawing the cannula.

expandable sheath positioned through the muscle complex. Serial dilation of the tract is accomplished by advancing progressively larger cannulas with blunt-tipped trocars through the radially expanding sheath. When a 10- or 12-mm cannula has been advanced through the muscle complex, a laparoscopic Allis clamp is advanced into the pelvis after placement of a reducing cap on the 12-mm cannula. The proximal end of the divided rectourethral fistula is positioned inside the jaws of the Allis clamp (Fig. 20-6). The surgeon then closes the jaws of the Allis clamp and pulls the proximal end of the fistula trailing behind the 12-mm cannula as it is removed from the central plane of the muscle complex. The edges of the fistula are freshened and secured to the perineal skin with 4-0 Vicryl (Ethicon, Inc., Somerville, NJ) suture. Adequate bites of fistula and skin along with subcutaneous tissues are taken to secure the fistula to the skin.

The rectum should then be hitched to the presacral fascia laparoscopically with two sutures. These hitch stitches pull the rectocutaneous junction in a cephalad direction to help prevent prolapse of the rectum, to lengthen the skin-lined anal canal, and to sharpen the anorectal angle. The abdominal cannulas are removed and the three small incisions closed.

POSTOPERATIVE CARE

Anorectal dilation is started 3 weeks after the laparoscopic-assisted anorectal pull-through. The anus and rectum are serially dilated from a size 6 Hegar dilator up to a size 12 to 14 Hegar dilator over a 6- to 8-week

period. The colostomy is closed after the neorectum is sufficiently dilated and compliant.

PEARLS

1. Before the pull-through, a distal colostogram should be performed with adequate pressure to exclude low anorectal anomalies and to identify the presence and position of a rectourethral fistula.
2. Hitching the posterior bladder wall to the anterior abdominal wall with a U-stitch improves visualization in the deep pelvis.
3. The vas deferens visually guides the surgeon to the prostate.
4. The rectal dissection should be kept immediately outside the muscle wall of the rectum.
5. Small nicks in the longitudinal and circumferential smooth muscle wall of the rectum do not need to be repaired.
6. Pushing the plastic guide of the pre-tied loop ligature to the caudal side of the rectourethral fistula simplifies flush ligation of the fistula.
7. Serial dilation of the plane inside the muscle complex is much simpler and safer with a cannula and blunt-tipped trocar inside an expandable sleeve than with Hegar dilators.
8. Opening the rectal fistula to confirm the position of its insertion into the urethra can be helpful in some patients.

PITFALLS

1. With the knees flexed onto the torso, the anorectal angle is straight. When introducing the Veress needle and expandable sheath from the perineum, the operator should not angle the Veress needle anteriorly or the urethra might be injured.
2. Because the levator muscles are angulated like a boat keel, when probing with the Veress needle and sleeve from the perineum, minimal deviations off the midline will appear to be much farther lateral than they actually are.

RESULTS

A study comparing laparoscopic-assisted anorectal pull-through and a posterior sagittal anorectal pull-through reported early satisfactory results after both procedures (Lin et al. 2003). The centrality of the pull-through was equal with both procedures. Sphincter asymmetry and irregularity were greater with the PSARP approach. Megarectum and constipation were also greater in the PSARP group. Development of an anorectal reflex was more common after the laparoscopic procedure. The patients were too young to evaluate for continence. Resting anorectal pressures were similar, but rectal compliance was greater in the laparoscopic-assisted group.

Laparoscopic-assisted anorectal pull-through appears to achieve some of its goals. It allows precise placement of the anorectum inside the external sphincter complex without dividing or weakening the sphincters. It diminishes scarring and allows for a safer primary procedure in the newborn, avoiding the morbidity associated with a colostomy. Long-term follow-up for continence is needed for further evaluation of this approach.

SELECTED REFERENCES

1. Langemeijer RA, Molenaar JC: Continence after posterior sagittal anorectoplasty. J Pediatr Surg 26:587-590, 1991
2. Bliss DP Jr, Tapper D, Anderson JM, et al: Does posterior sagittal anorectoplasty in patients with high imperforate anus provide superior fecal continence? J Pediatr Surg 31:26-30, 1996
3. Lin CL, Chen CC: The rectoanal relaxation reflex and continence in repaired anorectal malformations with and without an internal sphincter-saving procedure. J Pediatr Surg 31:630-633, 1996
4. Rintala RJ, Lindahl HG: Fecal continence in patients having undergone posterior sagittal anorectoplasty procedure for a high anorectal malformation improves at adolescence, as constipation disappears. J Pediatr Surg 36:1218-1221, 2001
5. Tsuji H, Okada A, Nakai H, et al: Follow-up studies of anorectal malformations after posterior sagittal anorectoplasty. J Pediatr Surg 37:1529-1533, 2002
6. Lin CL, Wong KK, Lan LC, et al: Earlier appearance and higher incidence of the rectoanal relaxation reflex in patients with imperforate anus repaired with laparoscopically assisted anorectoplasty. Surg Endosc 17:1646-1649, 2003
7. Wong KK, Khong PL, Lin SC, et al: Post-operative magnetic resonance evaluation of children after laparoscopic anorectoplasty for imperforate anus. Int J Colorectal Dis 20:33-37, 2005
8. Ichijo C, Kaneyama K, Okazaki T, et al: Mid-term postoperative clinico-radiological analysis of surgery for high type imperforate anus: Prospective comparative study between Georgeson and Peña Procedures. J Pediatr Surg 43:158-162, 2008

21
Laparoscopic Splenectomy

Frederick J. Rescorla

Laparoscopic splenectomy was popularized in the 1990s and has rapidly become the preferred method for splenectomy. Several techniques have been reported, including anterior and hand-assisted procedures, but most authors currently use a lateral, four-cannula approach. The laparoscopic technique offers the advantages of shorter length of stay, lower amounts of postoperative pain medication, and a more satisfactory appearance because very small incisions are used and the largest is placed in the umbilicus. Most children can be discharged on the first postoperative day.

INDICATIONS FOR WORKUP AND OPERATION

Splenectomy in childhood is most frequently required for hereditary spherocytosis (HS), idiopathic thrombocytopenic purpura (ITP), and sickle cell disease (SCD) with splenomegaly and splenic sequestration. Children with hemolytic disorders should undergo a preoperative gallbladder ultrasound examination to evaluate for associated cholelithiasis. If present, a concomitant laparoscopic cholecystectomy is performed. The hematologist and surgeon decide jointly whether and when the splenectomy will be performed, and the decision is influenced by several factors. One is the severity and duration of the thrombocytopenia in patients with ITP. In addition, a favorable but temporary response to medical management (steroids, intravenous IgG) can be predictive of a favorable and durable response to splenectomy. Severe splenic sequestration and splenomegaly are indications for the small group of children with SCD who require splenectomy. A hemoglobin of at least 10 g/dL is important before surgery in children with SCD. Children with HS who have severe anemia, chronic anemia, or aplastic crisis are usually referred for splenectomy. An attempt is made to defer splenectomy until age 5 or older. Moreover, in some young children with HS, partial splenectomy may be a reasonable consideration. The removal of accessory spleens is critical in children with ITP and HS, as the primary process may persist or recur because of residual splenic tissue. Some authors recommend preoperative computed tomography or scintigraphy to detect accessory splenic tissue. However, many have abandoned these imaging studies and have noted similar accessory spleen detection rates with laparoscopy. Detection of accessory spleens is usually quite easy in children at laparoscopy, whereas it may be more difficult in adults with more retroperitoneal adipose tissue.

Massive splenomegaly can be a relative contraindication to the laparoscopic approach for splenectomy. The Endocatch II retrieval bag (Covidien, Mansfield, MA) is 23 cm in depth, allowing removal of nearly all pediatric spleens. If splenosis from an intraperitoneal spill is not a concern, a large spleen may be divided and removed in two pieces. All children should be immunized preoperatively against *Streptococcus pneumoniae*, meningococcus, and *Haemophilus influenzae*.

OPERATIVE TECHNIQUE

General endotracheal anesthesia is administered with the child in the supine position. A urinary catheter and an orogastric tube are inserted, both of which are removed at the end of the procedure. The child is placed on the operating table with the left side up approximately 45 degrees. A small roll or raised kidney rest placed under the left flank helps to increase the distance between the left iliac crest and the 12th rib (Fig. 21-1). The table is tilted to the patient's left side to obtain a near supine position for port placement and then is rotated to the right to achieve a right lateral decubitus position for the operation (Fig. 21-2). The surgeon stands on the right side of the patient, with the surgical assistant cephalad. The monitor is situated over the patient's left abdomen, with the spleen between the surgeon and monitor (Fig. 21-3A).

Access is initiated with an open 15-mm vertical umbilical incision. A small umbilical fascial defect is usually present, allowing introduction of a hemostat

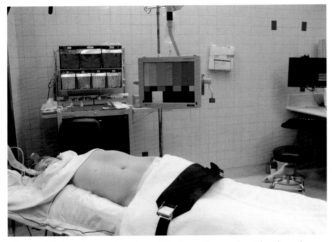

Figure 21-1. For optimal positioning, the patient is placed supine on the operating table with a small roll or raised kidney rest under the left flank to elevate the left side approximately 45 degrees off the table. Such positioning helps increase the distance between the iliac crest and the 12th rib.

that can then guide the fascial incision. A 15-mm cannula (chosen because of the 15-mm size of the retrieval bag) is inserted, and a pneumoperitoneum is created to 12 to 15 mm Hg with a CO_2 flow of 6 L/min. If the spleen is small, a 10- or 12-mm port can be placed for use with the 10-mm endoscopic bag (Endopouch, Ethicon Endosurgery, Inc., Cincinnati, OH). Diagnostic laparoscopy is performed with a 5-mm, 30-degree angled telescope using the 5-mm reducer attachment to the cannula. Three additional incisions are then created. A 5-mm port is placed in the left lower abdomen for insertion of the Harmonic Scalpel (Ethicon Endosurgery, Inc., Cincinnati, OH) or the Ligasure vessel-sealing device (Covidien, Mansfield, MA), and for the camera at the time of spleen removal. Two additional incisions are created in the midline, one just below the xiphoid process and the other midway between the xiphoid and the umbilicus (Fig. 21-3B). Because the instruments at these sites are not exchanged during the procedure, they may be inserted through small stab incisions without the use of a cannula. In children younger than 5 years and in older patients with small spleens, 3-mm instruments may be used at these sites. In patients with large spleens, usually one of these epigastric sites will need 5-mm instruments to provide adequate splenic elevation. If a concomitant cholecystectomy is needed, an additional incision is created on the patient's right flank for better traction of the gallbladder. In this instance, one of the midline ports is shifted to the right for use by the first assistant during the cholecystectomy.

The operating surgeon holds the camera in the left hand and either the ultrasonic scalpel or Ligasure in the right. The first assistant uses instruments inserted through the upper abdominal sites to provide elevation to the spleen and traction on surrounding structures (Fig. 21-4A). The table is rotated to the patient's right to achieve a right lateral decubitus position, leaving the spleen "hanging" in the left upper quadrant. Accessory

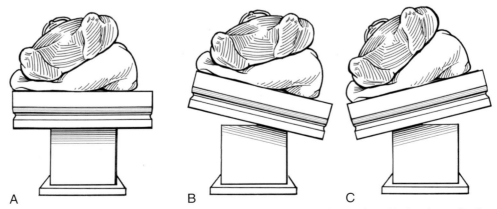

Figure 21-2. **A,** Initial positioning of the patient before any movement of the table. **B,** The table has been tilted to the patient's left to obtain a near supine position of the patient for port placement. **C,** The table is then rotated back to the patient's right to achieve a right lateral decubitus position for the operation.

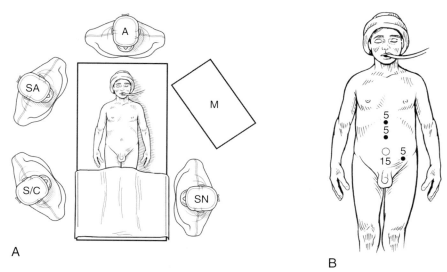

Figure 21-3. **A,** The personnel positions for a laparoscopic splenectomy. The surgeon (S/C) stands on the patient's right, with the surgical assistant (SA) cephalad. The surgeon also controls the camera. The monitor (M) is situated over the patient's left abdomen, with the spleen lying between the surgeon and the monitor. The scrub nurse (SN) stands opposite the surgeon. A, anesthesiologist. **B,** Placement of the ports. A 15-mm cannula is usually placed in the umbilicus because of the size of the endoscopic bag that is inserted. (If the spleen is small, a 10- to 12-mm port can be placed in the umbilicus for utilization of a 10-mm endoscopic bag.) Two 5-mm ports are placed in the midline above the umbilical port. The final port is 5 mm in size and is placed in the left lower abdomen. It is through this port that the Harmonic Scalpel or Ligasure is inserted during the operation.

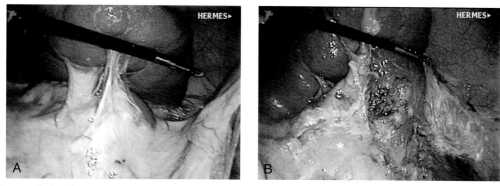

Figure 21-4. The surgical assistant usually manipulates instruments placed through the two cephalad cannulas. **A,** Initially, the inferior pole of the spleen is elevated to expose the lienocolic ligament. **B,** The Harmonic Scalpel or Ligasure has been used to divide the lienocolic ligament to expose the inferior portion of the spleen (*asterisk*).

spleens in the omentum, gastrosplenic ligament, or other sites can usually be removed through the umbilical port using the Harmonic Scalpel or Ligasure to divide the feeding vessel.

Either the Harmonic Scalpel or Ligasure can be used for most of the procedure. The splenocolic ligament is divided first, allowing the colon to fall away (Fig. 21-4B). There are frequently a few small attachments to the inferior pole, which can then be safely divided. Attention is then directed to the gastrosplenic ligament, in which a small opening is made. The assistant gently pulls the stomach to the right, providing excellent exposure, and the surgeon can divide all of these vessels with the Harmonic Scalpel or Ligasure (Fig. 21-5). The most

difficult aspect of this part of the operation is the uppermost short gastric vessels where the spleen and stomach are very close. The instrument in the surgeon's right hand maintains splenic elevation while the first assistant elevates the superior pole with the left-hand grasper and pulls the stomach to the right with the right-hand grasper. After these maneuvers, the splenophrenic ligament is divided, taking care to avoid injury to the diaphragm (Fig. 21-6). If a hole is made in the diaphragm, a figure-eight suture is placed, a catheter is inserted into the chest to aspirate the pneumothorax, and the suture is then tied.

At this point, the surgeon must decide whether to divide the hilum with the stapling device or with

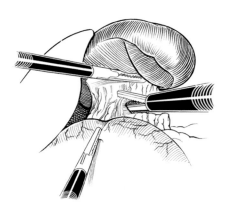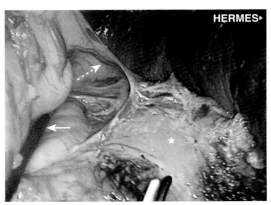

Figure 21-5. After division of the lienocolic ligament, the lesser sac is entered. In the photograph, the stomach is being retracted by an assistant's instrument (*solid arrow*). The Harmonic Scalpel, at the bottom of the photograph, is approaching one of the intact short gastric vessels (*dotted arrow*). The pancreas is marked with an *asterisk*.

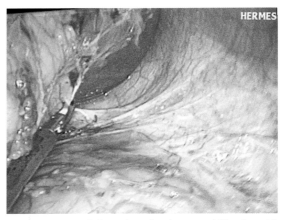

Figure 21-6. Most of the spleen has been mobilized at this point. The splenophrenic ligament is being incised from behind the hilum using scissors. At this point, great care is taken not to continue the dissection cephalad, as injury to the diaphragm can occur.

individual vessel division. If a stapling device is used, the posterior attachments are divided next so that circumferential control can be obtained at the hilum. The first assistant places both graspers under the inferior pole, with the left hand rotating the spleen slightly anteriorly. As the upper portion of the spleno-renal ligament is divided, both graspers are used to elevate the spleen with the left hand under the superior pole. When the hilum is isolated, the camera is rotated to the left lower quadrant port, and the stapler is inserted through the umbilical port. Care must be taken to make sure that the tail of the pancreas is not included in the stapler firing (Fig. 21-7). One application of the vascular load stapler is usually adequate for ligation and division of the vessels in the hilum.

Two alternative approaches for hilar division may also be used. The splenic vessels may be individually isolated, clipped, and divided with two clips on the portion of the vessel remaining in the patient. The other option is to divide the vessels using the Harmonic Scalpel or Ligasure. The Ligasure has a slight advantage in that the bipolar energy achieves a seal that, if placed across only part of a vessel, still seals it and does not allow bleeding. The 5-mm Ligasure is also approved for larger (8-mm) vessels. We have divided the hilar vessels using these devices.

If a partial splenectomy is planned, the vessels are divided close to the hilum, leaving one segmental vessel, usually to the upper pole. The intent with this procedure is to perform about 85% of a splenectomy. The splenic capsule and spleen are divided with the Harmonic Scalpel approximately 1 cm from the line of demarcation, thus leaving 1 cm of devascularized spleen with the viable remaining splenic fragment. This maneuver minimizes bleeding.

The spleen (total or partial) is then positioned in the left upper quadrant and held against the anterior abdominal wall. The Endocatch II retrieval bag is placed through the umbilical site with the telescope rotated to the left lower quadrant site. The bag is opened slowly under the spleen and the spleen is dropped into the open end of the bag (Fig. 21-8A). The spleen is allowed to gently fall into the bag. When it is below the metal ring, the drawstring ring is pulled to close the bag. The metal ring is removed first and the neck of the bag is then delivered through the umbilicus (Fig. 21-8B). The surgeon's index finger can usually fracture the splenic capsule, and a combination of the ring forceps and the surgeon's finger is used to remove the splenic fragments.

After the spleen is removed, completion laparoscopy is performed to inspect the hilum for bleeding and to check for the presence of accessory spleens. The umbilical fascial incision is closed with two figure-eight sutures. An attempt is made to close at least the anterior fascia at the 5-mm sites. Local anesthesia is injected at all sites and the skin is closed. The orogastric tube and bladder catheter are then removed.

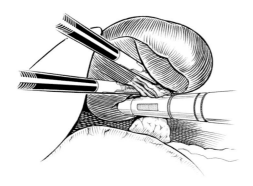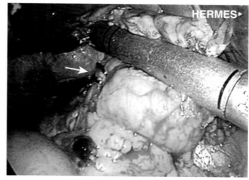

Figure 21-7. Once the spleen has been mobilized and is attached only through the hilar vessels, the camera is rotated to the left lower quadrant port and the stapler is introduced through the umbilical port. It is then placed across the hilar vessels, taking care not to incorporate a portion of the pancreas in the tissue to be divided. In the photograph, note that the splenic artery has been ligated with clips (*arrow*) before hilar division, because the spleen was extremely large.

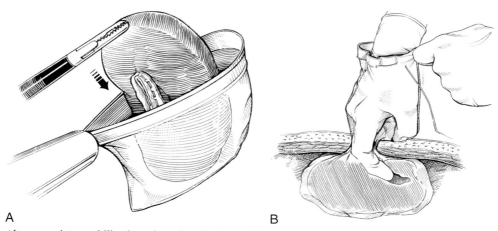

A   B

Figure 21-8. **A,** After complete mobilization, the spleen is dropped into an endoscopic retrieval bag. **B,** The neck of the bag is then exteriorized through the umbilicus, and the surgeon's finger is used to fracture the splenic capsule. A combination of ring forceps and the surgeon's finger is then used to remove the splenic fragments.

POSTOPERATIVE CARE

The children are admitted for a 23-hour observation. Pain control is achieved with a combination of intravenous ketorolac and narcotic, with transition to oral acetaminophen with codeine as liquids are tolerated. Postoperative cardiac and pulse oximetry monitoring is required to watch for the development of tachycardia. Children with SCD are maintained postoperatively on intravenous fluids at a slightly greater than maintenance dosage and are carefully monitored to avoid hypoxemia. Most children can be released on postoperative day 1, although the average stay for children with SCD in our experience is 2.5 days.

PEARLS

1. Utilize the 5-mm, 30-degree angled telescope for the entire procedure, as it allows use of the umbilical or left lower quadrant site without changing telescopes, and it allows visualization from various angles.
2. Place a 15-mm umbilical cannula initially, as this allows use of the 5-mm camera, EndoGIA stapler, and Endocatch bag through this site.
3. In older and large patients, the left lower quadrant port may need to be positioned higher to allow the instruments to reach the top of the spleen.
4. As the spleen falls into the open bag, gently rock the handle from side to side to promote unraveling of the bag as the spleen descends into it.

PITFALLS

1. The bag of the Endocatch device can easily separate from the ring. Make sure that the ring is fully deployed in the abdominal cavity before placing the spleen in the bag. Gently drop the spleen into the open bag

and allow the weight of the spleen to slowly unravel the bag. Do not push the spleen into the bag, as separation of the bag from the ring makes the entrapment of the spleen very difficult.

2. At the time of spleen removal, pull the bag up snugly against the anterior abdominal wall and attempt to break the splenic capsule with an index finger. This finger can then be used to fracture the spleen, and a ring forceps can be used to remove the fragments piecemeal. Be careful not to grab the bag with the ring forceps as a tear will lead to intraperitoneal spill or inadvertent bowel injury.

RESULTS

A review of our database at Riley Hospital for Children (1995-2006) identified 200 children (111 boys; 89 girls; average age, 7.69 years) undergoing laparoscopic splenic procedures. The number of children who underwent laparoscopic splenectomy by the lateral approach was 194 (188 total, six partial). The indications for splenectomy were HS (99), ITP (32), SCD (40), and other (23). Concomitant cholecystectomy was performed in 35. Four (2%) required conversion to an open operation. Accessory spleens were identified in 37 patients (19%). Six additional laparoscopic procedures were performed: splenic cystectomy for epithelial (two) or traumatic (two) cyst, and splenopexy for wandering spleen (two). The average postoperative hospitalization was 1.50 days. Complications included ileus (four), bleeding (four), acute chest syndrome (five), pneumonia (two), diaphragm perforation (two), missed accessory spleen (one), port-site hernia (one), and subsequent total laparoscopic splenectomy after an initial partial splenectomy (one). One traumatic cyst recurred and required reoperation. There were no deaths or wound infections.

SELECTED REFERENCES

1. Tulman S, Holcomb GW III, Karamanoukian HL, et al: Pediatric laparoscopic splenectomy. J Pediatr Surg 28:689-692, 1993
2. Katkhouda N, Hurwitz MB, Rivera RT, et al: Laparoscopic splenectomy: Outcome and efficacy in 103 consecutive patients. Ann Surg 228:568-578, 1998
3. Minkes RK, Lagzdins M, Langer JC: Laparoscopic versus open splenectomy in children. J Pediatr Surg 35:699-701, 2000
4. Walsh RM, Heniford BT, Brody F, et al: The ascendance of laparoscopic splenectomy. Am Surg 67:48-53, 2001
5. Velanovich V, Shurafa MS: Clinical and quality of life outcomes of laparoscopic and open splenectomy for haematological diseases. Eur J Surg 167:23-28, 2001
6. Rescorla FJ, Engum SA, West KW, et al: Laparoscopic splenectomy has become the gold standard in children. Am Surg 68:297-302, 2002
7. Rice HE, Oldham KT, Hillery CA, et al: Clinical and hematologic benefits of partial splenectomy for congenital hemolytic anemias in children. Ann Surg 237:281-288, 2003
8. Romano F, Caprotti R, Franciosi C, et al: The use of Ligasure during pediatric laparoscopic splenectomy: A preliminary report. Pediatr Surg Int 19:721-724, 2003
9. Winslow ER, Brunt LM: Perioperative outcomes of laparoscopic versus open splenectomy: A meta-analysis with an emphasis on complications. Surgery 134:647-655, 2003

22
Laparoscopic Cholecystectomy

Daniel J. Ostlie and George W. Holcomb III

The characteristics of biliary tract disease have been well documented in adults. However, many surgeons and pediatricians do not readily consider the possibility of cholecystitis or cholelithiasis in young patients who present with vague upper abdominal pain. Perhaps one reason for this hesitation has been the earlier belief that hemolytic disease was a prerequisite for gallstone formation in children and teenagers. A report in 1980 emphasized the increasing frequency of nonhemolytic gallbladder disease in the younger age group (Holcomb et al. 1980).

Gallbladder disease is being identified more frequently in the pediatric age group than in the past. The etiology of this increase is multifactorial and includes increased and prolonged use of total parenteral nutrition (TPN), biliary dyskinesia, more frequent and liberal use of diagnostic modalities (abdominal ultrasound [US], abdominal computed tomography scans), and diseases of anemia (especially sickle cell disease and hereditary spherocytosis). This has led to an increase in the number of cholecystectomies being performed in the pediatric and teenage population. As with adults, the gold standard approach for cholecystectomy in children is via laparoscopy. One should expect success and complication rates to be similar between the different population ages.

INDICATIONS FOR WORKUP AND OPERATION

The primary disease processes that lead to consideration for cholecystectomy include cholelithiasis, cholecystitis (acute, acalculous, and chronic), acute hydrops of the gallbladder, and biliary dyskinesia. Although the patients' histories may differ, usually the signs and symptoms are similar for all these conditions. Epigastric and right upper abdominal pain, with or without associated fever or jaundice, should immediately prompt the evaluating surgeon to consider a gallbladder condition as a possible diagnosis.

Symptomatic cholelithiasis is often but not always the result of impaired gallbladder emptying related to gallstone(s). Gallstones are generally classified as being either nonhemolytic or hemolytic (secondary to sickle cell disease, spherocytosis, and thalassemia) in composition. Nonhemolytic gallstones are nearly always cholesterolic, whereas hemolytic gallstones are usually composed primarily of calcium bilirubinate. Regardless, the signs and symptoms are identical, related to biliary colic, and sometimes seen in association with excessive fat intake. An abdominal US will reveal the presence of gallstones in the gallbladder. Should cholecystitis occur, the patient will develop fever, possibly jaundice, and the US may show gallbladder wall thickening or pericholecystic fluid, or both. Leukocytosis and right upper abdominal pain frequently occur. Patients with symptomatic cholelithiasis should undergo elective laparoscopic cholecystectomy. Those with acute, severe cholecystitis are usually treated with intravenous antibiotics and urgent cholecystectomy.

The finding of biliary ductal dilation with US or the development of jaundice raises the possibility of choledocholithiasis. A number of options exist at this point. We prefer to proceed with preoperative endoscopic retrograde cholangiopancreatography (ERCP) with sphincterotomy and stone removal, if indicated, because the surgeon is then better able to plan the subsequent operation. If the choledochal stone has been removed at

ERCP and sphincterotomy, the surgeon can proceed with routine laparoscopic cholecystectomy. However, if the stone could not be removed, the surgeon will know that laparoscopic choledochal exploration and stone removal should be planned. If that is not successful, then open exploration may be needed under the same anesthesia. Some surgeons prefer to wait and have the ERCP and sphincterotomy performed after the laparoscopic cholecystectomy. This is the strategy routinely used in adults. However, not every pediatric surgeon has an endoscopist experienced in ERCP or sphincterotomy in children, so the postoperative ERCP or sphincterotomy strategy is not likely to be as successful as in adults.

When the symptoms of epigastric and right upper abdominal pain, with or without associated fever or jaundice, are associated with a severe illness, trauma, burn, or sepsis, acalculous cholecystitis should be considered. The etiology of acalculous cholecystitis is, as its name implies, not due to gallstones. It is believed that this development is related to the association of events surrounding the disease under treatment. This includes gallbladder quiescence, excessive red cell hemolysis, TPN use with the absence of food intake, dehydration, and adynamic ileus. An abdominal US may reveal gallbladder distention, gallbladder wall thickening, and pericholecystic fluid. Occasionally, sludge or debris will be visualized in the gallbladder. Failure of medical management (nothing by mouth, parenteral antibiotics, and intravenous fluids) results in the need for laparoscopic cholecystectomy.

Biliary dyskinesia is rarely seen in infants. However this condition is being encountered more often in children and adolescents, and it is considered by some to be a valid reason for cholecystectomy in this age group. These patients often present with nonspecific abdominal pain that may be in the right upper abdomen or epigastrium. The pain may be associated with meals, which may be related to an excessively fatty diet. An abdominal US is invariably not diagnostic. In this instance, a technetium-99m radionuclide scan is diagnostic. In healthy individuals, the gallbladder ejection fraction should be greater than 35%. If a patient has symptoms consistent with biliary colic and a radionuclide gallbladder-emptying scan documenting an ejection fraction of less than 35%, laparoscopic cholecystectomy should be considered. Unfortunately, not all symptoms in these patients will be relieved. An ejection fraction of less than 15% usually results in good relief of symptoms.

OPERATIVE TECHNIQUE

Unless the patient is hospitalized for gallstone pancreatitis or acute cholecystitis, admission to the hospital is on the day of operation. The patient is asked to urinate just before going to the operating room, and a cephalosporin is administered before beginning the operation. The patient is endotracheally intubated, and gastric decompression is accomplished via an orogastric tube. The patient is placed in the supine position and the abdomen is prepped from the nipple line to the symphysis pubis. The operating surgeon stands to the patient's left and the assisting surgeon to the patient's right. The scrub nurse/camera holder is to the left of the surgeon. Viewing monitors are positioned at the head of the table on both the right and left sides (Fig. 22-1).

A vertically placed 10- to 12-mm incision is made directly through the umbilicus. Through this incision, a 10- to 12-mm cannula is inserted and the abdomen is insufflated. We generally use a 10-mm 45-degree operating telescope for visualization during the operation. The 10-mm telescope is used because a 10- to 12-mm umbilical cannula is needed for removal of the gallbladder. A second 5-mm cannula is inserted under direct vision in the epigastric region. In older patients, this cannula can be placed through or to the right of the falciform ligament and well above the liver edge. In younger patients, it should be to the left of the linea alba. Depending on the size and amount of subcutaneous fat, the remaining operating instruments are introduced directly through the abdominal wall via a stab incision (if the patient is thin), or through 5-mm cannulas. One instrument is placed in the right lower quadrant (RLQ) and the other is located in the right mid-abdomen (RMA), inferior to the right epigastric port and near the liver edge. These working sites need to be more widely separated in smaller patients (Fig. 22-2). In children less than 10 years of age, instruments

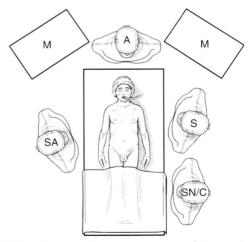

Figure 22-1.   The typical arrangement of monitors and personnel for a laparoscopic cholecystectomy. Two monitors (M) are usually placed at the head of the bed on each side of the patient's head. The surgeon (S) stands to the patient's left with the camera holder to the surgeon's left. In our hospital, the scrub nurse (SN/C) usually doubles as the camera holder. The surgical assistant (SA) stands to the patient's right and opposite the surgeon. A, anesthesiologist.

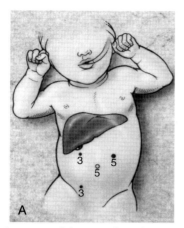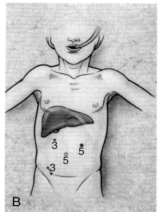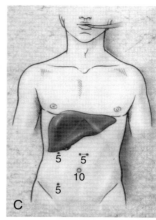

Figure 22-2. Placement of the ports for a laparoscopic cholecystectomy depends on the patient's age and size. There must be adequate working space between instruments. **A,** In small patients, it is necessary to place the primary working port for the surgeon in the patient's left epigastrium and the assistant's retracting port lower in the inguinal crease. **B,** In 5- to 10-year-old children, the primary working port should still be placed in the medial aspect of the patient's left epigastrium. The assistant's retracting port can be moved more cephalad. **C,** For teenagers, the orientation of the ports more closely resembles the orientation for adult patients, with the primary working port near the midline or right of midline, and the two right-sided ports more cephalad.

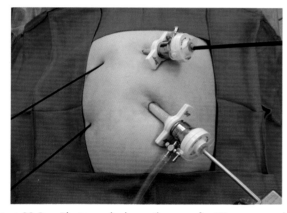

Figure 22-3. Photograph shows the use of a 10-mm cannula in the umbilicus and a 5-mm cannula in the epigastric region in a 10-year-old child. The two right-sided instruments have been placed using the stab incision technique.

inserted in these latter two sites may be 3 mm in size (Fig. 22-3).

Grasping the dome of the gallbladder with a locking grasper inserted through the RLQ incision and retracting the dome toward the right shoulder reveals the gallbladder infundibulum and porta hepatis. The infundibulum of the gallbladder (just distal to the cystic duct) is grasped with the surgeon's left-handed instrument using a nonlocking grasper. This grasping forceps is retracted inferior and laterally, creating a 90-degree angle between the cystic duct and the common bile duct (Fig. 22-4A). This helps avoid misidentification of these two structures. Using either a Maryland dissector or a spatula-tip cautery in the right hand, the peritoneum overlying the confluence of the cystic duct and infundibulum is incised. This peritoneum is then dissected toward the common duct in the triangle of Calot (Fig. 22-4B). The

cystic duct is then circumferentially dissected using the Maryland dissector in the right hand placed through the right epigastric cannula. Occasionally, a right-angled dissector is useful in completing the dissection. To avoid injury to the common duct, it is of paramount importance to clearly identify the cystic duct entering the gallbladder at the completion of this dissection. At this point, the cystic duct is ligated with two clips placed proximally and a single clip at the cystic duct–infundibulum junction, and it is then divided (Fig. 22-5). If an intraoperative cholangiogram is to be performed, a number of options are possible. The distal cystic duct near the infundibulum can be clip-ligated, and the cystic duct proximal to the clip is partially transected to expose its lumen. A cholangiocatheter is then inserted into the cystic duct to perform the study (Fig. 22-6A). Another option is to use the Kumar clamp technique, which involves an atraumatic clamp positioned across the infundibulum of the gallbladder. Through a side port in the clamp, a sclerotherapy needle is advanced into the infundibulum (Fig. 22-6B). The advantage of this technique is that a small cystic duct is not cannulated, which can sometimes be difficult. Thus, this technique is especially useful in smaller patients (Fig. 22-7).

In the absence of jaundice or evidence of choledocholithiasis, our current philosophy is to perform a cholangiogram only when the anatomy is unclear. With careful and thorough dissection in the triangle of Calot, this is rarely needed. Having clipped and divided the cystic duct, attention is turned to identification and dissection of the cystic artery, which generally lies beneath or adjacent to the cystic duct. Not uncommonly, the main cystic artery branches into its anterior and posterior branches proximal to the dissection plane.

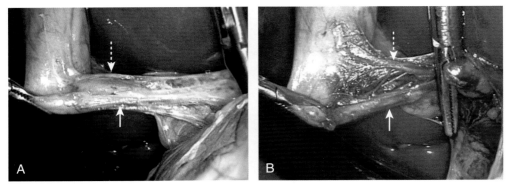

Figure 22-4.   **A,** To avoid misidentification of the cystic duct and the common bile duct, it is helpful to orient the cystic duct at a 90-degree angle to the common bile duct. **B,** Then, a Maryland dissecting instrument can be used to dissect the peritoneum off the cystic duct, allowing correct identification of this structure. In both photographs, the cystic duct is marked with a *solid arrow* and the cystic artery with a *dotted arrow*.

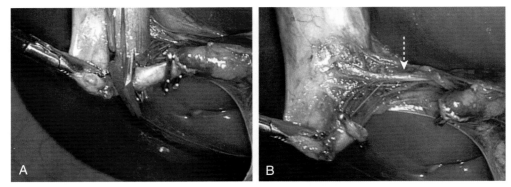

Figure 22-5.   **A,** After identification and exposure of the cystic duct, it is ligated with two clips placed proximally and a single clip placed at the cystic duct–infundibulum junction. **B,** After these clips are placed, the cystic duct is divided, leaving two clips on the proximal duct. Note the cystic artery (*dotted arrow*).

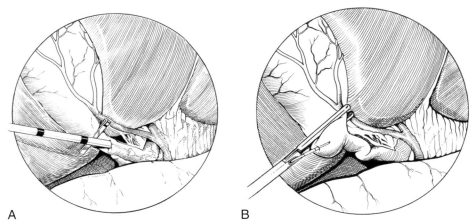

Figure 22-6.   If a cholangiogram is to be performed, several options exist. After ligation of the cystic duct near its junction with the infundibulum, the cystic duct proximal to the clip is partially transected to expose its lumen. **A,** A cholangiocatheter is then introduced into the cystic duct and the study is performed. **B,** Another option is to use the Kumar clamp technique. With this technique, an atraumatic clamp is positioned across the infundibulum of the gallbladder. Through a side port in the clamp, a sclerotherapy needle is advanced into the infundibulum and the cholangiogram is performed. The advantage of the Kumar clamp technique is that the small cystic duct is not cannulated, which can sometimes be difficult.
(Reprinted with permission from Holcomb GW III: Laparoscopic cholecystectomy. In Holcomb GW III [ed]: Pediatric Endoscopic Surgery. Norwalk, CT, Appleton and Lange, 1994.)

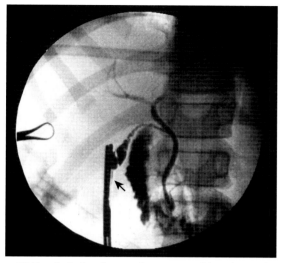

Figure 22-7. A cholangiogram in a 4-year-old patient using the Kumar clamp technique. The sclerotherapy needle has been introduced through a side port in the clamp and into the infundibulum (*arrow*).

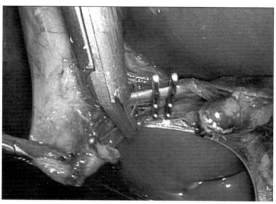

Figure 22-8. After ligation and division of the cystic duct and cholangiogram (if needed), the cystic artery is identified and controlled with 5-mm clips in the same way the cystic duct was secured.

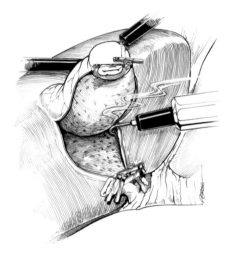

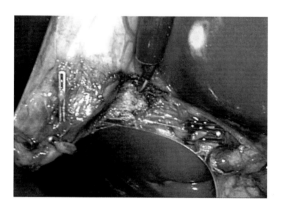

Figure 22-9. After ligation and division of the cystic duct and cystic artery, the connective tissue between the gallbladder and liver is divided using either the spatula-tip or hook-tip cautery.
(Reprinted with permission from Holcomb GW III: Laparoscopic cholecystectomy. In Holcomb GW III [ed]: Pediatric Endoscopic Surgery. Norwalk, CT, Appleton and Lange, 1994.)

When this occurs, the individual branches are dissected separately and controlled with 5-mm clips in the same way the cystic duct was secured (Fig. 22-8).

At this point, all that remains is removal of the gallbladder from its liver bed. Using a spatula tip or hook-tip cautery, the connective tissue between the gallbladder and liver is divided (Fig. 22-9). The most common time for the gallbladder to be perforated during its removal is at this point in the operation, when the infundibulum is being freed from the gallbladder fossa. Careful dissection from the hepatic bed will avoid spillage of its contents. Also, it is possible for the right hepatic artery to be lying superficially in the gallbladder fossa just beneath the wall of the gallbladder, and injury to it must be avoided. Once the gallbladder has been mobilized from

the majority of its attachments, the dome of the gallbladder is retracted inferiorly to allow improved visualization of its superior aspect so as to enhance separation from the liver. Before complete separation, the gallbladder fossa is inspected for hemostasis and bile leakage. Also, clips on the cystic duct and artery are visualized to ensure appropriate positioning.

Retrieval of the gallbladder from the abdominal cavity is easily accomplished through the umbilicus. A 5-mm laparoscope is inserted through the epigastric cannula (Fig. 22-10A). The gallbladder is grasped using a 10-mm toothed grasper inserted through the umbilical cannula and removed (Fig. 22-10B). If there is significant inflammation (acute or chronic cholecystitis), or if the gallbladder has been perforated during the dissection,

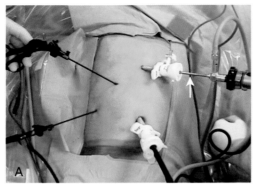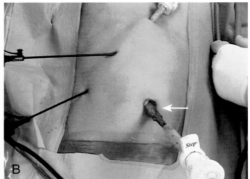

Figure 22-10. If a 10-mm cannula was introduced into the umbilical port and a 5-mm port was placed in the epigastric region, a 5-mm laparoscope is introduced through the epigastric port and a grasper is inserted through the umbilical cannula for removal of the gallbladder. **A,** The telescope (*arrow*) has been moved to the epigastric port, and a 10-mm grasping forceps has been introduced through the umbilical port. **B,** Often, the gallbladder cannot be extracted through the umbilical port, which needs to be removed to exteriorize the gallbladder (*arrow*) from the patient.

we recommend placing it into an endoscopic bag for extraction. Desufflation of the abdomen with occasional slight enlargement of the umbilical cannula site will facilitate its removal. The abdomen is re-insufflated and the gallbladder fossa is again inspected. The abdomen is irrigated if necessary. Instruments and cannulas are removed under direct vision with the laparoscope reinserted through the umbilical cannula. The fascia at the umbilical cannula and, if possible, the other cannula sites are closed using interrupted absorbable sutures. The skin is approximated with absorbable sutures. The subcutaneous tissues are injected with local anesthetic and sterile dressings are applied (Fig. 22-11).

Postoperatively, patients are allowed clear liquids once they have recovered from the anesthetic. Diet is advanced as tolerated, and most patients are discharged on the first postoperative day.

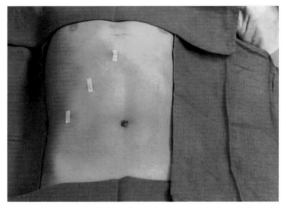

Figure 22-11. The incisions have been approximated with absorbable sutures and secured with Steri-Strips. The umbilical incision has been closed but a dressing has not been applied.

PEARLS

1. Preoperatively, if the patient presented with elevated hepatic enzymes or bilirubin levels, ensure that there is no biliary ductal dilation before embarking on laparoscopic cholecystectomy. If the US shows ductal dilation, an ERCP with sphincterotomy and stone removal should be considered before cholecystectomy.
2. If the patient is small, use of the stab incision technique avoids the presence of intra-abdominal cannulas, which can take up precious space and entail time and expense.
3. Intraoperative orogastric decompression greatly improves visualization and avoids possible injury to the stomach during dissection.
4. Positioning the right epigastric cannula to the right of the falciform ligament aids in retraction of the

inferior edge of the liver, and it gives added operating space for manipulation of instruments such as the clip applier, and for specimen removal.
5. Desufflation of the abdomen facilitates gallbladder extraction.

PITFALLS

1. Failure to retract the dome of the gallbladder toward the right shoulder results in suboptimal visualization and positioning of the gallbladder, with an increased risk of common duct injury.
2. Failure to retract the infundibulum of the gallbladder inferiorly and laterally results in lack of separation of the cystic duct and common duct and increases the risk of common duct injury.
3. Watch for both an anterior and a posterior branch of the cystic artery.

4. Remain cognizant of the possibility of a superficially lying right hepatic artery within the plane between the gallbladder and liver.
5. Careful dissection of the infundibulum from the gallbladder fossa avoids perforation and spillage of the gallbladder contents.
6. If there is significant inflammation, use an endoscope bag to avoid spillage of the gallbladder contents.

RESULTS

Between January 2000 and December 2006, 215 patients underwent laparoscopic cholecystectomy at Children's Mercy Hospital. The mean age was 12.4 years. Of these patients, 145 were female. Forty-seven patients underwent cholangiography. The mean operative time was 80 minutes.

Only one patient required common duct exploration. The reason for this low number was that all patients with suspected common duct involvement after either ultrasound or physical or chemical examination underwent preoperative ERCP with stone removal and sphincterotomy, if needed. Thus, the choledochus was usually cleared before laparoscopic cholecystectomy.

SELECTED REFERENCES

1. Holcomb GW Jr, O'Neill JA Jr, Holcomb GW III: Cholecystitis, cholelithiasis and common duct stenosis in children and adolescents. Ann Surg 191:626-635, 1980
2. Holcomb GW III: Laparoscopic cholecystectomy. In Holcomb GW III (ed): Pediatric Endoscopic Surgery. Norwalk, CT, Appleton and Lange, 1994
3. Newman KD, Powel DM, Holcomb GW III: The management of choledocholithiasis in children in the era of laparoscopic cholecystectomy. J Pediatr Surg 32:1116-1119, 1997
4. Holcomb GW III, Morgan WM III, Neblett WW III, et al: Laparoscopic cholecystectomy in children: Lessons learned from the first 100 patients. J Pediatr Surg 34:1236-1240, 1999
5. Mattioli G, Repetto P, Carlini C, et al: Medium-term results after cholecystectomy in patients younger than 10 years. Surg Endosc 15:1423-1426, 2001
6. Shah RS, Blakely ML, Lobe TE: The role of laparoscopy in the management of common bile duct obstruction in children. Surg Endosc 15:1353-1355, 2001
7. Alonso MH: Gall bladder abnormalities in children with sickle cell disease: Management with laparoscopic cholecystectomy. J Pediatr 145:580-581, 2004
8. Vegunta RK, Raso M, Pollock J, et al: Biliary dyskinesia: The most common indication for cholecystectomy in children. Surgery 138:726-731, 2006

23
Laparoscopic Adrenalectomy

George W. Holcomb III

The laparoscopic approach is ideal for patients with a well-circumscribed, benign-appearing lesion of the adrenal gland. Although neuroblastoma is the most common etiology for adrenal masses in children, these are usually identified late in the disease process and are seldom suitable for laparoscopic resection. However, a well-circumscribed neuroblastoma in the adrenal gland is certainly amenable to laparoscopic resection. Most patients undergoing laparoscopic adrenalectomy are ready for discharge on either the first or second postoperative day. This technique is ideal for the incidentally discovered lesion.

INDICATIONS FOR WORKUP AND OPERATION

The preoperative evaluation for an adrenal lesion is the same whether the mass is removed laparoscopically or with the open technique. In patients with incidentally discovered lesions, hormonal evaluation is required, including the dexamethasone suppression test and levels of aldosterone; cortisol, and adrenocorticotropic hormone, as well as evaluation for possible pheochromocytoma. Surgical removal is indicated for all functioning adrenocortical tumors and for pheochromocytoma. For incidentally discovered lesions, especially those larger than 3 cm, laparoscopic resection is also recommended. For patients with pheochromocytoma, preoperative suppression is indicated for the laparoscopic procedure and for the open operation. These patients should receive alpha adrenergic blockade with phenoxybenzamine before the operation to prevent the development of profound hypotension with removal of the catecholamine source.

OPERATIVE TECHNIQUE

General endotracheal anesthesia is used for this operation. Positioning of the patient for right and left adrenalectomies is the same, but the operative steps are different. The patient is placed on the operating room table in a true lateral position with the kidney rest situated just cephalad to the iliac crest. The kidney rest is then raised, accentuating the space between the iliac crest and the 12th rib. Also, to further enlarge this space, the operating table is flexed (Fig. 23-1). A urinary catheter is usually not needed. The abdomen and flank are prepared and draped sterilely. The umbilicus is not used for this operation, so the initial incision is 5 mm in length and is placed halfway between the umbilicus and the ipsilateral iliac crest. The Veress needle may be used, but the cutdown technique is preferred. After the skin is incised, the muscles of the anterior abdominal wall are divided using loupe magnification until the peritoneum is visualized and incised. The expandable Step sleeve (Covidien, Mansfield, MA) without the Veress needle is then introduced into the abdominal cavity, and a 5-mm blunt-tip cannula is inserted through the expandable sleeve. Pneumoperitoneum is created to 15 mm Hg with a flow of 4 to 6 L/min. Diagnostic laparoscopy is performed with a 5-mm, 45-degree angled telescope introduced through this cannula. At this point, the accessory 5-mm ports are inserted.

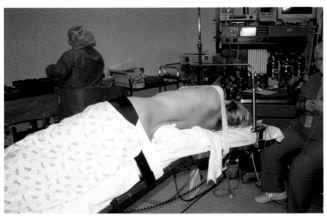

Figure 23-1. For laparoscopic adrenalectomy, the patient is placed on the operating table in a true lateral position, with the kidney rest situated just cephalad to the iliac crest. The kidney rest is then raised, accentuating the space between the iliac crest and the 12th rib. To further enlarge this space, the operating table is flexed. In this photo, the patient is positioned for a laparoscopic left adrenalectomy.

RIGHT ADRENALECTOMY

For a right adrenalectomy, the surgeon and camera holder stand at the patient's back and the surgical assistant stands opposite the surgeon so that the surgeon is actually working in a lateral-to-medial direction. The patient is positioned in a left lateral decubitus position (Fig. 23-2). After the initial 5-mm incision is created halfway between the umbilicus and the right iliac crest, a 5-mm cannula and an angled telescope are inserted. Because this operation is usually performed in larger children, ports rather than stab incisions are usually preferred. After insertion of the initial 5-mm cannula, a second port is positioned lateral to it, in the anterior axillary line. A third working port is placed lateral to this 5-mm port. It is important to place these cannulas close to the 12th rib, so that the iliac crest does not limit manipulation of the instruments inserted through the ports. (One of these 5-mm ports is usually enlarged later to 10 mm for extraction of the specimen. Alternatively, a 10-mm port can be introduced now at one of these working sites and used for extraction of the specimen.) The fourth cannula is for the liver retractor and is introduced above and slightly medial to the first 5-mm port (Fig. 23-3). The diamond-shaped flexible liver retractor (Snowden-Pencer, Tucker, GA) is used to retract the right lobe of the liver once it has been mobilized. The Thompson self-retaining instrument holder (Thompson Surgical Instruments, Traverse City, MI) is secured to the liver retractor so that another assistant is not needed to hold it.

The surgeon works through the two lateral 5-mm ports with a grasping forceps in the left hand and the Harmonic Scalpel (Ethicon Endosurgery, Inc., Cincinnati, OH) in the surgeon's right hand. The first step is

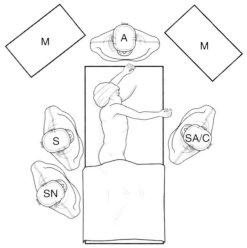

Figure 23-2. Positions of the surgeon, assistant, and scrub nurse depend on whether a right or left adrenalectomy is performed. In the diagram, the personnel are situated for a right adrenalectomy. Their positions are reversed for a left adrenalectomy. For a right adrenalectomy, as shown, the surgeon (S) stands behind the patient so that work proceeds in a posterior-to-anterior direction. The surgical assistant/camera holder (SA/C) stands on the patient's left. The scrub nurse (SN) is caudal to either the surgeon or the assistant, as preferred by the surgeon. If two monitors (M) are available, one is placed on either side of the anesthesiologist (A).

to incise the right triangular ligament of the liver so that the right lobe can be mobilized and retracted. This can be performed either with scissors connected to cautery or with the Harmonic Scalpel (Fig. 23-4). Once the right lobe has been mobilized so that the right adrenal gland is visualized, the liver retractor is secured to the Thompson self-retaining bar and the right lobe retracted medially. The general idea is to incise the peritoneum that lies lateral, cephalad, caudal, and finally anterior to the right adrenal gland, as well as the surrounding retroperitoneal tissue, containing the arterial supply to the gland, with the ultrasonic scalpel, and then to ligate the vein as the last step. The Harmonic Scalpel is used to perform this lateral, cephalad, caudal, and anterior peritoneal and retroperitoneal dissection, which can usually be completed in 20 to 30 minutes (Figs. 23-5 and 23-6). With lateral retraction of the adrenal gland, the vein can usually be visualized through the peritoneum overlying the medial portion of the gland. Dissection then proceeds in a caudal-to-cephalad direction toward the adrenal vein using the Harmonic Scalpel (Fig. 23-7). There is occasionally an accessory vein, so it is important to watch for this possibility. Once the adrenal vein is visualized, it is doubly clipped on both the vena cava side and the adrenal gland side and then divided between the middle clips (Fig. 23-8). The rest of the dissection can be completed with the Harmonic Scalpel quite easily.

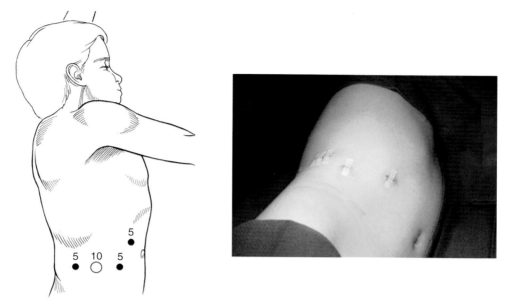

Figure 23-3.   Placement of the cannulas for a right adrenalectomy. The first working port, 5 mm in size, is positioned between the iliac crest and the umbilicus. This is the port through which the telescope and camera are placed. The second 5-mm port is placed lateral to the first cannula. This becomes one of the working ports for the surgeon. A 5-mm cannula is then placed above and medial to the initial port. This is the port through which a 5-mm liver retractor is introduced. The final 5-mm port is placed quite lateral, in the posterior axillary line. This cannula is placed last because sometimes the right colon needs to be mobilized to place this port in its proper position. Instruments inserted through the previously introduced cannulas can be used to help mobilize the right colon, if necessary. In the patient shown, the 5-mm incision in the midaxillary line was enlarged to extract the entire specimen.

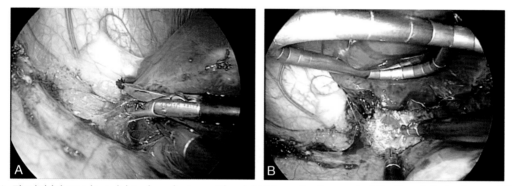

Figure 23-4.   **A,** The initial step in a right adrenalectomy. The right triangular ligament of the liver is incised to mobilize the right hepatic lobe. **B,** The liver retractor has been introduced and incision of the triangular ligament is being completed.

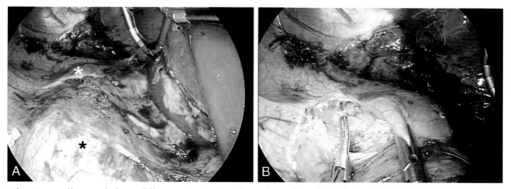

Figure 23-5.   **A,** The 5-mm diamond-shaped liver retractor has been introduced to elevate the liver anteriorly and medially. The adrenal gland (*white asterisk*) is seen cephalad to the kidney (*black asterisk*). **B,** Initial mobilization of the right adrenal gland begins at the inferolateral aspect of the gland. The peritoneum and adjacent tissues are being incised with the Harmonic Scalpel.

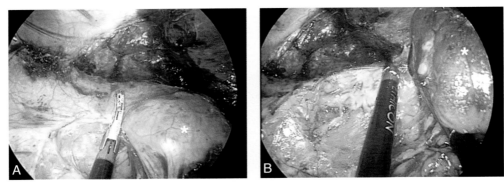

Figure 23-6.   **A,** The Harmonic Scalpel is being used to further incise the peritoneal attachments to the gland (*asterisk*) on its lateral border. **B,** The superior attachments of the peritoneum and retroperitoneal tissues to the gland (*asterisk*) are being incised with the ultrasonic scalpel.

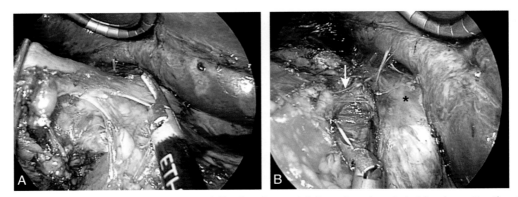

Figure 23-7.   After the right adrenal gland has been mobilized on its caudal, lateral, and cephalad borders, attention turns to dissection of the tissue between the gland and the vena cava. **A,** The tissues between the adrenal gland and the vena cava are being incised with the Harmonic Scalpel. **B,** The right adrenal vein (*arrow*) has been identified and isolated. The vena cava is marked with an *asterisk*.

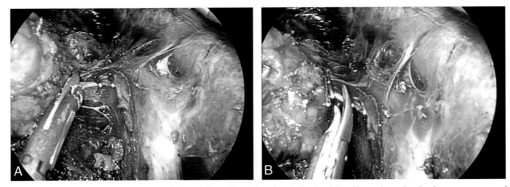

Figure 23-8.   After identification and isolation of the right adrenal vein, it is doubly clipped on both the vena cava side and the adrenal gland side (**A**), and then divided between the middle two clips (**B**). The rest of the dissection can be completed easily with the ultrasonic scalpel.

As adrenalectomy is usually performed for a mass lesion, we prefer to introduce an endoscopic retrieval bag and extract the specimen whole rather than piecemeal. Therefore, as previously mentioned, one of the 5-mm sites is enlarged to 10 mm, and the 10-mm endoscopic retrieval bag is inserted through this 10-mm cannula. The specimen is placed in the bag and the cannula and bag are exteriorized through the 10-mm

incision (Fig. 23-9). Occasionally, when the adrenal gland is large, the incision has to be enlarged, although the bag can usually be rocked back and forth and extracted without enlarging this incision. Having removed the specimen, the 10-mm port is replaced and the area of dissection is inspected for hemostasis. Once hemostasis is secure, the three 5-mm incisions are closed with 5-0 absorbable suture. The 10-mm incision is

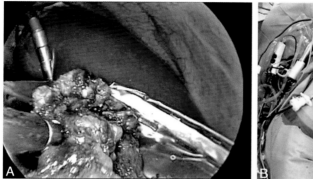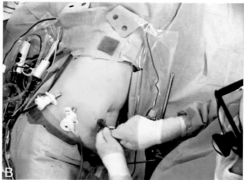

Figure 23-9. **A,** Usually, we prefer to extract the specimen whole and place it into an endoscopic retrieval bag. **B,** This bag is usually exteriorized after enlarging one of the 5-mm incisions.

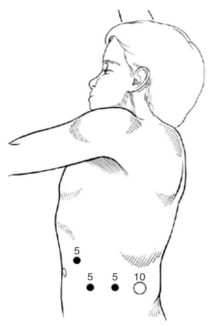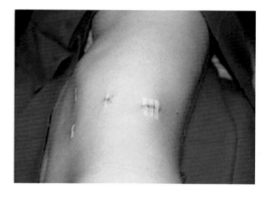

Figure 23-10. Placement of ports for a left adrenalectomy. The initial incision is made halfway between the umbilicus and the left iliac crest, and a 5-mm cannula is introduced. Two 5-mm working ports for the surgeon are placed lateral to this initial cannula. Often it is necessary to divide the lateral colonic peritoneal attachments before the most lateral of these two 5-mm cannulas can be introduced. The cannula for retracting the spleen and pancreas is placed cephalad and medial to the initial port. In this patient, the most lateral port was enlarged to 10 mm for extraction of the specimen.

closed in as many layers as possible with absorbable suture using loupe magnification. The skin is closed with 5-0 absorbable suture as well.

LEFT ADRENALECTOMY

Personnel placement for a left adrenalectomy is similar to that for a right adrenalectomy. The surgeon and camera holder stand at the patient's back. The surgical assistant stands opposite the surgeon so that the surgeon is working in a lateral-to-medial direction. The patient is placed in a right lateral decubitus position, and the initial 5-mm incision is made halfway between the umbilicus and the left iliac crest. Retraction of the liver

is not needed, as is the case for right adrenalectomy. However, it is important to retract the spleen and pancreas to expose the left adrenal gland. Two additional working ports are placed lateral to the initial 5-mm incision (Fig. 23-10). Sometimes it is necessary to divide the lateral peritoneal attachments to the colon before the most lateral cannula is introduced. The port for retracting the spleen and pancreas is placed cephalad and slightly medial to the initial port. The lateral peritoneal attachments of the colon are incised either with the Harmonic Scalpel or with scissors connected to cautery, as are the lateral peritoneal attachments to the spleen. The retracting instrument is then placed lateral to and somewhat under the spleen for better exposure

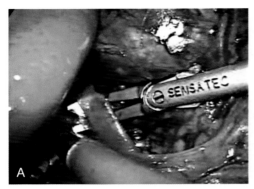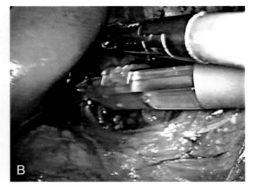

Figure 23-11. Although in a right adrenalectomy the vein is ligated as a final step, ligation of the adrenal vein is usually one of the early steps in a left adrenalectomy. **A,** The left adrenal vein entering the left renal vein is identified. **B,** It is doubly clipped on each side and will be divided between the middle clips.

of the left adrenal gland. Initially, the kidney is visualized, and the adrenal gland cephalad to the kidney can be identified.

Often, it is easier to ligate and divide the left adrenal vein early in the operative dissection rather than later. This is especially important when the adrenal gland contains a pheochromocytoma. Thus, the initial dissection starts at the inferolateral aspect of the left adrenal gland and moves medially across the superior pole of the kidney to where the left adrenal vein should be seen coursing toward the left renal vein. The vein is then doubly clipped on each side and divided between the two middle clips (Fig. 23-11). The remaining venous drainage from the adrenal gland as well as the arterial vasculature can usually be secured with the ultrasonic scalpel. To this end, dissection with the Harmonic Scalpel proceeds laterally around the left adrenal gland and toward its superior edge. The gland is then retracted inferiorly to gain better access to its cephalad portion. In a similar fashion as on the right side, the posterior attachments of the gland are also ligated and divided with the Harmonic Scalpel. The medial aspect of the gland is usually the last part ligated and divided, which is the final step and completes the adrenalectomy.

POSTOPERATIVE CARE

Patients are admitted after the operation and are usually ready for discharge the following day. Those with a pheochromocytoma usually require more postoperative attention but are often ready for discharge by the third or fourth postoperative day. Limited activity, usually for 1 to 2 weeks, is advised. The patient is usually seen for a postoperative clinic visit 2 weeks after the operation.

PEARLS

1. When performing a laparoscopic adrenalectomy for pheochromocytoma, ligate the adrenal vein first, even if it is on the right side.

2. Although cautery may be used, the Harmonic Scalpel is very useful for this operation, as it allows the surgeon to perform the operation efficiently without concern for hemostasis.
3. Always know where the right adrenal vein is, as this is the only part of a right adrenalectomy that is likely to cause problems.
4. Although piecemeal extraction of the specimen may be appropriate in some instances, such as in splenectomy, having the entire adrenal gland allows the pathologist to better evaluate whether the process is malignant or benign.

PITFALLS

1. For placement of the initial 5-mm cannula, use the cutdown technique rather than the Veress needle approach to prevent injury to underlying structures, as the umbilicus is not being used.

RESULTS

In 2002, a combined experience with laparoscopic adrenalectomy in children from Children's Mercy Hospital and from the University of California–San Francisco was reported (Miller et al. 2002). Subsequently, in 2005, the entire experience from two San Francisco area hospitals was published (Skarsgard and Albanese 2005). The entire experience of laparoscopic adrenalectomy from Children's Mercy Hospital is seen in Table 23-1. Eleven patients underwent operation at Children's Mercy from 2000 through 2006. The mean age was 10.4 years and the mean size of the lesion was 4.6 cm. Eight of the 11 patients underwent a left laparoscopic adrenalectomy. The 11 patients were hospitalized for 1.7 days (mean) after the operation. Their diagnoses are listed in the table. No complications have developed and no patient has required either another hospitalization or another operative procedure.

Table 23-1   Patients Undergoing Laparoscopic Adrenalectomy at Children's Mercy Hospital, 2000-2006

AGE (yr/sex)	Side	Size (max size in cm)	Operative Time (min)	Postoperative Hospitalization (days)	Diagnosis
12/M	L	4	140	2	Pheochromocytoma
13/F	L	3	120	2	Nonfunctioning adenoma
11/F	L	2.5	125	1	Nonfunctioning adenoma
16/F	L	8.5	180	1	Schwannoma
5/F	R	3.2	110	1	Nonfunctioning adenoma
12/M	R	3.5	120	1	Ganglioneuroma
14/F	L	4.0	130	1	Nonfunctioning adenoma
6/M	L	8.2	—	2	Virilizing adrenal cortical tumor
8/F	L	3.5	—	3	Ganglioneuroblastoma
16/F	R	4.9	150	1	Endothelial adrenal gland cyst
8 mo/F	L	5.2	120	4	Functioning adenoma (Cushing syndrome)

F, female; L, left; M, male; R, right.

SELECTED REFERENCES

1. Pretorius M, Rasmussen GE, Holcomb GW: Hemodynamic and catecholamine responses to a laparoscopic adrenalectomy for pheochromocytoma in a pediatric patient. Anesth Analg 87:1268-1270, 1998
2. Iwanaka T, Arai M, Ito M, et al: Surgical treatment for abdominal neuroblastoma in the laparoscopic era. Surg Endosc 15:751-754, 2001
3. Miller KA, Albanese CT, Harrison MA, et al: Experience with laparoscopic adrenalectomy in pediatric patients. J Pediatr Surg 37:979-982, 2002
4. Stanford A, Upperman JS, Nguyen N, et al: Surgical management of open versus laparoscopic adrenalectomy: Outcome analysis. J Pediatr Surg 37:1027-1029, 2002
5. Kaddah NM, Dessouky NM: Functioning adrenal tumors in children: A report of 17 cases. Saudi Med J 24:S46-S47, 2003
6. deLagausie P, Berrebi D, Michon J, et al: Laparoscopic adrenal surgery for neuroblastoma in children. J Urol 170:932-935, 2003
7. Kadamba P, Habib Z, Rossi L: Experience with laparoscopic adrenalectomy in children. J Pediatr Surg 39:764-767, 2004
8. Skarsgard ED, Albanese CT: The safety and efficacy of laparoscopic adrenalectomy in children. Arch Surg 140:905-908, 2005

24
Laparoscopic Orchiopexy

George W. Holcomb III

Most undescended testes are palpable at various levels in the inguinal canal. Approximately 10% are not palpable and are located in the abdomen. Surgical management of these nonpalpable testes has gradually evolved toward the laparoscopic route, with either a one-stage or a two-stage approach. The primary advantage of laparoscopy over initial inguinal exploration for a nonpalpable testis is that when the testis is in an intra-abdominal position, laparoscopy avoids the injury to the collateral vasculature that may occur with initial inguinal dissection. This collateral vasculature is necessary to nourish the intra-abdominal testis once the main testicular vessels are ligated and divided (Fowler-Stephens orchiopexy). Although I prefer a two-stage procedure, other surgeons find a one-stage laparoscopic orchiopexy to be as successful.

INDICATIONS FOR WORKUP AND OPERATION

An algorithm for boys older than 6 months with a non-palpable testis is shown in Figure 24-1. Because imaging studies are not universally accurate, they are not routinely used for this condition. Should a testis be visualized on the imaging study, initial laparoscopy is still indicated.

OPERATIVE TECHNIQUE

The patient is placed supine in a slight frogleg position on the operating room table, and general endotracheal anesthesia is administered. The abdomen and scrotum are prepared and draped widely. A vertical 5-mm incision is made in the umbilicus, and an expandable sleeve and a 5-mm Step cannula (Covidien, Mansfield, MA) are introduced directly through the skin and fascial incision. Diagnostic laparoscopy is then performed. Rarely, the vas deferens or testicular vessels end blindly in the retroperitoneum (Fig. 24-2A). In this situation, if the internal ring is closed and if there is no evidence of an intra-abdominal testis, inguinal exploration is not necessary. However, if the testicular vessels and vas deferens are seen to enter the inguinal canal, then inguinal exploration is performed (see Fig. 24-2B). Inguinal exploration is necessary, either to remove the remnant of a testis that torsed and subsequently atrophied or to perform an orchiopexy if a small, but viable, testis is found. In many cases, however, an intra-abdominal testis can be seen lying inside the internal ring associated with a patent processus vaginalis (Fig. 24-3). In this case, a staged laparoscopic approach is favored, with initial ligation and division of the vessels at the first stage followed by a second-stage laparoscopic orchiopexy 6 to 9 months later. This staged approach is favored to allow augmentation of the collateral vasculature that will eventually nourish the surgically relocated testis.

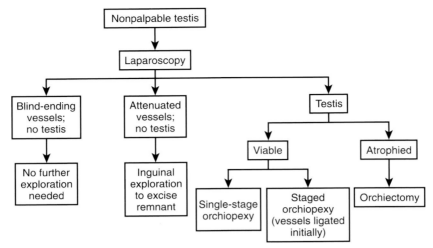

Figure 24-1.   The algorithm used for boys older than 6 months with a nonpalpable testis.

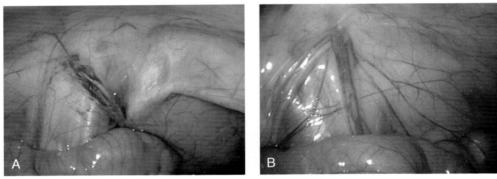

Figure 24-2.   **A,** The vas deferens and testicular vessels in this patient end blindly in the retroperitoneum. The internal ring is closed. In this very unusual situation, inguinal exploration is not necessary. **B,** In the more common scenario, the testicular vessels and vas deferens enter the inguinal canal. There is no evidence for a patent processus vaginalis. The vessels and vas deferens appear to be of relatively normal caliber. In this situation, inguinal exploration is necessary.

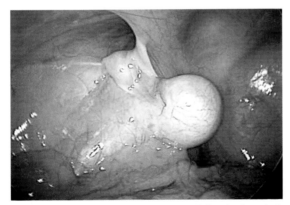

Figure 24-3.   In this patient, a left intra-abdominal testis is lying inside the internal ring, which is associated with a patent processus vaginalis.

FIRST STAGE

At the first stage of a planned two-stage approach, a stab incision is made on each side of the midline. A 3-mm atraumatic grasping forceps is introduced for use in the surgeon's left hand and a Maryland dissecting instru-

ment connected to cautery is inserted for use in the surgeon's right hand (Fig. 24-4). The patient is placed in a reverse Trendelenburg position, allowing the intestines to fall away from the area of dissection. The retroperitoneum overlying the testicular vessels proximal to the testis is then opened bluntly, and the testicular vessels are grasped with the atraumatic forceps. Being sure that the Maryland dissecting instrument is not in contact with any other structures, cautery is applied to the Maryland forceps to ligate and then divide the testicular vessels that are grasped by the atraumatic grasping forceps. This ligation and division is accomplished several centimeters away from the testis (Fig. 24-5). After ligation and division of these testicular vessels, the instruments are removed and Steri-Strips (3MCo., St. Paul, MN) are used to close the stab incisions. The umbilical cannula is then removed, the abdomen is desufflated, and the umbilical fascia is closed with interrupted 3-0 Vicryl (Ethicon, Inc., Somerville, NJ). The umbilical skin is closed with interrupted 5-0 plain catgut suture, and sterile dressings are applied.

The patient is awakened and is usually ready for discharge 1 to 2 hours after the operation. A clinic visit is scheduled for 2 weeks after the operation. Assuming that no postoperative problems have occurred, the patient is scheduled for a return visit in 6 to 9 months for assessment and to schedule the second-stage laparoscopic orchiopexy.

SECOND STAGE

Six to 9 months after laparoscopic ligation and division of the main testicular vessels to the intra-abdominal testis, the patient returns to the operating room for the laparoscopic orchiopexy. He is again placed in the frogleg position on the operating table, and general endotracheal anesthesia is administered. As occurred at the first operation, the umbilical skin and fascia are incised and the expandable sleeve is introduced, fol-

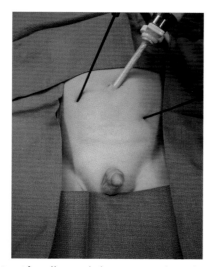

Figure 24-4. After diagnostic laparoscopy through a 5-mm umbilical cannula, if ligation and division of the testicular vessels are required, two accessory 3-mm instruments are introduced into the abdominal cavity using the stab incision technique. The surgeon stands on the side opposite the nonpalpable testis.

lowed by insertion of the 5-mm blunt cannula. Two stab incisions are again made near the previous stab incisions. As in the first operation, in the surgeon's left hand is an atraumatic grasping forceps and in the right hand is the 3-mm Maryland dissecting instrument connected to cautery. The ends of the testicular vessels near the testis are then grasped, and the peritoneum lateral to them is incised around the superior rim of the internal inguinal ring. The dissection is then carried medially from the testicular vessels over the ureter and toward the midline. When the ureter is approached, the cautery is no longer used, the Maryland dissecting forceps are removed, and scissors are inserted to incise the peritoneum. After the boundaries of the dissection are outlined, blunt dissection is performed to sweep caudally the peritoneum and the vasculature that it contains. At this point, using the atraumatic grasping forceps in the left hand, the surgeon grasps the gubernaculum in the inguinal canal and delivers it into the abdominal cavity (Fig. 24-6). The distal aspect of the gubernacular attachment is then incised with the Maryland dissecting instrument connected to cautery, thus freeing the testis of any distal attachments. With this maneuver, the testis is almost completely mobilized and is ready for delivery into the scrotum. During all this dissection, great care is taken to always visualize the vas deferens, the ureter, and the iliac vessels.

Having mobilized the testis intra-abdominally, attention is turned to the scrotum. A 10-mm incision is made transversely in one of the rugae of the scrotum, and dissection is continued to the dartos fascia. A dartos pouch is created in all directions and an incision is made in the dartos fascia. Using the Step cannula system, the Veress needle and its expandable sleeve are then introduced through the incision in the dartos fascia, advanced over the pubic tubercle, and visualized as they enter the abdominal cavity (Fig. 24-7A). Great care must be taken not to injure the bladder during introduction of this Veress needle and sleeve. For this reason, we usually do not place a catheter in the bladder, as we prefer to see the outlines of the bladder wall when inserting the

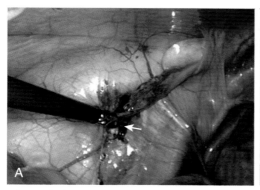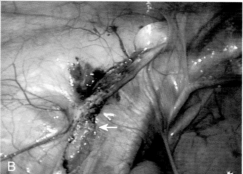

Figure 24-5. **A,** The testicular vessels to a left intra-abdominal testis are being cauterized with an atraumatic grasper (*arrow*) connected to cautery. **B,** The testicular vessels have been completely divided, and this cauterization (*arrow*) occurred several centimeters away from the testicle.

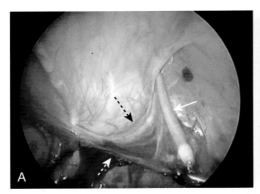
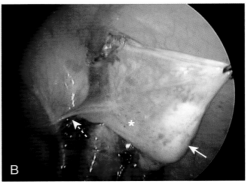

Figure 24-6. This patient is undergoing a laparoscopic right orchiopexy. **A,** The inferior portion of the peritoneal flap (*dotted white arrow*) containing the secondary vasculature to the testis is being mobilized. The testis has retracted into the right inguinal canal during this mobilization. The testicular vessels (*solid white arrow*) were divided previously and are retracted into the inguinal canal with the testis. The vas deferens is marked with a *dotted black arrow*. **B,** The right testis (*solid arrow*) is being mobilized for a laparoscopic orchiopexy. The peritoneum (*asterisk*), lying between the testis and vas deferens (*dotted arrow*), has been left intact. It is through this peritoneum that the accessory vasculature to the testicle lies.

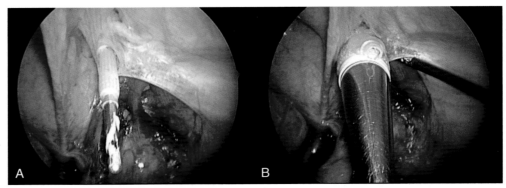

Figure 24-7. **A,** After mobilization of the testis and its secondary vasculature, a Veress needle and attached sheath are placed through an incision in the scrotum and directed over the pubic tubercle into the pelvis. **B,** The Veress needle has been removed. A 10-mm cannula with a blunt-tip trocar has been introduced through the expandable sheath and into the peritoneal cavity.

Veress needle and sleeve. Once the Veress needle and its sleeve are inserted into the abdominal cavity, the needle is removed and a 10-mm cannula with blunt trocar is introduced through the expandable sleeve (see Fig. 24-7B). It is important to use a 10-mm cannula, rather than a 5-mm size, as this larger cannula will create a soft tissue tract large enough for the testis to be delivered from the abdomen into the scrotum. Under direct visualization, a grasping instrument is introduced through the 10-mm cannula and into the pelvic cavity. The gubernaculum is delivered to this instrument and withdrawn into the 10-mm cannula. Sometimes the entire testis can be delivered into the 10-mm cannula, but sometimes it cannot (Fig. 24-8). It is helpful to reduce the intra-abdominal pressure to 5 mm Hg when exteriorizing the testis. After delivering the testis through the dartos fascia, the abdominal cavity is inspected for bleeding or injury to any structures (Fig. 24-9). The incision in the dartos fascia is then closed around the testis, and the testis is secured to the inferior portion of the scrotum with 3-0 PDS suture (Ethicon, Inc., Somerville, NJ). It is then placed in the dartos pouch and the scrotal skin closed over it with interrupted 5-0 chromic suture.

Attention returns to the abdominal cavity, and the area of dissection is inspected. The 3-mm instruments are withdrawn and the stab incisions closed with Steri-Strips. The umbilical fascia is approximated with 3-0 absorbable suture and the skin incision closed with 5-0 plain catgut suture (Fig. 24-10). Sterile dressings are applied, anesthesia is terminated, and the patient is transported to the recovery room. These boys are usually ready for discharge 1 to 2 hours later and return to the clinic for a postoperative visit in 2 weeks. An important postoperative instruction is to avoid a straddle toy for at least 2 weeks and preferably a month to allow the incisions to heal completely.

PEARLS

1. To manipulate the testis readily, grasp the gubernacular attachments securely, as this provides a good handle for manipulation.

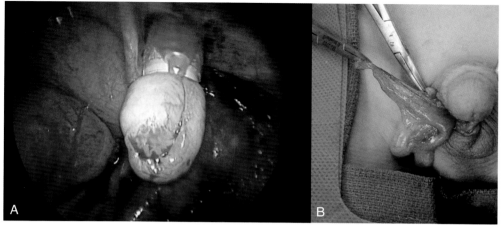

Figure 24-8.   A, The gubernaculum has been grasped with forceps introduced through the 10-mm cannula, and the testis is being withdrawn through the 10-mm cannula. Often, it is not possible to place the testis entirely into the 10-mm port. **B,** After removal of the cannula and with a secure hold on the gubernaculum, the testis is delivered over the pubic tubercle and into the right hemi-scrotum.

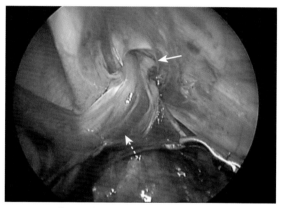

Figure 24-9.   The testis and secondary vasculature and the vas deferens have been transposed over the right pubic tubercle and into the right hemi-scrotum. Note the opening (*solid arrow*) in the peritoneum and lower abdominal wall as these structures (*dotted arrow*) exit the abdominal cavity.

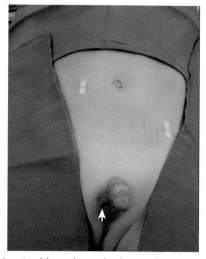

Figure 24-10.   In this patient who has undergone a laparoscopic right orchiopexy, the two stab incisions have been closed with Steri-Strips, and the umbilical fascia and skin have been closed with absorbable suture. Note the incision in the right hemi-scrotum (*arrow*).

2. Use the 10-mm cannula rather than the 5-mm one, as the tract that is developed by the 5-mm cannula is not large enough for the testis to be brought into the scrotum. As the cannula is withdrawn, the soft tissue collapses behind it and hinders the testis being brought into the scrotum.
3. If there are bilateral nonpalpable testes, treat each one separately. Make sure that the first is viable before embarking on the second.

PITFALLS

1. Use scissors when incising the peritoneum over the ureter so as not to injure the ureter with cautery.
2. Watch the border of the bladder when the Veress needle is introduced into the abdominal cavity from the scrotum, as the edge of the bladder is quite close to the path of the needle.
3. When making the stab incisions for the second operation, do not go directly through the previous incisions, as the scar will not heal as nicely. Try to go just near the previous stab incisions but not directly through them. These incisions will heal much better.

RESULTS

Over the past 7 years, 61 laparoscopic orchiopexies have been performed in 46 patients. The number of patients undergoing a single-stage orchiopexy (31) was almost equal to the number undergoing a two-staged orchiopexy (30). There was no significant difference in outcome between the two groups, nor was there a difference in the incidence of testicular atrophy. Three patients developed a postoperative wound infection. In two patients, entry into the bladder occurred during passage of the Veress needle and expandable sleeve over the pubic tubercle. This complication was noted intraoperatively and repaired, with an uneventful recovery in each patient.

SELECTED REFERENCES

1. Holcomb GH III, Brock JW III, Neblett WW III, et al: Laparoscopy for the nonpalpable testis. Am Surg 60:143-147, 1994

2. Esposito C, Garipoli V: The value of 2-step laparoscopic Fowler-Stephens orchiopexy for intra-abdominal testes. J Urol 158:1952-1954, 1997

3. Esposito C, Vallone G, Settimi A, et al: Laparoscopic orchiopexy without division of the spermatic vessels: Can it be considered the procedure of choice in cases of intra-abdominal testis? Surg Endosc 14:658-660, 2000

4. Radmayr C, Oswald J, Schwentner C, et al: Long-term outcome of laparoscopically managed nonpalpable testes. J Urol 170:2409-2411, 2003

5. Rodriguez A, Freire U, Orpez R, et al: Diagnostic and therapeutic laparoscopy for nonpalpable testis. Surg Endosc 17:1756-1758, 2003

6. Hanson GR, Castle EP, Ostlie DJ, et al: The use of stab incisions for instrument access in laparoscopic urological procedures. J Urol 172:1967-1969, 2004

25
Laparoscopic Ovarian Surgery

Mary L. Brandt

Laparoscopy is the approach of choice for many, if not most, ovarian lesions in adults and children. Understanding the expected pathologies of the ovary in children is important to planning and performing the optimal surgical procedure, particularly if ovarian pathology is discovered incidentally.

PREOPERATIVE EVALUATION OF A KNOWN OVARIAN MASS

The surgical treatment of ovarian lesions in children differs dramatically depending on whether the lesion is benign or malignant. Therefore, the preoperative workup is focused on differentiating between these conditions. In addition to asking about duration and type of symptoms, the history should reveal whether syndromes associated with ovarian lesions are present. For example, ovarian fibromas are associated with basal cell nevus syndrome, and sex cord tumors are associated with Peutz-Jeghers syndrome. The presence of signs and symptoms of hormonal activity, either isosexual or not, may also be helpful. Malignancy should be suspected if the patient has significant and persistent back, pelvic, or abdominal pain, bloating, or increasing abdominal girth, or if physical examination reveals the presence of a large adnexal mass, a fixed or irregular mass, or ascites.

Ultrasound (US) is the study of choice for evaluating ovarian masses. Signs that are suggestive of malignancy include size greater than 8 cm, complex masses, a lengthened utero-ovarian ligament, external ovarian vegetations, intracystic vegetations, an extra-ovarian spread, a thick wall in a cystic mass, and ill-defined, irregular borders and central necrosis in a solid mass. Computed tomography (CT) is indicated if the US is equivocal (Fig. 25-1). Additional findings on CT that are suggestive of malignancy include fine or coarse calcifications and direct extension to adjacent structures. Magnetic resonance imaging may be indicated to help differentiate uterine from ovarian masses.

Serum markers should be obtained in all patients with ovarian masses. Neoplasms of the ovary develop from one of the three embryologic cell lines: urogenital ridge (germinal epithelium), stroma, or yolk sac. Depending on the cell line of origin, different tumor markers are expressed. The germinal epithelium gives rise to epithelial cancers, which, although they are the most common tumor in adults, are rare in children. Sex cord–stromal tumors in children are most commonly granulosa–theca cell tumors.

Germ-cell tumors can be mature (teratomas), undifferentiated (germinoma), or differentiated malignancies (embryonal carcinoma, or mixed germ-cell tumor). An elevated alpha-fetoprotein level is often found with germ-cell tumors and yolk sac tumors. Beta–human chorionic gonadotropin is associated with dysgerminomas, choriocarcinoma, and occasionally embryonal carcinoma. Serum lactate dehydrogenase, which is increased with increased cell turnover, may be an indirect marker of malignancy. CA-125 is used as a serum marker for epithelial tumors and should be obtained in all children with tumors greater than 8 cm in diameter. CA-125 is elevated in 90% of women with advanced-stage ovarian carcinoma, but only 50% of those with early-stage cancers. Estrogen will be elevated and gonadotropins will be low in granulosa–theca cell tumors. Serum

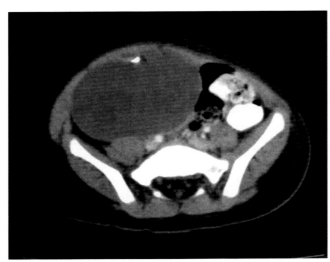

Figure 25-1. This CT scan shows a large (7- to 8-cm) mass arising from the pelvis. Anteriorly there is heterogeneous soft tissue with fat and possible calcification within the cyst that is suggestive of an ovarian teratoma. At operation, a teratoma was found and resected laparoscopically.

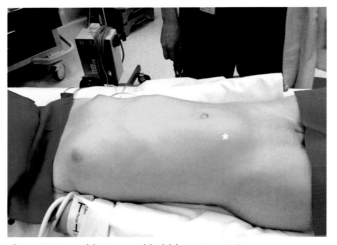

Figure 25-2. This 7-year-old girl has stage II Tanner development. In addition, she has a large lower abdominal/pelvic mass (*asterisk*). This patient has a granulosa–theca cell tumor.

inhibin, which is produced by granulosa cells, may be a useful tumor marker for granulosa–theca cell tumors. These patients often present with signs of precocious puberty (Fig. 25-2).

Sertoli-Leydig cell tumors are less common, but they should be suspected in the presence of virilization. Testosterone is elevated, and the degree of elevation correlates with tumor volume, making this a useful postoperative marker as well. Serum hormones are elevated in 10% of all ovarian lesions, both malignant and benign, and therefore are not helpful in differentiating malignant from benign tumors.

INDICATIONS FOR SURGERY

The majority of cystic masses can be followed if (1) there is no suspicion of malignancy (i.e., no solid component) and (2) they are asymptomatic. Follicular cysts are unilocular and can cause some pain with rupture. Corpus luteal cysts can rupture with significant hemorrhage. Prophylactic cystectomy to prevent torsion is more controversial. Because ovarian salvage is often difficult in the newborn period, many authors now recommend conservative management of asymptomatic cysts in newborns, regardless of size. In adolescents, cystic masses in the ovary are nearly always follicular cysts or corpus luteal cysts. Over 90% of these cysts will involute. In the adolescent, a large cyst (>5 cm) may be resected without sacrificing the ovary, and resection reduces the risk of torsion.

Any solid mass in the ovary should be resected. The type of resection depends on the suspicion of malignancy. Approximately 20% of ovarian masses in children and adolescents are malignant. If all tumor markers are negative, and imaging is supportive of a benign diagnosis, a laparoscopic approach or laparoscopic-assisted approach can be used.

OPERATIVE TECHNIQUE

Two principles underlie the decisions made in ovarian surgery. First, any solid mass should be presumed to be malignant in the absence of serum markers and imaging. Inadvertent spillage of a malignant tumor is a life-threatening complication. For example, in stage 1 granulosa cell tumors, survival is 80% to 95% with salpingo-oophorectomy. Spillage of the tumor, which changes the stage to stage 2, decreases survival to essentially zero. Because spillage of a malignant ovarian tumor has such significant consequences, most surgeons opt for resection using an open technique if there is a chance that the lesion is malignant.

The second principle is that staging before resection is critical in determining the appropriate treatment. If there is fluid in the pelvis, it should be aspirated and sent for cytology. If there is no fluid, lactated Ringer's solution should be instilled and washings obtained for cytology. The contralateral ovary should be inspected. The peritoneal surface and omentum should also be inspected. Any unusual implants should be biopsied. There is no need to perform an omentectomy or to biopsy the contralateral ovary unless a lesion is noted. However, in the rare case of an epithelial tumor, additional staging is necessary. If an epithelial tumor is suspected, a frozen section should be done after resection. An omentectomy and retroperitoneal lymph node biopsy should then be performed, as suggested by the Federation of Gynecology and Obstetrics in their staging system for primary carcinoma of the ovary.

For laparoscopic ovarian surgery, general anesthesia is used. The patient should be in a supine position, with the monitor at the patient's feet. Placing the patient in reverse Trendelenburg position facilitates visualization in the pelvis. Generally, a right-handed surgeon stands on the patient's left side, with the surgical assistant/camera holder opposite on the right. Port placement for ovarian surgery is dictated by the size of the patient and of the mass. The first cannula is inserted in the umbilicus. The placement of the two additional working ports is dictated by the best triangulation that can be achieved, usually with one port near the midline in the suprapubic area and the second one in the right or left lower abdomen (Fig. 25-3). The size of the cannulas should be the smallest that can effectively complete the objectives of the operation. In general, a 5- or 10-mm cannula is placed in the umbilicus and smaller (5- or 3-mm) ports are used as working ports.

CYSTECTOMY

When possible, the best surgical approach to cystic lesions of the ovary is to enucleate the cyst from the ovarian parenchyma. If the visceral peritoneum overlying the ovary is difficult to divide, the dissection can be facilitated with hydrodissection. A fine-bore needle is inserted under the visceral peritoneum and saline is injected to create a plane between the ovary and the peritoneum. The peritoneum is circumferentially incised to reveal the attachment of the cyst to the ovarian parenchyma, allowing resection with a hook cautery, ultrasonic scalpel, or Ligasure (Covidien, Mansfield, MA) (Fig. 25-4A,B). Once the cyst has been resected, it is

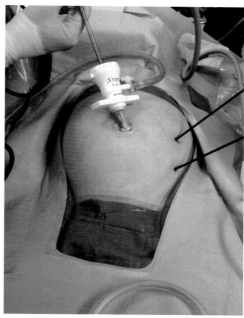

Figure 25-3. Port placements for excision of a left ovarian teratoma. For a right-handed surgeon, it is often helpful to place both ports on the patient's left side (as shown). In general, a 5- or 10-mm cannula is placed in the umbilicus and 3- or 5-mm instruments are used in the working ports. In this patient, 3-mm instruments were used for the working sites and were introduced through a stab incision.

Figure 25-4. Excision of an ovarian cyst. **A,** The peritoneum is circumferentially incised to reveal the attachment of the cyst to the ovarian parenchyma. **B,** Next, a plane is created between the cyst and the ovarian parenchyma. **C and D,** After removal of the cyst, the ovarian parenchyma is reconstructed by approximating the edges of the cortex together with fine absorbable suture.

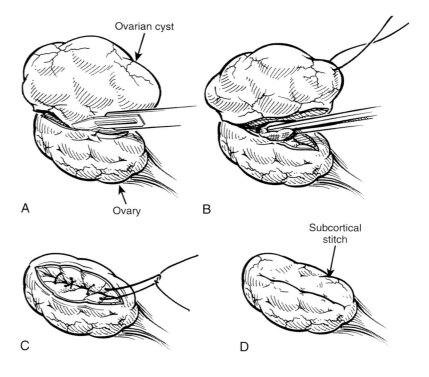

important to reconstruct the ovary by approximating the edges of the cortex together with very fine, absorbable suture (see Fig. 25-4C,D). If resection is not possible, and the diagnosis of a simple cyst is sure, the alternative approach is to unroof or marsupialize the cyst. The ovary should be handled gently, with the least amount of grasping and manipulation possible. Massive ovarian cysts can be aspirated preoperatively with ultrasound guidance before surgery, or intraoperatively and then mobilized through the umbilical cannula site (Fig. 25-5).

BENIGN TUMORS

Most benign tumors, like cysts, have a plane that can be developed between the ovary and the mass (Fig. 25-6). Using hydrodissection, as just described, often facilitates the resection. The overriding principle is to ensure complete resection of the mass while retaining the maximal amount of ovarian tissue. The mass should always be removed from the abdomen in an endoscopic retrieval bag to avoid any spillage. It is impressive how thin and fragile-appearing the ovary can be after resection of the mass. At the borders, it may appear only as

a slight thickening in the visceral peritoneum. Regardless of how little tissue appears to be present, it should be retained. The ovary should be reconstructed by approximating the cortical edges. If there is a significant amount of dead space in the center of the ovary, it can be obliterated with deep, absorbable sutures. The cortical edges are then approximated with a running suture of fine, absorbable suture. This ensures that the cortex is to the "outside" of the ovary, allowing ovulation to occur normally.

OOPHORECTOMY

Oophorectomy is indicated in pediatric patients for malignant lesions and abnormal gonads associated with intersex states. The streak gonads of intersex patients and the testes present in girls with testicular feminization syndrome are easily removed laparoscopically (Fig. 25-7). In general, malignant lesions should be resected with the fallopian tube (salpingo-oophorectomy). In children, because of the dramatic change in outcome for germ-cell tumors, malignant lesions can be staged laparoscopically, but they should be resected using an open technique to avoid spillage.

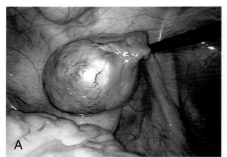 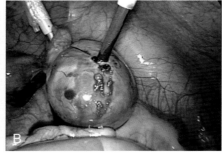 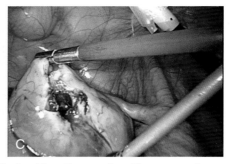

Figure 25-5.   Often, massive ovarian cysts can be aspirated intraoperatively to reduce their size. Then they can be either removed laparoscopically or mobilized through the umbilical cannula site for extracorporeal resection. **A,** A large ovarian cyst is visualized. **B,** A suction device is introduced into the cyst to aspirate it. **C,** The cystostomy is well visualized.

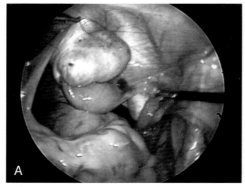 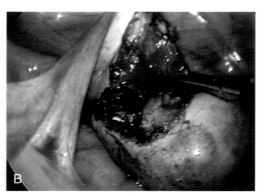

Figure 25-6.   Most benign tumors have a plane that can be developed between the ovary and the mass. **A,** A left ovarian teratoma is visualized. **B,** The mass is being separated from the ovary. After excision of the mass, the ovarian edges were reapproximated with interrupted absorbable sutures.

Figure 25-7.   This four-quadrant view depicts streak gonads in a baby with Turner syndrome. **A,** The streak gonads are visualized. **B,** The right gonad is being removed. **C,** The uterus is visualized after excision of the streak gonads (*arrows*) bilaterally. **D,** This photograph depicts port placement for the laparoscopic gonadectomy. The stab incision technique was used and the incisions are marked with the *arrows*. A 5-mm port was introduced in the umbilicus.

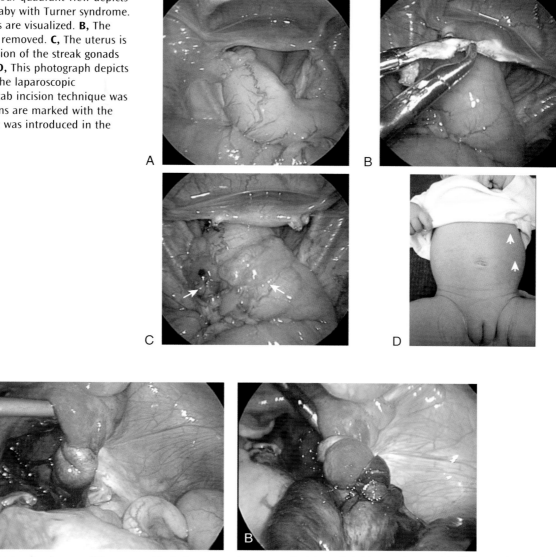

Figure 25-8.   Ovarian torsion is a condition amenable to laparoscopic surgery. **A,** A torsed right ovary is seen. **B,** The torsed ovary has been manipulated into the lower abdomen, and the torsion is well visualized.

PARAOVARIAN LESIONS

Paraovarian cysts arise from epoöphoron and are usually present on the leaves of the mesosalpinx. Lesions that are 3 cm or greater should be resected or enucleated. If they are less than 3 cm and difficult to resect, the anterior cyst wall can be obliterated with bipolar coagulation.

INCIDENTALLY DISCOVERED OVARIAN MASSES

The treatment of incidentally discovered masses is dictated by whether there is an associated solid component. A single, loculated cyst with clear fluid can be enucleated, or unroofed as described previously.

Solid ovarian masses that are incidentally discovered are a completely different problem. In the absence of imaging and tumor markers, there is no easy way to differentiate benign from malignant tumors. For that reason, in the absence of a clear indication for surgery (rupture with hemorrhage, e.g.), these should be left in place, staging performed, and markers drawn. Once the results of the staging and serum markers are known, a second procedure can be planned to resect the lesion.

OVARIAN TORSION

Ovarian torsion is a condition amenable to laparoscopic surgery (Fig. 25-8). However, if there is suspicion of a mass in a torsed ovary, the principles of ovarian surgery should be followed. First, ovary sparing is the goal if the

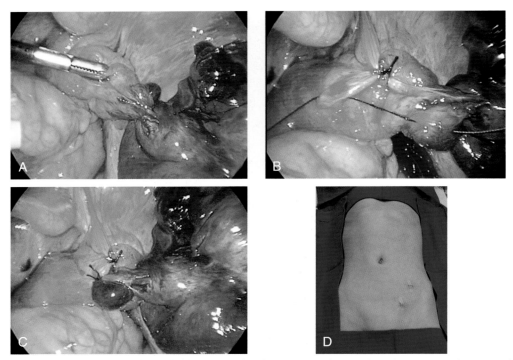

Figure 25-9. A, The ovary in the patient shown in Figure 25-8 has been detorsed. Note the edematous and congested right ovary. **B,** After detorsion, an oophoropexy is performed by shortening the length of the adnexa to help prevent another torsion. **C,** The two sutures that were used to reduce the length of the adnexa have been tied. **D,** The incisions used for this operation are visualized. A 5-mm port was inserted in the umbilicus.

mass is not malignant. Second, oncologic principles must be followed if the mass is malignant. And, third, if there is uncertainty, treat it as malignant. In the setting of an ovarian torsion with a mass, it is probably best to leave the ovary in place (after detorsion) with plans to return for a second operation. If this option is taken, staging should be accomplished by performing washings and inspecting the other ovary and the peritoneum. If, after the ovary is detorsed, it is clear that the ovary is ruptured, the procedure should be converted to an open operation so as to perform an oophorectomy with minimal intra-abdominal spillage. An ovary that looks necrotic can be left in place (see Fig. 25-8). It is clear that the appearance of the ovary after detorsion is not predictive of subsequent survival (Fig. 25-9). Histologic review of ovaries surgically removed for suspected nonviability has shown that the majority had clearly viable ovarian tissue. More importantly, detorsion with a second procedure later increases ovarian salvage and reproductive potential, without leading to complications. The issue of oophoropexy is also controversial. Bilateral asynchronous ovarian torsion has been reported and is one of the arguments used to support oophoropexy. Most surgeons reserve oophoropexy for patients who clearly have anatomically elongated adnexa that appear to lead to a higher risk for torsion. Others feel that oophoropexy, both ipsilateral and contralateral, is indicated in all cases of torsion.

SELECTED REFERENCES

1. Skinner MA, Schlatter MG, Heifetz SA, et al: Ovarian neoplasms in children. Arch Surg 128:849-853; discussion 853-854, 1993
2. Luzzatto C, Midrio P, Toffolutti T, Suma V: Neonatal ovarian cysts: Management and follow-up. Pediatr Surg Int 16:56-59, 2000
3. Strickland JL: Ovarian cysts in neonates, children and adolescents. Curr Opin Obstet Gynecol 14:459-465, 2002
4. Morowitz M, Huff D, von Allmen D: Epithelial ovarian tumors in children: A retrospective analysis. J Pediatr Surg 38:331-335, 2003
5. Abes M, Sarihan H: Oophoropexy in children with ovarian torsion. Eur J Pediatr Surg 14:168-171, 2004
6. Aziz D, Davis V, Allen L, et al: Ovarian torsion in children: Is oophorectomy necessary? J Pediatr Surg 39:750-753, 2004
7. Beaunoyer M, Chapdelaine J, Bouchard S, Ouimet A: Asynchronous bilateral ovarian torsion. J Pediatr Surg 39:746-749, 2004
8. Modlin IM, Kidd M, Lye KD: From the lumen to the laparoscope. Arch Surg 139:1110-1126, 2004
9. Anders JF, Powell EC: Urgency of evaluation and outcome of acute ovarian torsion in pediatric patients. Arch Pediatr Adolesc Med 159:532-535, 2005
10. Brandt ML, Helmrath MA: Ovarian cysts in infants and children. Semin Pediatr Surg 14:78-85, 2005
11. Breech LL, Hillard PJ: Adnexal torsion in pediatric and adolescent girls. Curr Opin Obstet Gynecol 17:483-489, 2005

12. Cass DL: Ovarian torsion. Semin Pediatr Surg 14:86-92, 2005

13. Celik A, Ergun O, Aldemir H, et al: Long-term results of conservative management of adnexal torsion in children. J Pediatr Surg 40:704-708, 2005

14. Enriquez G, Duran C, Toran N, et al: Conservative versus surgical treatment for complex neonatal ovarian cysts: Outcomes study. AJR Am J Roentgenol 185:501-508, 2005

15. Ghezzi F, Cromi A, Colombo G, et al: Minimizing ancillary ports size in gynecologic laparoscopy: A randomized trial. J Minim Invasive Gynecol 12:480-485, 2005

16. Hayes-Jordan A: Surgical management of the incidentally identified ovarian mass. Semin Pediatr Surg 14:106-110, 2005

17. von Allmen D: Malignant lesions of the ovary in childhood. Semin Pediatr Surg 14:100-105, 2005

18. Ates O, Karakaya E, Hakguder G, et al: Laparoscopic excision of a giant ovarian cyst after ultrasound-guided drainage. J Pediatr Surg 41:E9-11, 2006

19. Hilger WS, Magrina JF, Magtibay PM: Laparoscopic management of the adnexal mass. Clin Obstet Gynecol 49:535-548, 2006

20. Templeman C, Fallat M: Ovarian tumors. In Grosfeld J, O'Neill J, Coran A, Fonkalsrud E (eds): Pediatric Surgery. Philadelphia, Mosby, pp 593-621, 2006

26
Laparoscopic Portoenterostomy (Kasai Operation)

Marcelo Martinez-Ferro

Biliary atresia (BA) is a progressive sclerosis of the extrahepatic biliary tree that occurs within the first 3 months of life. It is one of the most common causes of neonatal cholestasis and accounts for over half of children who undergo liver transplantation. The management in the majority of cases consists of a primary portoenterostomy (Kasai procedure) to restore bile flow and alleviate jaundice.

Although the Kasai portoenterostomy remains the initial definitive surgical procedure for infants with BA, it invariably leads to the formation of intra-abdominal adhesions, particularly in the supracolic compartment. In the eventuality of a liver transplantation months or years later, the presence of adhesions with profuse vascularization resulting from portal hypertension, together with coagulation defects associated with liver dysfunction in end-stage liver disease, adds considerable technical difficulties and risks to the already complex transplant procedure.

The rationale for laparoscopic portoenterostomy relies on the proven advantages of minimally invasive surgery plus an often ignored attribute: the absence of postoperative adhesions.

INDICATIONS FOR WORKUP AND OPERATION

Most of the patients with BA develop an insidious jaundice by the second week of life. The infant often looks active, not acutely ill, but progressively develops acholic stools, choluria, and hepatomegaly. Persistent conjugated hyperbilirubinemia (greater than 20% of total, or 1.5 mg/dL) should be urgently evaluated. Initial evaluation should include a careful history and physical examination, partial and total bilirubin determinations, blood type and group, a Coombs test, reticulocyte cell count, and a peripheral smear. The diagnostic evaluation of the cholestatic infant should include laboratory tests that can exclude perinatal infectious (toxoplasma, rubella, cytomegalovirus, herpes virus [TORCH] titers, hepatitis profile), metabolic (alpha-1-antitrypsin levels), systemic, and hereditary causes.

The total bilirubin in infants with BA is around 6 to 10 mg/dL, with 50% to 80% conjugated. Liver function tests are nonspecific. Lipoprotein-X levels greater than 300 mg/dL and gamma glutamyl transpeptidase (GGT) above 200 units/dL suggest this diagnosis.

An ultrasound study of the abdomen should be the first diagnostic imaging study done in cholestatic infants to evaluate for the presence of a gallbladder, and to identify intrahepatic or extrahepatic biliary ductal dilation and liver parenchyma echogenicity. BA sonographic characteristics include an absent or small gallbladder that does not contract with hormonal stimuli, and increased liver echogenicity. Nuclear studies of bilioenteric excretion (99m-technetium di-isopropyl-iminodiacetic acid [DISIDA] scan) after prestimulation of the microsomal hepatic system with phenobarbital for 3 to 5 days is the diagnostic imaging test of choice. Patients with BA show an increased hepatic uptake during early injection without significant bilioenteric excretion in delayed films (24 hr). A percutaneous liver biopsy should be the next diagnostic step if previous studies suggest BA, and the infant has no associated coagulopathy. The histologic findings of BA are bile duct proliferation and fibrosis. Unfortunately, these changes are nonspecific and can also be found in neonatal hepatitis. Once the diagnosis of BA is suspected, laparoscopic cholangiography is indicated. The confirmation of BA during this study should be followed by a laparoscopic portoenterostomy.

OPERATIVE TECHNIQUE

The infant is placed in a supine position across the table or at the lower end of the table. The surgeon stands at the patient's feet, with assistants on the left and right. To increase the range of movement of the instruments, patients are raised up by means of a custom-made, 10-cm-high platform (Fig. 26-1).

Four cannulas are introduced (Fig. 26-2). Technical specifications and diameters of the cannulas are detailed in Table 26-1. For the insertion of the first port, access to the peritoneal cavity is accomplished by an open infraumbilical approach. A purse-string suture is tied around the umbilical opening and a 6-mm cannula is introduced. The purse-string suture is tightened around the cannula, and extra fixation of the port is achieved using the Shah-Neto technique, which involves rubber suction tubing placed around the cannula. A stay suture is tied around the tubing and then around the insufflation stopcock. This cannula stabilization technique is used for all ports, thus avoiding dislodgment of the cannula and development of CO_2 subcutaneous emphysema.

The umbilical port is used for insertion of a short (18-cm) 4-mm, 30-degree angled telescope. We recommend using a wide angle telescope, because it provides better vision in a limited working space. This umbilical

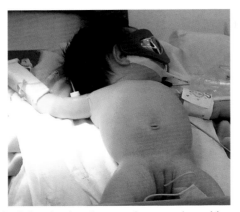
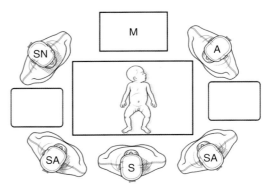

Figure 26-1.   The infant is placed across the operating table and positioned over an elevated platform to achieve maximal instrument mobility. The surgeon (S) and both surgical assistants (SA) are situated at the patient's feet, facing the monitor (M). One of the surgical assistants holds the camera. A, anesthesiologist; SN, scrub nurse.

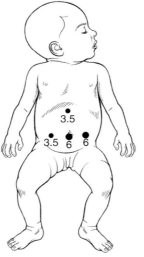
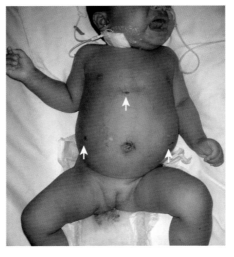

Figure 26-2.   Cannula placement. A 6-mm port is introduced in the umbilicus, and through it the camera is inserted. The two main working ports are in the left lower abdomen and the right flank. The subcostal 3.5-mm port is used for an irrigation or suction device. The locations of the ports are seen in the photograph (*arrows*). Note the green stool in the diaper 1 month postoperatively.

cannula is also used for CO_2 insufflation. A pressure of 8 mm Hg with a flow of 4 to 6 L/min provides excellent visualization and is well tolerated by these patients.

A second cannula is inserted in the left flank via a 6-mm port with a 3-mm reducer cap. If possible, we prefer a threaded cannula that enhances the fixation to the abdominal wall. This cannula must have a silicone leaflet valve or a similar device for insertion of a curved needle. A third port (3.5 mm) is introduced in the right flank and is used for the introduction of grasping and dissection forceps. The fourth port (3.5 mm) is inserted in the subcostal region and is used mainly for the introduction of a 3-mm aspiration or irrigation device.

Liver stay sutures are very convenient for adequate exposure of the biliary tree. As originally described by Esteves and colleagues (2002), two percutaneous transhepatic stitches are inserted through the abdominal wall near the border of the left and right costal margins and pass through the liver parenchyma. These sutures exit the abdominal cavity 1 cm away from their entrance point (Fig. 26-3). In our experience, no patients have bled after this maneuver, regardless of the diagnosis or the degree of liver fibrosis.

Initial inspection of the atretic biliary tree is important for determining if there is a real need to perform cholangiography. In most cases, no study is needed, as experienced surgeons can determine precisely whether the biliary tree is patent or atretic. If cholangiography is needed, a 22-gauge angiocatheter is used to percutaneously access the gallbladder and to perform a contrast study using diatrizoate meglumine contrast under fluoroscopy. Once the presence of an atretic biliary tree is confirmed, dissection is started at the fundus of the gallbladder using a 3-mm hook cautery. The atretic gallbladder and cystic duct are dissected free from the liver and the dissection is carried toward the fibrous remnant of the common bile duct and hepatic duct (Fig. 26-4A). The dissection then proceeds to the duodenum and pancreas distally, following the choledochal remnants, which are transected using the monopolar hook cautery. Proximally, the atretic biliary tree leads directly to the portal plate. At this point, careful resection of enlarged hilar lymph nodes is usually needed to access the hilar vessels. Once both hepatic arteries and the portal vein are recognized, the portal plate is gently dissected using

Table 26-1 Cannulas for Laparoscopic Portoenterostomy

Cannula	Diameter (mm)	Length (cm)	Accessories (Extra)	Position
1	6	8.5	3-mm rubber sealing cap (reducer)	Umbilicus
2	6	6	3-mm rubber sealing cap (reducer)	Left flank
3 and 4	3.5	5	—	Subcostal and right lower quadrant

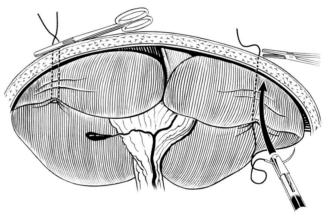

Figure 26-3. The liver is elevated and retracted as described by Esteves. A percutaneous transhepatic stay suture is introduced into the left lobe and into the right lobe. If needed, another percutaneous suture introduced just below the xiphoid process can be used to snare the round ligament and retract the liver cephalad. (From Esteves E, Neto EC, Neto MO, et al: Laparoscopic Kasai portoenterostomy for biliary atresia. Pediatr Surg Int 18:737-740, 2002.)

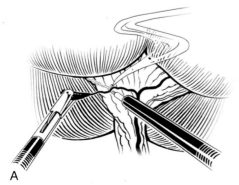
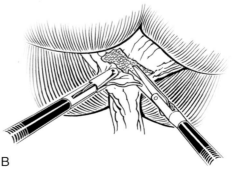

A   B

Figure 26-4. **A,** Most of the dissection as well as the resection of the atretic biliary tract is performed using a 3-mm monopolar hook instrument. **B,** The portal plate is carefully sectioned and excised with 3-mm scissors.

a 3-mm Kelly dissector. Special care must be taken with the small portal vessels that emerge vertically from the portal vein to the portal plate. It is advantageous to coagulate them with the hook cautery to increase the portal plate surface. The main hepatic arteries (left and right) and the portal vein are the anatomic landmarks that establish the boundaries of the portal plate. Finally, the fibrous remnant of the portal plate is excised sharply with 3-mm curved endoscopic scissors (Fig. 26-4B). In the majority of the cases, one can see bile flowing from small bile ducts still patent at the portal plate (Fig. 26-5). Often, profuse bleeding appears after cutting the plate. The use of monopolar cautery should be avoided, as the patent microscopic bile ducts can be destroyed. We recommend stuffing the plate site with Surgicel (Ethicon, Inc., Somerville, NJ) and waiting while the Roux-en-Y jejunojejunostomy is performed. The hemostatic pack must be retrieved later, before starting the anastomosis.

To perform the Roux-en-Y jejunostomy, the ligament of Treitz is identified and the proximal jejunum is grasped at a point 20 to 40 cm distal to the ligament; it is marked and subsequently exteriorized through the umbilical incision. Marking the bowel correctly is crucial for accurate identification of the proximal and distal ends of the jejunum after exteriorization. We mark the proximal end with one dot and mark the distal end with two dots. These marks are placed by gently applying the tip of the monopolar hook to the seromuscular surface of the jejunum. The marked jejunum is exteriorized through the umbilical incision and divided. The previously marked area (1 to 2 cm long) must be completely resected to avoid potential complications. The umbilical fascia should be enlarged to 15 mm, so that the anastomosis can be performed without tension (Fig. 26-6). A 30-cm Roux limb is created, and treatment of the proxi-

mal end varies with the diagnosis. In patients with BA, the end is left open and returned to the peritoneal cavity for an end-to-end portal anastomosis. (In patients with a choledochal cyst, the end is closed manually or by means of a mechanical stapler.) After the extracorporeal jejunal anastomosis, the small bowel is returned to the abdominal cavity and a new purse-string suture of thicker thread (0 or 1 nylon) is placed around the umbilical site to avoid leakage of CO_2. Finally, the Roux limb is passed either antecolic or retrocolic to the porta hepatis.

The laparoscopic anastomosis to the portal plate is performed with 5-0 PDS (Ethicon, Inc., Somerville, NJ) with a C1 needle. Because it has a silicone leaflet valve, all the sutures are passed in and out the peritoneal cavity through the 6-mm left flank port. Also, we recommend passing two initial percutaneous stay sutures at both posterior corners of the anastomosis (Fig. 26-7). These stay sutures facilitate the precise placement of the posterior central stitches, which must enter the portal plate near its posterior border and exit very close to the portal

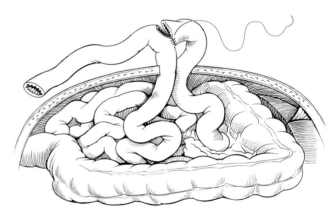

Figure 26-6. The jejunojejunostomy is performed outside the peritoneal cavity by exteriorizing the jejunum through the dilated umbilical fascia and skin incision.

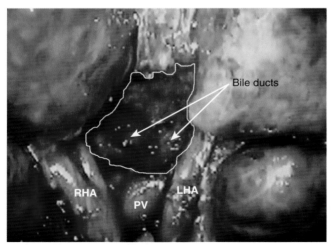

Figure 26-5. Bile can be seen flowing from the incised portal plate as seen in this magnified view. The Roux-en-Y limb will be placed at the encircled area. LHA, left hepatic artery; PV, portal vein; RHA, right hepatic artery.

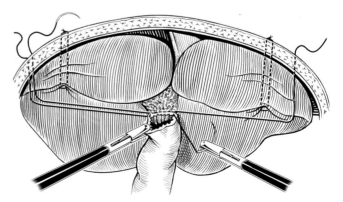

Figure 26-7. Percutaneous stay sutures are placed at each corner of the posterior wall of the anastomosis. This maneuver facilitates the correct placement of the rest of the posterior anastomotic stitches as they pass close to the portal vein.

vein. For the anastomosis, we use the extracorporeal Roeder knot-tying method. The anterior face of the portojejunostomy is easily performed by means of interrupted PDS sutures.

POSTOPERATIVE CARE

The patients are admitted after the operation and allowed to drink clear liquids or formula approximately 8 hours after the operation at a low volume and low concentration. The volume and concentration can be advanced over 24 hours. Over 80% of our patients are ready for discharge the day after the operation, and the remaining 20% are discharged on the second postoperative morning. No patient who was admitted the day of the operation has required hospitalization longer than 48 hours. We ask the parents to collect a sample of all stools and bring these samples to the first postoperative clinic visit (Fig. 26-8). With these samples, we are able to evaluate the bile flow through the portoenterostomy.

PEARLS

1. If massive intestinal distention impedes an optimal view of the surgical field, selective transperitoneal aspiration of the bowel (STAB) is encouraged. Using a 25- or 21-gauge needle and a 20- or 60-cc syringe, the dilated intestinal loops are punctured under endoscopic vision and the contents aspirated. The procedure can be repeated as many times as needed until an adequate surgical field is achieved.
2. For additional liver retraction, another percutaneous stitch placed extracorporeally just below the xiphoid

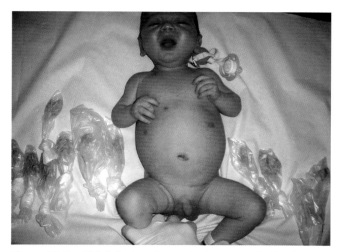

Figure 26-8. This infant underwent a laparoscopic Kasai portoenterostomy 3 weeks earlier. His mother was asked to collect a sample of each stool for the past week to evaluate the bile flow. The stool samples indicated good bile flow through the portoenterostomy.

process can be used to snare the falciform ligament and retract the liver anteriorly and superiorly.
3. Always start by resecting the atretic gallbladder. The atretic remnant will take you directly to the portal plate.
4. In older patients with advanced liver fibrosis, hepatic segment IV may protrude into the porta hepatis, thus occluding the laparoscopic view. In these cases, a fifth cannula can be placed just under the right costal margin at the midclavicular line to aid in retraction of the liver.
5. Dissection of the portal vein must be performed with the Maryland dissector. The small portal vein tributaries can be coagulated with the monopolar hook. If bleeding develops, do not panic. Apply gentle pressure with a dissector and grasper while the assistant aspirates the field.
6. When performing the jejunojejunostomy, be very generous in enlarging the umbilical port site. Use your thumb as a reference. Your whole thumb should pass through the enlarged umbilical incision.

PITFALLS

1. Avoid wasting time in dealing with cannula displacement. Fixation of all the cannulas must be done in all cases.
2. Avoid aggressive use of the monopolar hook when dissecting the portal plate.
3. Watch for injury to the hepatic arteries while dissecting enlarged lymph nodes in the area. Lymph nodes must be resected after dissection to obtain optimal visualization of the portal plate.
4. Watch for small portal vein tributaries to the portal plate, and gently surround them with the monopolar hook and coagulate them using this device.
5. Ask the anesthesiologist not to ventilate the patient while placing the posterior portal plate stitches. This helps avoid an accidental portal vein puncture.
6. Securely close all the incisions to avoid leaking of biliary ascites.

RESULTS

Twenty-two patients have undergone this operation at two institutions: the J. P. Garrahan National Children's Hospital (JPGNCH) and the Fundación Hospitalaria Private Children's Hospital, Buenos Aires. Only patients operated on or supervised by me were included in this analysis. The mean age at surgery was 79.1 days (range, 20 to 135). No conversion to an open operation has been needed. Two intraoperative complications were observed: an accidental injury to the left hepatic artery without clinical consequences, and an intraoperative pneumothorax not related to the surgical procedure but rather to airway anesthetic instrumentation.

The mean operating time was 3.5 hours (range, 2.5 to 4.5). After operation, the mean time to oral feedings was 48 hours (range, 20 to 600). The mean hospital stay was 5 days (range, 2 to 40). Only two patients received postoperative prednisolone. Immediate bile flow recovery was defined by the presence of bile-colored stools by 1 month after operation, and this was observed in 89% of the cases. On long-term assessment, 7 of 22 (32%) had good flow, 9 of 22 (41%) had partial flow, and 6 of 22 (27%) had poor flow. Patients with good and partial flow represent 73% of the series. From this entire group, 10 of 22 patients have required liver transplantation at a mean age of 13 months. Excellent cosmetic results were observed in all patients. Four patients developed an umbilical hernia, and two required further surgical repair. Table 26-2 summarizes this experience.

This series was compared to a retrospective analysis of 29 patients who received a conventional open Kasai procedure at the JPGNCH from 1997 to 2001. No difference in age at surgery was observed. As seen in Table 26-3, overall bile flow was better for the laparoscopic

group. A similar number of patients required liver transplantation in both groups and at a similar age.

As a second part of this analysis, further data were collected in a prospective study regarding the presence or absence of adhesions at the moment of laparotomy for liver transplantation. Adhesions were classified as solitary or multiple. Multiple adhesions were subclassified in nine groups depending on the compromised organs. In this study, six patients received a laparoscopic Kasai procedure and were transplanted by the same transplant team at the JPGNCH. They were compared with six patients who received a conventional open Kasai procedure elsewhere and were transplanted in the same period at the JPGNCH. Both groups had similar characteristics of age, weight, and type of transplant. As seen in Table 26-4, although surgical time and blood loss were better for the laparoscopic group, statistical analysis revealed no statistical difference. However, when analyzing for the presence of peritoneal adhesions, there were no adhesions seen in the patients who had undergone a laparoscopic portoenterostomy (Fig. 26-9). When compared with the open group, a highly significant difference was observed (see Table 26-4).

Table 26-2 Results of Laparoscopic Kasai Procedure at the JPGNCH (2001-2006)

Patients (n)	Age at Kasai (days)	Conversions	Operating Time (mean, hr)	Good or Partial Bile Flow	Steroids Needed?	Liver Transplant Performed?	Age at Transplant (mo)
22	79.1	0	3.5	73%	2/22 (9%)	10/22 (45.4%)	13

JPGNCH, J. P. Garrahan National Children's Hospital.

Table 26-3 Comparison between Conventional Kasai Procedures (1997-2001) and Laparoscopic Cases at the JPGNCH (2001-2006)

	Conventional Kasai (n = 29)	Laparoscopic Kasai (n = 22)
Age at Kasai (days)	82.4	79.15
Good or partial bile flow	52%	73%
Poor bile flow	48%	27%
Liver transplant	15/29 (51.7%)	10/22 (45.45%)
Age at liver transplant (mo)	14	13

JPGNCH, J. P. Garrahan National Children's Hospital.

Table 26-4 Complications at Liver Transplantation in Patients with Biliary Atresia: Comparison between Prior Conventional Open Kasai and Prior Laparoscopic Kasai Procedures

	Conventional Kasai	Laparoscopic Kasai	P value
Blood loss (mL)	370	170	0.07
Operative time (min)	180	120	0.1
Multiple adhesions	6/6 (100%)	0	0.015
Simple adhesions	0	1/6 (16.6%)	

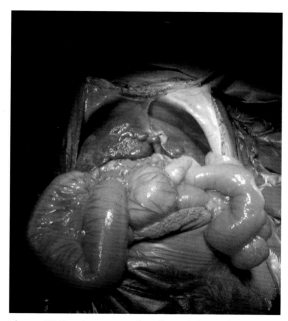

Figure 26-9.   Intraoperative view of the peritoneal cavity at the time of liver transplantation in a patient who had previously undergone a laparoscopic portoenterostomy. The absence of adhesions is characteristic of these patients. Notice the tortuous aspect of the revascularized umbilical vein resulting from portal hypertension.

SELECTED REFERENCES

1. Shah R, Neto PN: An innovative technique for reusable laparoscopic cannula stabilization and fixation. Pediatr Endosurg Innov Tech 1:59-61, 1997
2. Esposito C, De Petra MR, Palazzo G, et al: Is there a reduction of postoperative adhesion formation in the pediatric age group after laparoscopy compared with open surgery? Pediatr Endosurg Innov Tech 2:115-119, 2000
3. Esteves E, Neto EC, Neto MO, et al: Laparoscopic Kasai portoenterostomy for biliary atresia. Pediatr Surg Int 18:737-740, 2002
4. Petersen C, Ure BM: What's new in biliary atresia? Eur J Pediatr Surg 13:1-6, 2003
5. Lee H, Hirose S, Bratton B, et al: Initial experience with complex laparoscopic biliary surgery in children: Biliary atresia and choledochal cyst. J Pediatr Surg 39:804-807, 2004
6. Martínez M, Questa H, Gutierrez V: Operación de Kasai laparoscópica: Detalles técnicos y resultados iniciales de una técnica promisoria. Cir Pediatr 17:36-39, 2004
7. van Heurn ELW, Saing H, Tam PKH: Portoenterostomy for biliary atresia: Long term survival and prognosis after esophageal variceal bleeding. J Pediatr Surg 39:6-9, 2004
8. Martinez-Ferro M, Esteves E, Laje P: Laparoscopic treatment of biliary atresia and choledochal cyst. Semin Pediatr Surg 14:206-215, 2005

27
Laparoscopic Resection of Choledochal Cyst

Hanmin Lee and Raul Cortes

Complex biliary surgery has been one of the last frontiers for minimal-access pediatric surgery. Improvements in optics and instrumentation have allowed pediatric surgeons to perform laparoscopic portoenterostomies and resections of choledochal cysts. These procedures remain technically challenging, but several tricks make performing these operations feasible. The technique of laparoscopic resection of the common type of choledochal cyst with Roux-en-Y reconstruction is detailed in this chapter.

INDICATIONS FOR WORKUP AND OPERATION

Increasingly, the diagnosis of a choledochal cyst is made prenatally by sonography. Most often, the infants are well at birth and can be followed as outpatients. We recommend an ultrasound shortly after birth to confirm the diagnosis, and a magnetic resonance cholangiopancreatogram (MRCP) at 3 to 6 months of age to better delineate the anatomy. Ideally, we perform the laparoscopic resection and biliary reconstruction between 6 and 12 months of age.

OPERATIVE TECHNIQUE

General endotracheal anesthesia is used for this operation. The patient is placed in a frogleg position at the foot of the bed. An orogastric or nasogastric tube is inserted to decompress the stomach. A Credé maneuver is performed to empty the bladder. The abdomen is widely prepared and draped. The surgeon stands at the foot of the bed while the first assistant stands just to the surgeon's right, controlling the endoscope (Fig. 27-1).

The umbilicus is incised vertically, and the peritoneal cavity is entered using the Veress needle approach with an expanding Step sleeve (Covidien, Mansfield, MA). A pneumoperitoneum is created to 12 mm Hg with a flow of 0.5 to 2 L/min. A 5-mm short Step port is then introduced through the Step sleeve. Diagnostic laparoscopy is performed with a 4- or 5-mm 30-degree angled telescope. Although a 2.7- or 3-mm endoscope can be used for infants, we generally find that the larger telescope has better optics, which is critical for dissection and for the biliary reconstruction. Three additional cannulas are then introduced: a 3-mm port in the right lower quadrant, a 5-mm port in the left abdomen in the midclavicular line just superior to the umbilicus, and a 3-mm port in the midclavicular line just below the costal margin (Fig. 27-2). In older children, 5-mm ports and 5-mm instruments are used.

After introduction of the endoscope, the table is placed in reverse Trendelenburg position to allow the intestines to fall caudally. With a grasping instrument inserted through the left subcostal port, the assistant secures the gallbladder and retracts it and the liver cephalad. (In older children, this liver retraction port can be positioned in the right lower abdomen. However, in younger children, the right hip and thigh of the child may interfere with attempts to retract the liver through a right lower quadrant port.) The gallbladder and choledochal cyst can usually be visualized easily (Fig. 27-3).

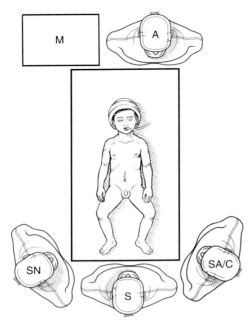

Figure 27-1. For laparoscopic resection of a choledochal cyst, the patient is usually placed at the foot of the bed. An older child can be placed in stirrups. The surgeon (S) stands at the foot of the bed while the surgical assistant/camera holder (SA/C) stands to the surgeon's right and controls the telescope and camera. The scrub nurse (SN) is usually positioned to the surgeon's left. A single monitor (M) can be placed above the patient's right shoulder. If two monitors are used, they are positioned on either side of the head of the bed. A, anesthesiologist.

A cholangiogram can be performed if preoperative imaging or intraoperative visualization is unclear. Also, the gallbladder can be divided at the infundibulum–cystic duct junction between 5-mm clips, which allows the gallbladder to be retracted farther cephalad (Fig. 27-4). In turn, the liver is retracted even more cephalad to better expose the porta hepatis. Another option is to place large transcutaneous sutures through either the falciform ligament or the gallbladder to assist in retraction of the liver.

With the porta hepatis and triangle of Calot well-exposed, the cystic duct is dissected to the choledochal

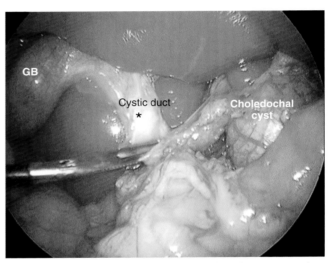

Figure 27-3. This intraoperative view depicts the anatomy that the surgeon initially sees for a typical choledochal cyst. The cystic duct and choledochal cyst are well visualized. GB, gallbladder.

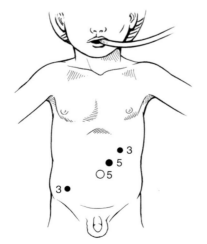

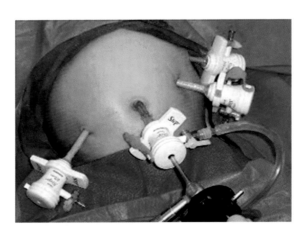

Figure 27-2. Port placement for laparoscopic resection of a choledochal cyst. A 5-mm port is inserted through the umbilicus for introduction of a 4- or 5-mm, 30-degree angled telescope. In an infant or young child, a 3-mm port is placed in the right lower quadrant, through which an instrument is used in the surgeon's left hand. The main working port is a 5-mm cannula in the left abdomen in the midclavicular line, just cephalad to the umbilicus. A grasping instrument for retraction is inserted through the 3-mm left subcostal port for use by the assistant. In older children, 5-mm ports and 5-mm instruments are employed.

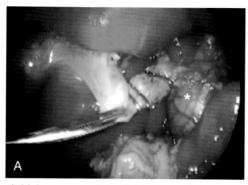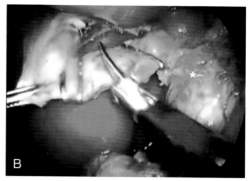

Figure 27-4.   An initial maneuver is to divide the cystic duct to further retract the gallbladder and then the liver for better exposure of the porta hepatis. **A,** The cystic duct has been ligated with endoscopic clips. **B,** The cystic duct is being divided so that the gallbladder and liver can be retracted further. In both photographs, an *asterisk* identifies the choledochal cyst.

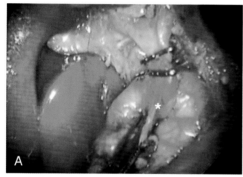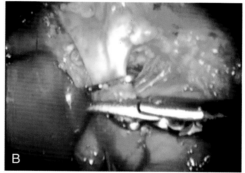

Figure 27-5.   Generally, dividing the hepatic duct just proximal to the cystic dilation allows the best exposure to the posterior surface of the choledochal cyst for dissection and mobilization of the cyst down to the duodenum. **A,** The common hepatic duct just caudal to the confluence of the hepatic ducts is visualized, and clips have been applied to the common hepatic duct. The cyst is marked with an *asterisk.* **B,** The common hepatic duct is being divided between the clips.

cyst. Care is taken to avoid the right hepatic artery or an accessory branch, either of which can be mistaken for the cystic artery. Dissection of the cyst begins on its medial and lateral aspects. Retracting the cyst using the cystic duct attachment may be helpful. After the hepatic artery and its branches and the portal vein and its branches are identified, division of the choledochal cyst either proximally or distally is necessary to complete the dissection of the cyst off the full length of the hepatic artery and portal vein. Generally, dividing the hepatic duct just proximal to the cystic dilation allows the best exposure to the posterior surface of the choledochal cyst (Fig. 27-5). Dissection of the cyst is then carried down to the duodenum. To avoid injury to the pancreas, care is now taken to carry out the dissection on the cyst wall. This dissection of the caudal portion of the cyst is continued until the cyst narrows (Fig. 27-6). A high-quality MRCP is useful for this part of the dissection, as it allows the surgeon to know how much distance exists in the narrowed portion of the distal common bile duct before the pancreatic duct enters it. The distal common bile

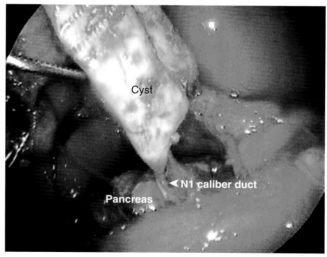

Figure 27-6.   After mobilization of the cyst circumferentially, the dissection is carried caudally toward the duodenum. Here, the cyst and pancreas have been identified. The point of narrowing of the cyst into a normal-size common bile duct is seen.

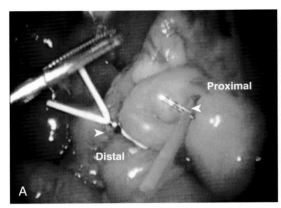
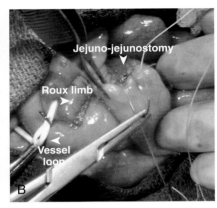

Figure 27-7. After resection of the cyst, attention is turned to creating the Roux limb. **A,** The endoscopic view shows that the proximal jejunum has been marked with two colored vessel loops. The red vessel loop identifies the proximal portion of the jejunum, and the white vessel loop identifies the distal portion of the jejunum. This is important so that the correct orientation is understood once the jejunum is exteriorized through the small umbilical incision for an extracorporeal jejunojejunostomy. **B,** The jejunum has been delivered through the umbilicus, and the jejunojejunostomy is being performed extracorporeally.

duct is then divided between clips or ligated with ties. The cyst is then free and is placed to the right of the liver for later removal.

The surgeon's attention now turns toward identification of the proximal jejunum. This is best found by identifying the transverse colon and retracting it anteriorly. The proximal jejunum can then be easily identified coming through the base of the transverse mesocolon. The jejunum is grasped gently, and the site where it will be divided is identified (approximately 15 cm from the ligament of Treitz). A small incision is made bluntly in the mesentery of the jejunum, and a colored vessel loop is passed around the jejunum. It is secured using a 5-mm clip so that it will not slip off the bowel. Two to 3 cm distal to this first vessel loop, a second vessel loop of another color is similarly placed to identify the distal aspect of the bowel (Fig. 27-7A). The ligament of Treitz is then once again identified to make sure the orientation of the bowel is correct.

The umbilical incision is then enlarged to approximately 1.5 cm, and the umbilical port is removed. The segment of jejunum marked by the vessel loops is then eviscerated through the umbilical incision. Failure to mark the bowel as just described makes identifying proximal and distal aspects quite challenging once the bowel has been exteriorized through the small umbilical incision. The jejunum is then divided with a stapler between the two vessel loops. The Roux-en-Y limb is measured to 30 to 45 cm, according to surgeon preference. The end-to-side anastomosis to reestablish continuity of the small bowel is performed (Fig. 27-7B). We usually hand-sew this anastomosis, but it can be stapled as well. The mesenteric defect is then closed. The proximal vessel loop is removed, and the distal vessel loop is left in place. The bowel is then returned to the peritoneal cavity.

The umbilical cannula is then reinserted. Towel clips or sutures can be used to make the incision airtight to allow adequate abdominal insufflation. After identification of the Roux limb, it is brought either retrocolic or antecolic, according to surgeon preference. The hepatic duct stump is identified and the clip occluding it is removed. A longitudinal incision on the antimesenteric aspect of the Roux limb is made slightly longer than the diameter of the hepatic duct stump. Either 4-0 or 5-0 absorbable monofilament sutures are used for the biliary–enteric anastomosis. Stay sutures are placed on the lateral aspects of the anastomosis to approximate the Roux limb to the hepatic duct. These stay sutures are inserted posterior to the equator line of the hepatic duct to facilitate approximating the posterior wall. A running suture is used on the posterior wall, tying it to the stay sutures. All sutures are tied on the outside of the anastomotic lumen to minimize the development of possible biliary sludge or stones. The lateral and anterior walls are approximated with interrupted sutures (Fig. 27-8). In some cases, the cyst extends to the bifurcation of the hepatic duct. In these instances, the two ducts can be sewn together and a single anastomosis to the Roux limb can be performed. Alternatively, the two ducts can be sewn separately to the Roux limb. A drain may be left, at the surgeon's discretion.

Occasionally, it may be necessary to convert to an open procedure if dissection of the choledochal cyst or the anastomosis cannot be completed safely, as these are challenging operations.

POSTOPERATIVE CARE

The patients are admitted after the operation and are usually ready for discharge within 4 to 5 days postop-

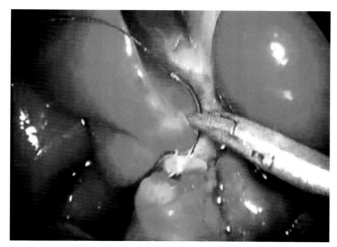

Figure 27-8. This operative view shows placement of one of the interrupted sutures used to approximate the common hepatic duct to the Roux limb.

eratively, after return of bowel function. Patients are monitored for the possibility of a bile leak. They are usually seen for a postoperative clinic visit 3 to 4 weeks after the operation. Total and direct bilirubin levels are checked at that time.

PEARLS

1. Use a 4- or 5-mm, 30-degree telescope in a smaller child, or a 10-mm, 30-degree scope in an older child. Optimal visualization is important.
2. Several techniques can be used to retract the liver. Some surgeons place sutures through the liver transcutaneously. Others use a liver retractor. We advocate leaving the gallbladder attached to the liver, dividing the gallbladder from the cystic duct, and then using the gallbladder to retract the liver cephalad, much as occurs in a laparoscopic cholecystectomy. This is best done from a port in the left subcostal region. A right lower quadrant cannula may seem to be an optimal site for gallbladder or liver retraction, but in little children, the right thigh and hip may interfere with optimal manipulation of the instruments.
3. Divide the choledochal cyst proximally or distally early in the dissection. This allows better exposure for the dissection of the cyst off the portal vein and hepatic artery.
4. Create the Roux-en-Y limb extracorporeally. To accomplish this easily, laparoscopically place two vessel loops of different colors around the area of the jejunum to be divided for creation of the Roux limb (Fig. 27-7A). Note which color represents proximal and which represents distal. Enlarge the umbilical incision to accommodate evisceration of the marked

segment of bowel (about 1.5 cm in a 6-month-old). The vessel loops will allow identification of the proximal and distal limbs of bowel to facilitate creation of the Roux limb. Leave the vessel loop on the Roux limb to easily identify it once the bowel has been returned into the abdomen.
5. Use a running suture to create the posterior wall of the hepaticojejunostomy. Use interrupted sutures anteriorly and laterally.

PITFALLS

1. Identify the portal vein early to avoid injury.
2. Be aware of the variations of the hepatic artery branches.

RESULTS

Since 2001, we have attempted nine laparoscopic repairs of choledochal cysts in infants and children. Eight of the nine were completed laparoscopically. The single conversion occurred early in our series and involved an infant with a choledochal cyst that extended to the bifurcation of the hepatic duct. We performed two separate anastomoses of the right and left hepatic ducts to the Roux limb with a limited open incision. In future cases, we would probably perform this laparoscopically.

There were no postoperative complications. All children are well, with normal bilirubin levels and no evidence of cholangitis or pancreatitis. The mean operative time was approximately 5 hours, and the postoperative hospitalization was 3 to 4 days.

SELECTED REFERENCES

1. Shimura H, Tanaka M, Shimizu S, et al: Laparoscopic treatment of congenital choledochal cyst. Surg Endosc 12:1268-1271, 1998
2. Tanaka M, Shimizu S, Mizumoto K, et al: Laparoscopically assisted resection of choledochal cyst and Roux-en-Y reconstruction. Surg Endosc 15:545-552, 2001
3. Tan HL, Shankar KR, Ford WD: Laparoscopic resection of type I choledochal cyst. Surg Endosc 17:1495-1497, 2003
4. Lee H, Hirose S, Bratton B, et al: Initial experience with complex laparoscopic biliary surgery in children: Biliary atresia and choledochal cyst. J Pediatr Surg 39:804-807, 2004
5. Li L, Feng W, Jing-Bo F, et al: Laparoscopic-assisted total cyst excision of choledochal cyst and Roux-en-Y hepatoenterostomy. J Pediatr Surg 39:1663-1666, 2004
6. Martinez-Ferro M, Esteves E, Laje P: Laparoscopic treatment of biliary atresia and choledochal cyst. Semin Pediatr Surg 14:206-215, 2005

28
Minimally Invasive Diaphragmatic Plication

Steven S. Rothenberg

Paralysis or eventration of the diaphragm is a relatively uncommon problem in infants and children but one that may cause significant respiratory distress. Eventration may be congenital in nature, or it may result from iatrogenic injury, either from birth trauma or from injury to the phrenic nerves during cardiac surgery. When there is significant compromise to pulmonary function, diaphragmatic plication should be considered to allow better expansion of the affected lower lobe. Both laparoscopic and thoracoscopic plication are minimally invasive approaches for dealing with this problem and significantly decrease the morbidity of an open approach. I prefer a laparoscopic approach because the abdomen affords increased workspace, whereas the rigid thoracic cage restricts movement of the instruments.

INDICATIONS FOR WORKUP AND OPERATION

The indication for surgery is an elevated hemidiaphragm with evidence of lung compression or atelectasis, which may be segmental or lobar. The elevated diaphragm is usually associated with some degree of respiratory compromise, which can be quite severe in some patients. The goals of intervention range from an attempt to improve pulmonary function enough to allow a patient to be weaned from a ventilator, to improving function enough to relieve dyspnea on exertion. The advent of minimally invasive surgery has allowed a more liberal use of this procedure.

The workup includes a routine chest radiograph that shows an elevated hemidiaphragm, as well as pulmonary function testing (in older patients) that shows a restrictive pattern. Confirmation of a paralyzed diaphragm can be obtained with ultrasound or fluoroscopy, with demonstration of paradoxical motion of the diaphragm. In some cases, it can be difficult to differentiate an eventration from a diaphragmatic hernia with a thick sac. However, these are probably variations of the same developmental defect, and they are often treated similarly.

OPERATIVE TECHNIQUE

LAPAROSCOPIC APPROACH

An infant is placed supine on or across the operating table (depending on age and size) near the foot of the bed (Fig. 28-1). Larger patients are placed in stirrups so that the surgeon can stand between the legs, which allows good access to the upper abdomen and diaphragm. An orogastric tube is inserted to decompress the stomach, and the bladder is manually emptied.

The abdomen is insufflated through a 5-mm cannula inserted in the umbilicus. The upper abdomen and diaphragm are then evaluated, and the diagnosis of eventration is confirmed. If a diaphragmatic hernia is present, a laparoscopic repair can be performed, with or without resection of the sac. Generally, two additional ports (3

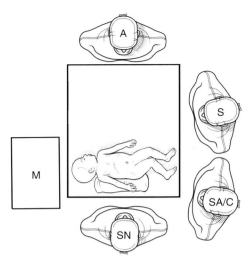

Figure 28-1. For a minimally invasive diaphragmatic plication, the laparoscopic approach is preferred. Infants are placed either supine or across the operating table (depending on age and size) near the foot of the bed. The surgeon (S) and surgical assistant/camera holder (SA/C) are positioned at the feet of the patient. The monitor (M) is above the patient's head. If the patient is placed supine across the operating table, the scrub nurse (SN) can be positioned at the foot of the operating table. In this diagram, a small roll has been placed under an infant undergoing plication of the right hemidiaphragm. A, anesthesiologist.

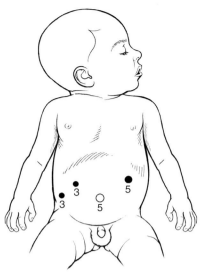

Figure 28-2. Port placement for plication of an eventration of the right hemidiaphragm. The umbilical port, usually 5 mm, is the site for insertion of the telescope attached to the camera. The two main working ports are the 3-mm and 5-mm ports in the upper epigastric regions. The lateral 3-mm port near the infant's right flank is used for an instrument to push down on the liver for improved exposure.

or 5 mm) are needed and are situated in the right and left epigastrium, slightly above the umbilical port. If the eventration is on the right, the left port should be slightly higher, and vice versa. Occasionally, if the eventration is on the right, a fourth port or instrument is necessary to hold down the dome of the liver (Fig. 28-2).

The initial step is to break the surface tension and collapse the diaphragm, reducing the tension on the plication stitches. This is accomplished with the first stitch. In most infants, 2-0 Ethibond (Ethicon, Inc., Somerville, NJ) on an RB-1 needle is used. Starting medial and anterior on the affected diaphragm, two or three bites are taken, going front to back, imbricating the attenuated muscle (Fig. 28-3). This not only starts to plicate the diaphragm but also removes a considerable amount of the tension on the diaphragmatic muscle. Because these sutures can be under tension and because the area under the diaphragm is at an awkward angle to sew, it can be helpful to exteriorize the first stitch through the abdominal wall and use this suture to remove tension on the diaphragm while the other sutures are placed. The other option is to use a knot pusher and tie the sutures extracorporeally. This is the preferred technique in most cases. A series of interrupted sutures is then placed going from medial to lateral, each one taking two or three bites of diaphragm going from anterior to posterior (Fig. 28-4). Generally,

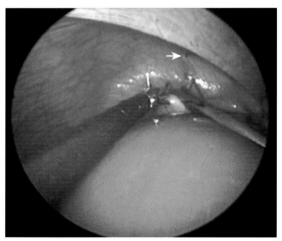

Figure 28-3. Starting medial and anterior on the affected diaphragm, two or three stitches are taken going from anterior to posterior on the diaphragm to imbricate it. Here, the suture has already been taken through the anterior aspect of the diaphragm (*arrow*) and is now taking a portion of the posterior aspect of the diaphragm.

seven or eight stitches are required. If the diaphragm is still lax, then a second row of sutures can be placed (Fig. 28-5). Sutures should be placed until the diaphragm is taut. This is important because some laxity in the plication will develop over time.

THORACOSCOPIC APPROACH

The patient is placed in a lateral decubitus position and the working ports are situated in the seventh or eighth

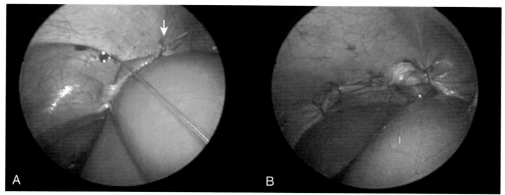

Figure 28-4.   A, This view shows the second of the interrupted sutures being used to imbricate the diaphragm. The initial suture has been tied (*arrow*). **B,** The imbricated diaphragm is visualized. In this patient, a total of five sutures were used to plicate this diaphragm.

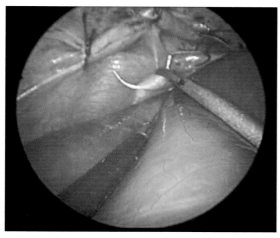

Figure 28-5. Here, a second layer of sutures is being placed to make the diaphragm more taut. This is important, as some laxity in the plication will develop over time.

intercostal space in the anterior and posterior axillary lines. The telescope is introduced in the midaxillary line in an interspace just above the previously mentioned ports. Sutures are placed as described previously, progressing from medial to lateral. The restricted working space in the chest can create a more difficult suturing environment.

Unless there has been trauma to the lung parenchyma, there is no need to leave a chest drain after either a laparoscopic or a thoracoscopic approach. If a thoracoscopic approach is used, the valve on the cannula can be used to evacuate the air. The lung is then inflated under positive pressure. The cannula is removed, and an occlusive dressing is applied.

POSTOPERATIVE CARE

Unless the patient was ventilated preoperatively, extubation is done in the operating room. A chest radio-graph is obtained in the recovery room to check the position of the diaphragm and to look for a pneumothorax. No treatment is required for a small residual pneumothorax. A patient who was ventilator dependent is slowly weaned as tolerated over the next few days. Once the patient is extubated, a diet is started. The patient is discharged as soon as the diet and oral analgesics are tolerated. A follow-up chest radiograph and pulmonary function tests are obtained at 1 month.

PEARLS

1. Piercing the diaphragm can relieve the tension on the diaphragm and make suturing easier.
2. An extra instrument can be inserted laterally in the left upper abdomen to push down on the liver and improve visualization if exposure is difficult. It can be introduced using the stab incision technique.
3. If the diaphragm is so attenuated that it is transparent, it may be better to resect a portion of it and treat it as though it was a diaphragmatic hernia.
4. If there is excessive tension, the knots can be tied extracorporeally using a knot pusher. This is safe, as the sutures do not tend to tear out of the diaphragm.

PITFALLS

1. The diaphragm can be plicated too much and create a chest wall deformity.
2. Inadequate plication results in inadequate repair. Expect to lose 15% to 20% of the repair over time.
3. It is possible that a small pneumothorax will be created while suturing the diaphragm, but this is usually not clinically significant. The surgeon and anesthesiologist should be aware of this possibility.

RESULTS

Nineteen infants, weighing between 1.7 and 6.2 kg, along with two children of ages 3 and 8 years, have required laparoscopic diaphragmatic plication. The indication in the infants was diaphragmatic eventration in 14 and (iatrogenic) diaphragmatic paralysis in five. In the two children, one had an eventration and the other had a phrenic nerve injury secondary to resection of a giant mediastinal teratoma. All procedures were successfully completed laparoscopically. Before the plication, 18 of the infants were ventilator dependent. The average operative time was 46 minutes. There were no operative complications, and no patient required a chest tube. All infants were successfully extubated within 10 days of surgery. Chest radiographs immediately postoperatively and at 1 month showed successful plication. The two older patients showed significant clinical improvement.

SELECTED REFERENCES

1. Partrick D, Rothenberg SS: Laparoscopic plication of the diaphragm in infants. Pediatr Endosurg Innov Tech 5:175-182, 2001
2. Huttl TP, Wichmann MW, Reichart B, et al: Laparoscopic diaphragmatic plication: Long-term results of a novel surgical technique for postoperative phrenic nerve palsy. Surg Endosc Surg 18:547-551, 2004
3. Becmeur F, Talon I, Schaarschmidt K, et al: Thoracoscopic diaphragmatic eventration repair in children: About 10 cases. J Pediatr Surg 40:1712-1715, 2005

29
Laparoscopic-Assisted Donor Nephrectomy

Maria Alonso, Frederick Ryckman, and Greg Tiao

In children with end-stage renal disease, the treatment that will best maintain growth and development is renal transplantation. Because many parents are readily willing to donate a kidney, living related transplantation is the most common method by which renal transplantation occurs in these children. In the past, open nephrectomy was often used to procure a kidney from a living related donor; however, it is associated with significant discomfort and, on occasion, prolonged recovery. With the development of minimally invasive technology, laparoscopic techniques have been applied to the living donor nephrectomy. As the benefits of this procedure have become apparent, laparoscopic-assisted donor nephrectomy (LDN) has replaced open nephrectomy as the most common method used to obtain a living-donor kidney.

INDICATIONS FOR WORKUP AND OPERATION

The preoperative evaluation for a living kidney donor is extensive. HLA typing and cross-matching of the donor and the recipient is performed. If these tests are satisfactory, the donor undergoes a workup including a medical evaluation by a physician who is independent from the transplant program, serum biochemical analysis, urinalysis, and radiographic imaging of both kidneys. In the past, radiographic imaging consisted of ultrasonography and renal angiography. With the improvement in high-resolution contrast-enhanced computerized tomography (CT), CT angiography has become our preferred modality in the assessment of the donor's renal anatomy. If the medical evaluation reveals a suitable candidate, discussion is undertaken to ensure that the risks and benefits of the procedure are clearly understood.

The ideal kidney to be procured is one in which there is a single renal artery and renal vein. If both of the donor's kidneys have this vascular configuration, the left kidney is preferred because its renal vein is longer. If the left kidney has more than one artery and the right kidney has a single artery, procurement of the right kidney is considered. It is important to discuss the anatomic configuration of the donor kidney with the recipient's transplant surgeon, as there may be anatomic aspects of the recipient that make one side favorable to the other. For example, in older recipients (e.g., teenagers), the maturation of the pelvis results in an iliac artery and vein that lies deeper within the pelvis. A deep iliac vein may make the use of a right kidney less than ideal, as its short renal vein will make the venous anastomosis challenging.

Patients are admitted on the day of surgery, and two units of packed red blood cells are cross-matched.

OPERATIVE TECHNIQUE

Patients undergo general anesthesia. Two large-bore intravenous lines, a urinary catheter, a nasogastric (NG) tube, and pneumatic compression boots are placed. Intravenous antibiotics are administered. The patient is positioned on the operating table in a supine position, with the side from which the kidney is to be removed elevated by a gel roll placed parallel to the spine, and with the kidney rest situated just cephalad to the iliac crest. The table is flexed and the kidney rest is raised, accentuating the space between the iliac crest and the 12th rib (Fig. 29-1A). The surgeon stands facing the patient with the surgical assistant/camera holder on the left. The monitor is positioned beyond the table, so that the area of dissection is in line between the surgeon and the monitor (see Fig. 29-1B). When possible, we use AESOP (Intuitive Surgical, Sunnyvale, CA), a robotic arm, to hold and move the camera.

The abdomen and flank are prepared and draped sterilely. The first port is placed lateral to the umbilicus on the side from which the kidney is to be removed. Although a Veress needle approach can be utilized, we prefer the open Hassan technique. After the skin incision, the anterior rectus fascia is opened and the rectus sheath and muscle are separated until the posterior rectus sheath is visualized and incised. Two stay sutures are placed, and a blunt-tip 12-mm port is introduced. Pneumoperitoneum to a pressure of 15 mm Hg is generated via CO_2 insufflation at a flow rate of 20 L/min. Diagnostic laparoscopy is performed with a 5-mm, 30-degree angled telescope. Two additional 5-mm ports are inserted superior to the first port and just to the side of midline on the side from which the kidney is to be removed (Fig. 29-2). The telescope and camera are introduced through the superior-most port.

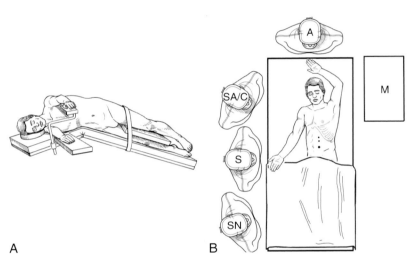

Figure 29-1. **A,** For a laparoscopic-assisted left donor nephrectomy, the patient is placed supine on the operating table with a roll underneath the left flank to rotate the patient to the right. The table is flexed and the kidney rest is raised, thereby accentuating the space between the iliac crest and the 12th rib. **B,** Placement of operating personnel. The surgeon (S) stands facing the patient, with the surgical assistant/camera holder (SA/C) standing to the left of the operating surgeon. When possible, the robotic telescopic holder is used. The scrub nurse (SN) is situated caudal to the surgeon. The monitor (M) is over the patient's left side, so that the area of dissection is between the surgeon and the monitor. A, anesthesiologist.

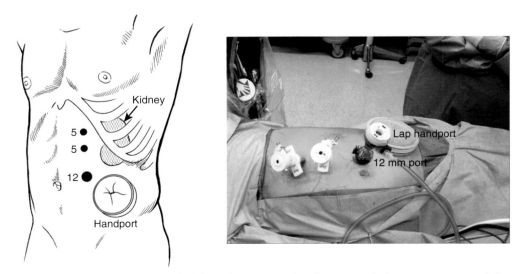

Figure 29-2.   Placement of ports for a laparoscopic left nephrectomy. Using the open technique, a 12-mm port is introduced through the left rectus muscle as the initial port. After insufflation and diagnostic laparoscopy, two additional 5-mm ports are inserted cephalad to this first port and to the left of midline. The telescope/camera is introduced through the most cephalad port, and the surgeon works through the caudal 5-mm port and the initial 12-mm port. The HandPort is introduced later to aid in mobilization of the kidney, and it is the site through which the kidney is removed.

LEFT NEPHRECTOMY

The surgeon, using a grasping forceps in the left hand and the Harmonic Scalpel (Ethicon Endosurgery, Cincinnati, OH) or laparoscopic scissors connected to electrocautery in the right hand, mobilizes the left colon by dividing its lateral retroperitoneal attachments from the splenic flexure to below the pelvic inlet. This mobilization includes freeing the colon from its attachments to the inferior aspect of the spleen. When mobilizing the colon, care must be taken to avoid dissection within the colonic mesentery. After the colon has been mobilized, the retroperitoneal attachments of the spleen to the diaphragm are divided. On occasion, a long 5-mm scissor is needed to free the superior-most attachments of the spleen to the diaphragm. This allows the spleen to fall medially, thereby exposing much of Gerota's fascia. In addition to the spleen, the tail of the pancreas is often adherent to Gerota's fascia and must be freed so that the hilum of the left kidney can be visualized.

Mobilization of the colon and its mesentery inferior to the kidney allows identification of the left gonadal vein and left ureter. The gonadal vein is followed cephalad to locate the renal vein. The gonadal vein is freed and divided between endoclips several centimeters distal to its insertion point on the inferior aspect of the left renal vein. The adventitia over the left renal vein is opened, exposing the renal vein and, on its superior edge, the left adrenal vein. The adrenal vein is mobilized. This vein is typically short and often has small side branches inserting along its course. Once adequate length has been obtained, the adrenal vein is divided between endoclips. Once the adrenal vein is divided, the renal vein is circumferentially dissected free. On occasion, there are short lumbar veins inserting into the posterior aspect of the renal vein. These can be divided with the Harmonic Scalpel if they are less than 3 mm;

endoclips are preferred to secure larger lumbar veins. Once the vein is completely mobilized, attention is turned toward identifying the renal artery at its origin from the aorta. It is often embedded within lymphatic tissue that must be divided. This mobilization is best accomplished with blunt dissection and, if necessary, electrocautery. After the artery has been visualized, the adrenal gland is freed from the superior aspect of the kidney. It is important to review the angiographic location of the renal artery before doing this dissection to ensure there is no superior branch of the renal artery that could be damaged during this mobilization.

Once the adrenal gland is free, an incision is made at the level of the anterior iliac crest, and the laparoscopic HandPort (Ethicon Endosurgery, Cincinnati, OH) is inserted. The assistant stands at the patient's back and inserts the left hand into the abdomen. Using the left hand, blunt mobilization of Gerota's fascia from the retroperitoneum is performed. The assistant also mobilizes the ureteral bundle off the psoas muscle. When dense bands are encountered, they are divided either with electrocautery or the Harmonic Scalpel. Once the kidney is mobilized, it is elevated between the first and second fingers of the assistant's hand, exposing the renal artery and vein (Fig. 29-3). The hilar dissection is completed by dividing connective tissue attachments and lymphatics from the kidney to the aorta and inferior vena cava (IVC) up to the level of the artery and vein.

At the time of the placement of the HandPort, the recipient is placed under general anesthesia in an adjacent operating room and the operative exposure is begun. The donor kidney is left in situ until the recipient is adequately prepared, so that the cold ischemia time is minimized. When both teams are ready, completion of the donor nephrectomy is performed. We administer heparin intravenously to minimize the likelihood of small-vessel thrombosis during the division of the artery

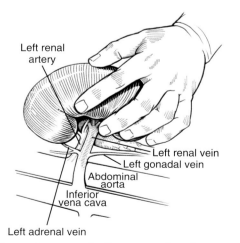

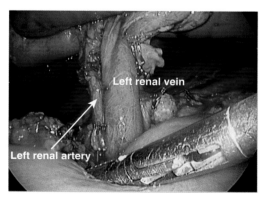

Figure 29-3. The anatomy seen by the surgeon for a laparoscopic left donor nephrectomy before ligation and division of the artery and vein. The hand (blue glove, top of photograph) is being used to elevate the kidney for maximal visualization and access to the left renal hilum. The left adrenal and gonadal veins have been ligated with clips and divided.

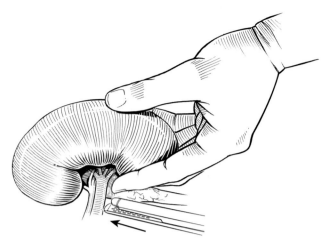

Figure 29-4. Placement of the stapler across the hilum for ligation and division of the left renal vessels. The artery is divided first, followed by ligation and division of the vein. The kidney is then delivered through the HandPort.

and vein. An endovascular stapler placed through the 12-mm port is used to divide the renal artery (Fig. 29-4). The stapler is reloaded and used to divide the renal vein. The kidney is delivered through the HandPort. A large clamp is placed across the ureteral bundle, and it is divided. The kidney is placed in slush, the staple lines of the artery and vein are removed, and the kidney is flushed with 1 L of refrigerated University of Wisconsin (UW) solution. The fat overlying the kidney is removed, and the vessels are dissected so that adequate length is available for revascularization. The donor kidney is now ready for reimplantation. Once the kidney has been removed, protamine is administered intravenously to reverse the effects of the heparin.

RIGHT NEPHRECTOMY

The surgeon stands facing the patient's front with the camera holder toward the patient's head. When possible, we use AESOP, the robotic arm, to hold the camera; however, because a right nephrectomy often requires the placement of a fourth port through which a self-retaining retractor is introduced to elevate the liver, positioning of the robotic arm may be difficult, as it may interfere with the self-retaining retractor. The right colon is mobilized from its lateral retroperitoneal attachments beginning at the hepatic flexure and working inferiorly toward the cecum. This mobilization includes freeing the colon from its attachments to the inferior aspect of the liver. Once again, care must be taken to avoid dissection within the colonic mesentery. Mobilization of the right colon exposes the duodenum. A Kocher maneuver is used to expose the infrahepatic IVC. A portion of the right triangular ligament and the retroperitoneal attachments of the liver are divided, which allows the liver to fall medially. This exposes the superior aspect of the right kidney. Although the liver falls medially, a

fourth port is usually required so that a retractor can be placed to elevate the liver superiorly and allow complete visualization of the right kidney. We place this 5-mm port along the midaxillary line. Either a fan or a triangle retractor is used to elevate the underside of the liver. A self-retaining arm is situated on the right side of the table and is used to hold the liver retractor in place.

The right gonadal vein is identified on the anterior surface of the IVC. Adequate length is mobilized and the vessel is divided. Inferior dissection of the ureteral bundle is performed, proceeding along the psoas muscle and ensuring that the ureter and its blood supply are not damaged. The termination point of the right renal vein is identified where it enters the vena cava. The renal vein is circumferentially dissected from adventitial tissue. On occasion, short lumbar vessels insert into the posterior aspect of the renal vein. Once adequate length is obtained, the right renal artery is identified. It is typically found in a retrocaval position, but, on occasion, it can be found on the anterior surface of the IVC. Once it has been identified, the right adrenal gland is dissected free from the superior pole of the kidney with great care taken so as not to damage the right adrenal vein.

Once the artery has been identified, a HandPort is introduced at the level of the anterior iliac crest. The assistant surgeon stands at the patient's back and places the right hand through the port. Once again, blunt dissection is used to mobilize Gerota's fascia from the retroperitoneum. Once the kidney is mobilized, the hilar dissection is completed, releasing the hilum of the kidney from its attachments to the IVC and retroperitoneum. The remainder of the procedure is completed as described earlier for the left nephrectomy.

POSTOPERATIVE CARE

The NG tube is removed before extubation in the operating room. However, the urinary catheter is left to document urine output. Good hydration is maintained, and patient-controlled analgesia is administered. We avoid the use nonsteroidal anti-inflammatory agents. A renal profile is obtained the following day. The urinary catheter is usually removed within 24 hours. Compression boots are continued to minimize the risk of deep vein thrombosis. The patients are often ready for discharge within 48 hours after surgery. As most of our donors are parents, many stay for 4 to 5 days after surgery to make visitations with the recipient more convenient. Limited activity for 1 to 2 weeks is advised. A postoperative visit is scheduled 2 weeks after discharge.

PEARLS

1. When performing a left nephrectomy, divide the gonadal vein several centimeters from its termination

point on the renal vein. The remnant gonadal vein can then be used as a handle to rotate the renal vein to look for lumbar veins that insert on its posterior aspect.

2. The renal artery often lies immediately behind the renal vein. Circumferential mobilization of the vein allows traction to be applied to the vein, exposing the artery. On occasion, placement of the HandPort may be necessary so that the artery can be localized by direct palpation.

3. Locate the renal artery before the kidney is mobilized from its retroperitoneal attachments. Once these attachments are divided, the kidney tends to fall forward, making the hilar dissection more difficult.

4. Avoid superior dissection along the vena cava on the right, as the right adrenal vein is short and can easily be torn.

5. In patients in whom dissection is difficult, early insertion of the HandPort may be helpful. However, if the patient has a small amount of abdominal domain, the hand reduces the intra-abdominal space, making dissection more difficult.

PITFALLS

1. For placement of the initial 12-mm cannula, use the cutdown technique rather than the Veress needle technique to prevent injury to underlying structures.

2. Mobilization of the ureter can be performed bluntly once the HandPort has been placed, but care should be taken not to strip the ureter of is blood supply.

3. The spleen should be mobilized completely when performing a left nephrectomy, as it can be torn if its retroperitoneal attachments are left in place.

RESULTS

Recent studies have documented the efficacy of laparoscopic-assisted donor nephrectomy in adult renal transplant patients. LDN has improved donor satisfaction and is thought to have increased the frequency of living donation. As a result, it has become the most common approach for procuring a living related kidney. Although LDN is widely accepted in the adult population, its role in the pediatric population requires further study. A recent analysis based on data obtained from the United Network Organ Sharing (UNOS) registry suggested that in the young recipient, LDN-procured organs were associated with delayed graft function and increased risk of rejection. The basis for delayed graft function was thought to be caused by a combination of the laparoscopy-associated alterations in renal hemodynamics and the lower perfusion

pressures that occur in young children because of their lower systemic blood pressures. The authors of this study cautioned about using LDN in recipients less than 3 years of age. These findings are controversial, as other groups have reported no impact of LDN on recipient renal function.

At Cincinnati Children's Medical Center, LDN has been attempted in 57 patients. Ten patients required conversion to open nephrectomy. Most of these cases occurred early in our experience. The indications to convert to open nephrectomy were bleeding in two patients and technical difficulty in eight patients. Donor survival has been 100%. There has been one major complication: a patient required splenectomy for bleeding. The mean length of hospitalization was 5.5 days, but much of this resulted from parental desires to stay with their hospitalized children. One-year recipient-patient and graft survival rate has been 98%. The one recipient mortality resulted from dysequilibrium syndrome. The average 30-day and 1-year creatinine levels were 0.8 and 1 mg/dL, respectively. LDN is now our technique of choice in the procurement of a living related kidney for transplantation.

SELECTED REFERENCES

1. Seikaly M, Ho PL, Emmett L, et al: The 12th annual report of the North American pediatric renal transplant cooperative study: Renal transplantation from 1987 through 1998. Pediatr Transplant 5:215-231, 2001

2. Kayler LK, Merion RM, Maraschio MA, et al: Outcomes of pediatric living donor renal transplant after laparoscopic versus open donor nephrectomy. Transplant Proc 34:3097-3098, 2002

3. Troppmann C, Pierce JL, Wiesmann KM, et al: Early and late recipient graft function and donor outcome after laparoscopic vs. open adult live donor nephrectomy for pediatric renal transplantation. Arch Surg 137:908-915, 2002

4. Hsu TH, Su LM, Trock BJ, et al: Laparoscopic adult donor nephrectomy for pediatric renal transplantation. Urology 61:320-322, 2003

5. Abrahams HM, Meng MV, Freise CE, et al: Laparoscopic donor nephrectomy for pediatric recipients: Outcomes analysis. Urology 63:163-166, 2004

6. Kim DY, Stegall MD, Prieto M, et al: Hand-assisted laparoscopic donor nephrectomy for pediatric kidney allograft recipients. Pediatr Transplant 8:460-463, 2004

7. McDonald SP, Craig JC: Long-term survival of children with end-stage renal disease. N Engl J Med 350:2654-2662, 2004

8. Singer JS, Ettenger RB, Gore JL, et al: Laparoscopic versus open renal procurement for pediatric recipients of living donor renal transplantation. Am J Transplant 5:2514-2520, 2005

9. Darido E, Alonso M, Ryckman F, et al: Laparoscopic donor nephrectomy for pediatric renal transplantation: A retrospective review. J Pediatr Surg (in press)

30
Laparoscopic Roux-en-Y Gastric Bypass

Thomas H. Inge

O ver the past 30 years, childhood obesity has become an unmistakable problem. Current estimates suggest that up to 3% of teenagers are actually morbidly obese (body mass index [BMI], >40 kg/m^2), a problem that was certainly not apparent before this decade. The health benefits and safety of bariatric surgery for adults are increasingly being documented. At the same time, nonoperative treatment regimens for adolescents are largely ineffective. Therefore, teenagers are now being considered for bariatric treatment. Numerous bariatric operations are currently available, but the procedure that has been used for weight loss in more than 90% of all adolescents and adults in the United States is the Roux-en-Y gastric bypass (RYGBP). RYGBP effectively allows adolescents to lose a third or more of bodyweight and reverses most of the comorbidities of obesity.

RYGBP is perhaps the most technically challenging laparoscopic operation to perform, even for experienced minimally invasive surgeons. Laparoscopic skills used in other procedures are not directly transferable to bariatric surgery, primarily because of the more limited visibility associated with excess intra-abdominal fat, and because the thick abdominal pannus affords a distinctly limited range of cannula and instrument move-

ment. Guidelines for training in bariatric surgery can be obtained from a number of professional societies including the American Society for Bariatric Surgery (www. asbs.org) and the Society of American Gastrointestinal and Endoscopic Surgeons (www.sages.org).

INDICATIONS FOR WORKUP AND OPERATION

Although the Bariatric Consensus Development Conference of the National Institutes of Health, which sanctioned adult weight loss surgery in 1991, did not include recommendations for morbidly obese individuals less than 18 years old, many pediatric specialists have now come to recognize the need to intervene surgically when an adolescent's health is compromised or threatened by marked obesity. For those adolescents with a BMI of greater than 40 kg/m^2 and severe obesity-related comorbidities such as type 2 diabetes, obstructive sleep apnea syndrome, or pseudotumor cerebri, laparoscopic RYGBP is a reasonable consideration. In addition, for those with BMI values of greater than 50 kg/m^2, even the presence of less severe comorbidities of obesity (e.g., dyslipidemia, hypertension, degenerative joint disease, asthma, venous stasis, intertriginous infections, gastroesophageal reflux, polycystic ovary syndrome, interference with activities of daily living, and social discrimination) should prompt consideration of a surgical option.

The studies obtained preoperatively vary widely. In essence, the evaluation is based largely on the review of systems and physical examination. In the broadest sense, individuals who have become morbidly obese can manifest this disease as dysfunction in any number of organ systems, and it is incumbent on the multidisciplinary weight-management team to thoroughly assess patients for obesity-related comorbidities both before and after any planned operation for weight loss.

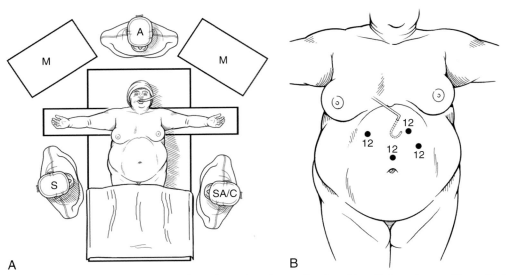

A

B

Figure 30-1. **A,** Personnel positioning for the operation. The patient is usually placed in a flat, supine position with the arms abducted and legs together. Care should be taken to secure the thighs and lower legs. The operation can usually be performed with a single surgeon (S) on the patient's right side and a surgical assistant/camera holder (SA/C) on the patient's left side. Two monitors (M) are used and are placed on either side of the anesthesiologist (A). **B,** Port placement for the operation. The initial cannula is 12 mm in size and is positioned 5 to 10 cm cephalad to the umbilicus. The three other port sites are also shown. The liver retractor is inserted below the xiphoid and is usually the last instrument to be inserted.

Patients are limited to clear liquids on the day before RYGBP. There is no need for a bowel preparation. Preoperative medications include low-molecular-weight heparin for deep venous thrombosis (DVT) prophylaxis (40 mg subcutaneously and continued twice a day postoperatively while in the hospital) and a second-generation cephalosporin. Additional DVT prophylaxis includes sequential compression boots, which must be used intraoperatively and postoperatively.

OPERATIVE TECHNIQUE

The patient is usually placed in a flat, supine position with arms abducted, legs together. Care should be taken to secure the thighs and lower legs. The procedure can usually be performed with a single surgeon (patient's right side) and an assistant (patient's left side) (Fig. 30-1A). Two monitors are used and are placed near the patient's shoulders. A urinary catheter and orogastric tube are inserted before the operation. The anesthesiologist is encouraged not to titrate fluid administration to urine output, but rather to replace overnight nothing-by-mouth deficits and then provide only maintenance fluids plus replacement of ongoing insensible losses.

Standard 32-cm-length adult instrumentation is commonly used for laparoscopic RYGBP. Abdominal access can be achieved safely using a bladeless, direct-viewing, 12-mm cannula with the laparoscope positioned in center of the cannula (Optiview, Ethicon Endosurgery, Cincinnati, OH). The skin incision for the first port is transverse and is positioned 5 to 10 cm cephalad to the

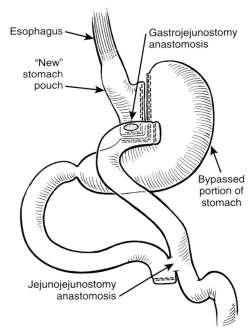

Figure 30-2. The final reconstructed anatomy for a laparoscopic gastric bypass.

umbilicus. The three other 12-mm ports sites are shown in Figure 30-1B.

Many surgeons begin the procedure by first creating the gastric pouch. Others create the Roux-en-Y anastomosis first, so that, in the event that dense small bowel adhesions (e.g., from prior surgery) are encountered, the more challenging portion of the procedure is completed first. Figure 30-2 shows the final reconstructed anatomy. To create the Roux-en-Y anastomosis, the duodenojejunal flexure is identified. The assistant secures a portion of adjacent transverse mesocolon to hold and expose the small bowel. If a retrocolic Roux limb is planned, the jejunum is divided 25 cm beyond the duodenojejunal flexure (Fig. 30-3) using two firings of the 45-mm endoGIA (Ethicon Endosurgery, Cincinnati, OH) with white load. The biliopancreatic limb or afferent limb transmits biliopancreatic secretions to the Roux limb. Some surgeons use a longer (50- to 75-cm) biliopancreatic limb of jejunum, especially if the antecolic technique has been chosen. Bipolar electrocautery is often needed for hemostasis in the mesentery.

A 75- to 150-cm Roux limb is used for most patients. The Roux is created by measuring 75 to 150 cm beyond the previously described jejunal transection and then creating a side-to-side jejunojejunostomy between the biliopancreatic jejunal limb and the Roux limb, using the 45-mm endoGIA with white load (Fig. 30-4). The resulting enterotomy defect is closed either by a running suture (Fig. 30-5) or with another firing of the stapler. The mesenteric defect is carefully closed with a running 2-0 silk suture to avoid an internal hernia.

If the Roux limb is to be retrocolic in location, the mesocolon is opened just anterior and left of the duodenojejunal junction. Once the Roux limb is deposited through the defect and directed into the lesser sac, the

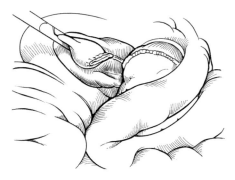 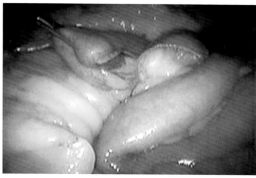

Figure 30-3. The jejunum is divided 20 cm beyond the duodenojejunal flexure.

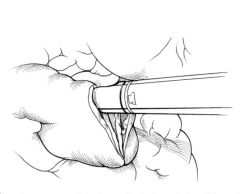 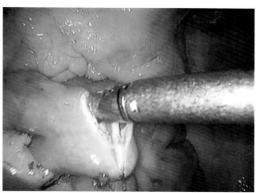

Figure 30-4. After the appropriate Roux limb length is achieved, a side-to-side jejunojejunostomy is created using an endoscopic stapler.

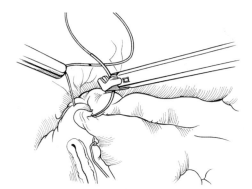 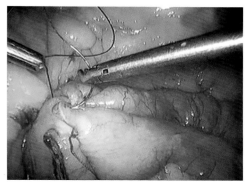

Figure 30-5. After the stapled jejunojejunostomy anastomosis has been created, the remaining enterotomy is closed using the hand-sewn technique.

mesocolic defect is closed around the Roux limb using silk sutures. Additionally, Petersen's defect between the small bowel mesentery and the mesocolon is closed to prevent the well-described postoperative internal hernia in this location.

The liver retractor is next inserted below the xiphoid and used to elevate the left lateral hepatic segment, exposing the gastroesophageal junction, as in a fundoplication. A vertical, tubular gastric pouch based on the lesser curve is then created using a 34 French orogastric tube as a guide. The pouch creation begins with perigastric dissection along the lesser curve approximately 8 to 10 cm inferior to the gastroesophageal junction (usually just below the second lesser curve vessel) using the ultrasonic dissector. This dissection is continued posteriorly in close proximity to the gastric wall until the plane reaches the lesser sac behind the stomach.

The pouch is crafted using the endoGIA 35-mm stapler with blue loads. The first transverse cut across the lesser curvature is achieved by bringing the stapler into the right upper quadrant port while subsequent firings are achieved with the stapler introduced through the left upper quadrant port. Once the angle of His is reached, the pouch has been completed (Fig. 30-6).

The numerous techniques for performing the gastrojejunostomy include a hand-sewn technique, the end-to-end stapled technique with the anvil inserted into the pouch laparoscopically, the end-to-end stapled technique with the anvil inserted orally, and the linearly stapled technique. We have found the hand-sewn approach to be preferable. The remainder of this chapter focuses on details and pearls for performance of the hand-sewn gastrojejunostomy.

If the Roux limb was placed in a retrocolic location, the stapled end is located in the lesser sac and directed anterior to the antrum for the gastrojejunal anastomosis. The two-layer anastomosis between the pouch and the side of the jejunum is begun by first running a posterior seromuscular 3-0 Vicryl (Ethicon, Inc., Somerville, NJ) suture to bring the antimesenteric border of the Roux to the edge of the small gastric pouch (Fig. 30-7). A gastrotomy and enterotomy (1 to 1.5 cm) are next created in the pouch and the jejunum, respectively, using the ultrasonic scalpel. Running full-thickness suture lines are used to close the anastomosis over a 40 Fr calibration dilator (Fig. 30-8). The final anterior seromuscular suture line is then made (Fig. 30-9). The integrity and patency of the anastomosis is

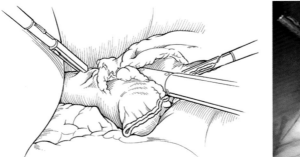
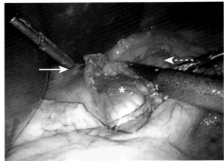

Figure 30-6. A 30-mL gastric pouch (*asterisk*) is created along the lesser curve of the stomach just beyond the gastroesophageal junction using a linear cutting stapler. The esophagogastric junction is labeled (*solid arrow*) to show that the distal-most portion of the pouch is typically located within several centimeters of the gastroesophageal junction. The first transverse application of the stapler that creates the distal-most portion of the vertically oriented, tubular gastric pouch is shown. Also shown is the remnant stomach (*dotted arrow*), which will be left in situ beside the gastric pouch. The Roux limb will be brought anterior to this remnant stomach, hence the term *antegastric*.

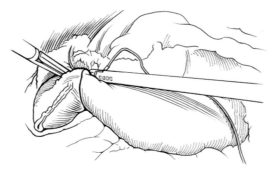
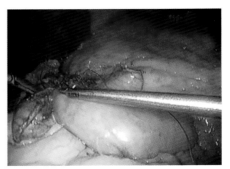

Figure 30-7. The gastrojejunostomy is performed by first running the posterior "outer" layer using 3-0 absorbable braided suture to approximate the antimesenteric border of the end of the Roux limb to the distal-most staple line of the vertically oriented, tubular gastric pouch.

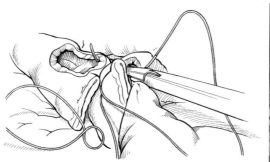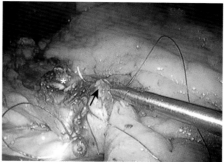

Figure 30-8.   The inner posterior running layer of the gastrojejunostomy is performed next. This full-thickness suture line unites small bowel and gastric pouch tissue, resulting in a mucosa-to-mucosa approximation. The lumen of the gastric pouch is marked by an *asterisk* and the jejunal wall by an *arrow*.

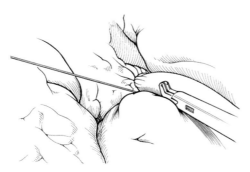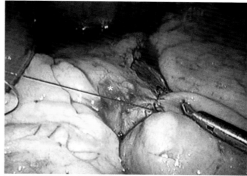

Figure 30-9.   The two-layer hand-sewn gastrojejunal anastomosis has been completed. The gastric pouch is marked with an *asterisk*. A leak test is then performed under saline, using air insufflated into an orogastric tube (not shown).

assessed laparoscopically with intraluminal air insufflation under saline.

A closed suction drain to prevent fluid from collecting within the abdomen and for early identification of an anastomotic leak is left near the anastomosis. It is exteriorized through the patient's upper left cannula site. A temporary gastrostomy can be created in the remnant stomach if the surgeon is concerned about the possibility of postoperative anastomotic complications or the development of the afferent limb syndrome (obstruction or ileus of the biliopancreatic limb). Cannula sites in these patients do not require fascial closure.

POSTOPERATIVE CARE

Patients are typically extubated in the operating room. They usually recuperate in a nonintensive care setting, with 24-hour oxygen saturation and electrocardiographic monitoring. Maintenance fluids are administered at a rate of 75 mL/hr. A nasogastric tube is not used. Patient-controlled analgesia with intravenous narcotics is employed for the first 24 to 48 hours. Early signs of complications include fever, tachycardia, tachypnea, increasing oxygen requirement, oliguria, hiccoughs, regurgitation, left shoulder pain, worsening abdominal pain, a feeling of anxiety, or an acute alteration in mental status. Vigilance is required, as these signs may signal a gastrointestinal leak, a pulmonary embolus, a bowel obstruction, or an acute dilation and impending rupture of the bypassed gastric remnant, and they warrant aggressive attention and appropriate investigation.

A water-soluble upper gastrointestinal contrast study is routinely obtained on the first postoperative day. After satisfactory passage of contrast is documented without evidence of an anastomotic leak, patients are begun on clear liquids and subsequently advanced to a high-protein liquid diet for the first month after operation. Patients are discharged most commonly by the postoperative day 2 or 3. In the event of a leak or obstruction early (days) after operation, laparoscopic intervention is usually performed. Although discussion of these issues is beyond the scope of this text, an excellent resource is cited in the bibliography.

PEARLS

1. It is advantageous for the operating team to stand on a platform 20 to 40 cm above the floor because of

the height of the abdominal surface resulting from the exaggerated sagittal abdominal diameter of a morbidly obese patient.

2. Typical intravenous fluid requirements during a procedure are in the range of 2 to 3 L. When greater quantities are administered without clear justification, postoperative recovery can be more prolonged and complicated.

3. The positioning of the port for the laparoscope is critical. It should be sited in the midline, above the umbilicus. The incision should be made by measuring from the nipples down to the point on the abdominal wall corresponding to the length of the laparoscope being used. When this reference is used, being able to see the uppermost areas of dissection well is ensured.

4. The transverse colon and small bowel are best exposed by first lifting the omentum and tucking it beneath the liver edge.

PITFALLS

1. The antegastric position of the Roux limb is preferable to a retrogastric position because, if complications occur (e.g., anastomotic hemorrhage, pouch dilation, gastrogastric fistula, recalcitrant anastomotic stricture) and the pouch or anastomosis requires revisional surgery, it is much more easily found and exposed when the Roux is antegastric.

2. When performing a retrocolic Roux limb placement, significant bleeding from the mesocolon can be avoided if a loose, avascular area is identified above and to the left of the duodenojejunal flexure for entry into the lesser sac. Regardless of the degree of obesity, a thin, safe area of mesocolon is present in most of these patients and should be sought.

3. Bipolar electrocautery should be readily available to control mesenteric and other bleeding in these cases while avoiding the degree of collateral damage often seen with monopolar cautery.

4. If intraoperative complications occur that portend a potentially complicated postoperative recovery, it is preferable to place a gastrostomy tube in the excluded stomach at the time of the bypass procedure. This will provide a route to vent the afferent limb (biliopancreatic system) as well as to feed and hydrate the patient postoperatively if there is a leak or stricture at the gastrojejunostomy.

5. Patients should be moved from the operating table to the bed before extubation to reduce the risk of falling from the table during emergence from anesthesia.

6. Postoperatively, the risk of DVT can be minimized with early ambulation, prophylactic use of subcutaneous heparin (low molecular weight), and sequential compression devices. Not uncommonly, the sequential compression devices are either not on the nonambulatory patient or, if they are on, they are not plugged in and working.

RESULTS

Seventy adolescent patients (BMI range, 43 to 96 kg/m^2; mean, 58 kg/m^2) have undergone laparoscopic gastric bypass in Cincinnati. After this procedure, weight loss occurs at a rate of approximately 2.5 kg/wk over the first 6 months, after which time the rate decreases. On average, weight loss after gastric bypass is approximately 25% at 6 months, and 35% at 1 year. Significantly greater fat than lean mass loss occurs, with percent fat in these patients falling from a mean of 47% preoperatively to 36% at 1 year.

Significant improvements are seen in sleep apnea and metabolic parameters in adolescents after gastric bypass. Approximately half of adolescents referred for bariatric surgery have obstructive sleep apnea (OSA) syndrome. Sleep apnea resolves completely in more than 90% of patients, with severity indices decreasing from 9.1 obstructive events per hour to 0.65 per hour. Thus, although sleep apnea is highly prevalent in adolescents with extreme obesity meeting eligibility criteria for bariatric surgery, a marked reduction in OSA severity is achieved after gastric bypass.

From the metabolic standpoint, a significant (33%) decrease in triglyceride levels has been seen after surgical weight loss in adolescents (137 to 98 mg/dL, $P < .02$). Perhaps more important are the endocrine changes that have been recognized. Mean preoperative fasting glucose significantly decreases after operation as well (95 to 86 mg/dL, $P < .02$). Preoperative fasting insulin levels are almost always abnormally elevated, and dramatic postoperative improvements are common (30 to 9 μU/mL, $P < .0002$). These findings strongly suggest that sleep apnea, cardiovascular risk factors, and insulin resistance all reverse in adolescents after bariatric surgery.

SELECTED REFERENCES

1. Strauss RS, Bradley LJ, Brolin RE: Gastric bypass surgery in adolescents with morbid obesity. J Pediatr 138:499-504, 2001

2. Buchwald H, Avidor Y, Braunwald E, et al: Bariatric surgery: A systematic review and meta-analysis. JAMA 292:1724-1737, 2004

3. Inge T, Krebs N, Garcia V, et al: Bariatric surgery for severely overweight adolescents: Concerns and recommendations. Pediatrics 114:217-223, 2004

4. Inge TH, Donnelly LF, Vierra M, et al: Managing bariatric patients in a children's hospital: Radiologic considerations and limitations. J Pediatr Surg 40:609-617, 2005

5. Inge TH, Zeller M, Lawson L, et al: Critical appraisal of the evidence supporting bariatric surgery for weight management in adolescence. J Pediatr 147:10-19, 2005

6. Kalra M, Inge T, Garcia V, et al: Obstructive sleep apnea in morbidly obese adolescents: Effect of bariatric surgical intervention. Obes Res 13:1175-1179, 2005

7. Lawson L, Harmon C, Chen M, et al: One year outcomes of roux en Y gastric bypass in adolescents: A multicenter report from the Pediatric Bariatric Study Group. J Pediatr Surg 41:137-143, 2006

31

Laparoscopic Adjustable Gastric Band Placement

Allen F. Browne and Mark J. Holterman

Approximately 15% of adolescents in the United States are morbidly obese. Thus, their body mass index (BMI) is above the 95th percentile for age and they are suffering from, or are at risk for, a number of significant comorbidities. In 1991, the National Institutes of Health recommended that morbidly obese patients consider bariatric surgery to improve their health. Nonsurgical means of weight loss therapy such as behavioral therapy, nutritional education, and physical activity programs result in 30% of the patients losing about 20% of their excess weight. In contrast, bariatric surgery combined with the other modalities results in 60% to 80% of the patients losing 50% to 60% of their excess weight, with resolution or improvement of their comorbidities. With the surgical approach, caloric restriction in bariatric surgery is achieved by inducing malabsorption or restricting food intake, or both. In the United States, the two most commonly performed operations for morbid obesity are the adjustable gastric band (or AGB, a restrictive operation) and the Roux-en-Y gastric bypass (a restrictive and malabsorptive operation). Although the long-term results and durability of these two procedures are similar, we prefer the AGB because it is adjustable, it is removable, it causes no malabsorption, and it is 10 to 100 times safer (mortality rate, 0.05% to 0.01%). Finally, it has one half to one third of the morbidity rate (5% to 10%).

INDICATIONS FOR WORKUP AND OPERATION

We currently restrict the use of the AGB operation to those adolescents who have a BMI of greater than 40, or greater than 35 with at least one significant comorbidity. In addition, they should have been obese for over 5 years and have documented weight loss attempts with diet, behavioral therapy, and activity.

Our patients meet with a nutritionist to establish an understanding of the dietary expectations after they have the AGB placed. Moreover, an exercise trainer or physical therapist works with the patients to custom design an activity program. It is essential that the patients be evaluated by a psychologist or psychiatrist, and that a strong psychological support system be available to assist before and after surgery. The involvement of the parents is extremely important in this regard.

Patients are carefully screened for obesity-related comorbidities—especially sleep apnea. Preferably, this preoperative evaluation is accomplished by a multidisciplinary adolescent weight-management program that includes a pediatric surgeon trained in the placement of the AGB, a pediatrician, a pediatric psychologist or psychiatrist, a pediatric AGB dietitian, and a pediatric trainer or physical therapist. Before surgery, all of our patients are placed on a low-calorie, high-protein diet for 2 weeks to lose 10 to 15 pounds. This reduces the size and fragility of the liver and reduces the risk of retraction injury during surgery.

OPERATIVE TECHNIQUE

Obese adolescents frequently have sleep apnea caused by the adipose tissue in their neck and oropharynx. This can result in significant perioperative airway problems. Anesthesiologists with experience in adult bariatric surgical patients provide excellent perioperative care for these adult-sized adolescents. The position of the patient is changed during the operation, and an orogastric tube is passed and removed during the operation. The patient receives 5000 U of heparin subcutaneously and 2 gm cefazolin intravenously before the operation.

The operating table must be able to support up to 700 pounds and to be raised, lowered, and placed into steep reverse Trendelenburg position. The patient is positioned supine, both arms are out on arm boards, and the legs are in stirrups. The patient has sequential compression devices on either the calves or the feet. The patient is placed on a pneumatic "sand-bag" device. A pocket is made for the patient's torso by positioning the sand bag up into the perineum and around the sides before the air is evacuated. The patient's pelvis is further secured to the table with strong 3-inch tape wrapped around the table and the patient's inguinal crease. All these steps are very important to keep the patient from moving when the steep Trendelenburg position is used.

There should be either one video screen over the patient's head or one on either side of the head of the table. An adjustable locking-arm system is fastened to the right side of the bed to hold the liver retractor. To place the ports, the surgeon starts on the patient's left side and then moves between the patient's legs for the procedure. The assistant starts on the patient's right side

for port placement and then moves to the left side for the procedure (Fig. 31-1).

Access to the peritoneal cavity is obtained with a 5-mm Endopath dilating cannula (Ethicon Endosurgery, Cincinnati, OH) and a 5-mm, 0-degree telescope under direct vision. This initial port (#1) is positioned to the left of the midline and halfway between the xiphoid process and the umbilicus (Fig. 31-2). The abdomen is insufflated to 20 mm Hg through this initial port, and the telescope is changed to a 5-mm, 30-degree telescope.

The second port (#2) is placed subcostally on the left in the midclavicular line. The incision is 5 to 6 cm in length to accommodate the reservoir pocket later in the procedure. A 15-mm dilating port is placed under direct vision at the medial end of this skin incision and angled cephalad toward the gastroesophageal junction.

The third port (#3) is a 5-mm dilating port placed under direct vision through the left lateral abdominal wall subcostally at the anterior axillary line and angled toward the gastroesophageal junction. At this point, the telescope is switched to port #3.

The fourth port is for the liver retractor (a 5-mm Nathanson retractor, Mediflex Surgical Products, Islandia, NY) and is inserted under direct vision through a 5-mm subxiphoid incision that is just to the left of the midline. The liver retractor is positioned underneath the left lobe of the liver, so that the diaphragm above the gastroesophageal hiatus is visible. It is held in place by the adjustable arm system attached to the right side of the table.

The fifth port (#5) is a 12-mm dilating port placed through the mid right upper quadrant at the level of port #2 and angled toward the gastroesophageal junc-

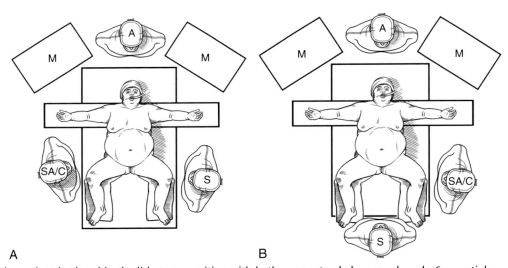

A   B

Figure 31-1. The patient is placed in the lithotomy position with both arms extended on arm boards. Sequential compression devices are placed on the calves or feet. Either one video monitor (M) is placed above the patient's head, or two are used, one on either side of the anesthesiologist (A) at the head of the table. The surgeon (S) stands on the patient's left side for port placement (**A**) and then moves between the patient's legs for the procedure (**B**). The surgical assistant/camera holder (SA/C) starts on the patient's right side for port placement and then moves to the left side for the procedure.

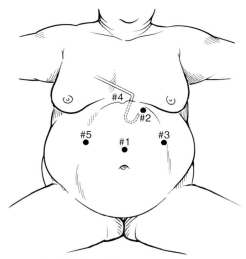

Figure 31-2. The initial working port (#1) is situated just to the left of the midline and half-way between the xiphoid process and the umbilicus. Port #2 is a 15-mm port placed in the midclavicular line in the left subcostal region. This will be the site for the reservoir pocket at the end of the operation. The third accessory port (#3) is a 5-mm port introduced through the left lateral abdominal wall in the anterior axillary line. The fourth port (#4) is for a 5-mm Nathanson liver retractor, which is inserted through a 5-mm subxiphoid incision just to the left of the midline. This liver retractor is held in place by an external liver-retractor holder attached to the right side of the table. Port #5 is a 12-mm port situated in the right subcostal region in the right mid-epigastrium and about the same level as port #2.

tion. Because of the thickness of the anterior abdominal wall, all cannulas are 15 mm in length.

Once all the cannulas are inserted, the telescope is moved back to port #1, the surgeon moves between the patient's legs, and the assistant moves to the patient's left side. All instruments need to be 45 cm in length. A 4 × 4 sponge is introduced into the abdomen through the 15-mm left subcostal port (#2). The assistant manipulates the telescope through port #1 with the left hand.

To start the operation, the assistant grasps the 4 × 4 sponge with a grasper in the right hand, and retracts the greater curvature of the stomach inferiorly with the sponge, exposing the angle of His and the greater curvature of the stomach over to the gastrosplenic ligament. The surgeon uses a grasper in the left hand through port #5 and a Maryland dissector in the right hand through port #3. The surgeon divides the peritoneum between the greater curvature of the stomach and the diaphragm over to the gastrosplenic ligament using blunt dissection.

The epiphrenic fat pad is then evaluated. If it descends to the level of the anterior wall of the stomach and obscures the serosal surface of the cardia of the stomach, it will need to be elevated, or excised with the Harmonic Scalpel (Ethicon Endosurgery, Cincinnati, OH). This is important because the anterior plication of the stomach around the band must be done with secure sutures from gastric wall to gastric wall. Care must be taken to avoid injury to the anterior vagus nerve.

The avascular portion of the gastrohepatic ligament overlying the caudate lobe of the liver (pars flaccida) is opened with blunt dissection, and any bleeding is controlled with the electrocautery via the Maryland dissector. If there is a significant fat pad along the lesser curvature, it should be excised to limit the amount of fat that will be encircled by the AGB. This step is often necessary in the patients with a BMI of greater than 60. Care must be taken to recognize and preserve an aberrant left hepatic artery if it is present. The greater curvature is retracted laterally by the assistant to expose the inferior extent of the right diaphragmatic crus. The surgeon uses a Maryland dissector in the right hand (through port #2) to open the peritoneum anterior to the inferior extent of the right diaphragmatic crus. The Maryland dissector is then used to retract the stomach laterally. Through port #5, the surgeon's left hand gently advances a blunt grasper (or the band passer) to a point behind the greater curvature of the stomach and medial to the spleen. Care is taken to stay anterior to the left diaphragmatic crus and posterior to the stomach. It is a short distance, only 2 to 3 cm, and no resistance should be encountered. The stomach is then reflected medially to expose the tip of the blunt grasper. The tunnel behind the stomach should be just large enough to accept the grasper to ensure good posterior fixation of the AGB in the areolar tissue.

Once the grasper is visible in a position cephalad and lateral to the medially reflected greater curvature, the AGB is inserted into the abdomen through port #2 and the tubing is handed to the grasper (Fig. 31-3). The tubing and AGB are pulled behind the stomach with the grasper, and the tubing is pulled out through port #5 to allow manual traction on the band as it dilates the narrow retrogastric tunnel (Fig. 31-4A). Once the thick band portion emerges from behind the stomach, the tubing is reintroduced through port #5 and threaded through the hole in the AGB buckle (see Fig. 31-4B). The buckle is then locked in place. The band should be loose around the stomach, with the buckle located on the anteromedial aspect of the stomach.

The plication of the anterior wall of the stomach over the AGB is done with three to four sutures of permanent 2-0 suture material (Fig. 31-5). The sutures are placed starting very laterally at the greater curvature and working medially. They should be deep and full thickness. The plication should be loose and should not be over the

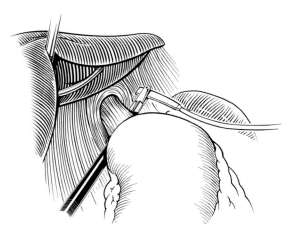

Figure 31-3. Through port #5, the surgeon's left hand gently advances a blunt grasper or the band passer behind the greater curvature of the stomach and medial to the spleen to grasp the tubing of the adjustable gastric band.

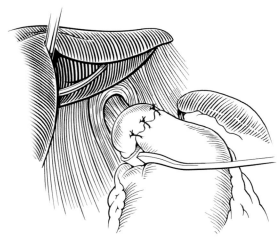

Figure 31-5. Plication of the anterior wall of the stomach over the gastric band is accomplished with three or four sutures of 2-0 permanent suture material. These sutures should be deep and full thickness. It is important to remove the orogastric tube before placement of these sutures, so that the tube is not incorporated in these plication sutures.

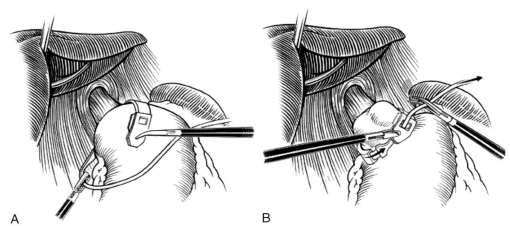

A   B

Figure 31-4. **A,** The tubing and the adjustable gastric band are pulled behind the stomach with the grasper. The tubing is pulled out through port #5 to allow manual traction on the gastric band as it dilates the narrow retrogastric tunnel. Once the thick portion of the gastric band emerges from behind the stomach, the tubing is reintroduced into the abdomen through port #5 and threaded through the hole in the buckle of the gastric band. **B,** The buckle is locked in place.

buckle of the AGB. The orogastric tube should be removed before placement of these sutures.

The tubing is then brought out port #2 along with the 4 × 4 sponge. The tubing is attached to the reservoir. A pocket on top of the muscle fascia and inferior to the incision is formed with blunt dissection. The fascial opening is not sutured. The reservoir is sutured into the pocket with four nonabsorbable sutures from the fascia to the holes in the port. The excess tubing is returned to the abdominal cavity. The site for port #2 is closed in layers over the reservoir, and the other incisions are closed with subcuticular sutures. The area around each incision is infiltrated with local anesthetic at the end of the procedure. No fluid is left in the AGB at this time.

POSTOPERATIVE CARE

After extubation, the patient is sent to the recovery room and soon after surgery is started on sips of liquids and encouraged to ambulate. Patients with sleep apnea or other serious comorbidities are observed for 23 hours in a monitored bed. Inpatient pain management consists of scheduled intravenous nonsteroidal anti-inflammatory medication, and supplemental intravenous narcotics as needed. All patients undergo a fluoroscopic swallowing evaluation with barium before discharge from the hospital. Patients are discharged on ibuprofen, acetaminophen, or Naprosyn, as well as acetaminophen with codeine. For the first week, they remain on a liquid diet and then return for a postoperative

Table 31-1   Laparoscopic Adjustable Gastric Band Placement at the University of Illinois at Chicago: FDA Study 2005-2006

Patient	Sex	Age (yr)	Race	Baseline Weight (kg)	Baseline EW (kg)	Baseline BMI (kg/m²)	Current Weight (kg)	Current BMI (kg/m²)	Current % EW Lost	Follow-up Time (mo)
1	F	17	C	114.8	57.27	40.8	89.8	32	43.65	12
2	F	17	AA	113.2	51.64	38	90.7	30.4	43.66	6
3	F	16	H	178	118.00	61	161	55	15.25	6
4	F	15	AA	227	165.91	81	208	72	11.34	6
5	F	15	C	133.9	42.73	41	97	30	85.10	6
6	F	17	C	118	62.00	43.7	116	42	3.23	3
7	F	17	C	130	76.45	49	113	43	23.00	1.5
8	F	17	C	129	75.00	49	114	43	20.00	1.5
9	F	17	C	117	65.00	44	110	43	11.00	0.25
10	F	16	C	146	91.82	54	—	—	—	—

AA, African-American; BMI, body mass index; C, Caucasian; EW, excess weight; FDA, U.S. Food and Drug Administration; H, Hispanic.

evaluation. Then the diet is advanced to a soft, blenderized diet for 4 to 5 weeks before they return for the first adjustment of the gastric band.

PEARLS AND PITFALLS

1. Access to the peritoneal cavity under direct vision with the Endopath dilating system is safer than the Veress needle technique and avoids the larger incision required for the open (Hasson) technique.
2. The very thick abdominal wall places a premium on passing the cannulas at the correct angle toward the gastroesophageal junction. This reduces surgeon and instrument strain caused by the torque applied by the heavy abdominal wall.
3. Evaluate and act on the epiphrenic fat and lesser curvature fat before going behind the stomach. It is much harder to work on these fat pads once the AGB has been passed.
4. Go gently behind the stomach. The maneuver is somewhat blind, and posterior perforations of the stomach are difficult to recognize and repair.
5. The tunnel behind the stomach must be narrow to prevent posterior prolapse. Usually, a 5-mm blunt tipped grasper works well. If there is a problem or question, the 10-mm band passer should be used.
6. Remove the orogastric tube before plication. The plication sutures should be deep and can catch the tube if it is in the stomach.
7. To reduce the incidence of band erosion, the plication should be loose and not over the buckle.

8. Place the reservoir away from the fascial opening of port #2. This avoids an acute angle and possible tube obstruction.
9. Fix the reservoir securely to the fascia to prevent migration and flipping.

RESULTS

Results of laparoscopic adjustable gastric band placement at the University of Illinois at Chicago, compiled in the U.S. Food and Drug Administration study of 2005-2006, can be seen in Table 31-1.

ACKNOWLEDGEMENT

We thank Dr Santiago Horgan for sharing his expertise and mentoring us, and also for allowing us to modify his illustrations of the surgical technique.

SELECTED REFERENCES

1. Epstein LH, Myers MD, Raynor, HA, et al: Treatment of pediatric obesity. Pediatrics 10:554-570, 1978
2. Dixon JB, O'Brien P: Changes in comorbidities and improvements in quality of life after LAP-BAND placement. Am J Surg 184:51S-54, 2002
3. Fielding GA, Allen JW: A step-by-step guide to placement of the LAP-BAND adjustable gastric banding system. Am J Surg 184:26S-30, 2002

4. Ogden CL, Flegal KM, Carroll MD, et al: Prevalence and trends in overweight among U.S. children and adolescents, 1999-2000. JAMA 288:1728-1732, 2002

5. Abu-Abeid S, Gavert N, Klausner JM, et al: Bariatric surgery in adolescence. J Pediatr Surg 38:1379-1382, 2003

6. Chapman AE, Kiroff G, Game P, et al: Laparoscopic adjustable gastric banding in the treatment of obesity: A systematic literature review. Surgery 135:326-335, 2004

7. Dolan K, Fielding G: A comparison of laparoscopic adjustable gastric banding in adolescents and adults. Surg Endosc 18:45-47, 2004

8. Gortmaker SL, Must A, Perrin JM, et al: Social and economic consequences of overweight in adolescence and young adulthood. N Engl J Med 329:1008-1012, 2004

9. Holloway JA, Forney FA, Gould DE: The Lap-Band is an effective tool for weight loss even in the United States. Am J Surg 188:659-662, 2004

10. Garcia VF: Should adolescents have weight-loss surgery? Contemp Surg 61:378-381, 2005

11. Horgan S, Holterman MJ, Jacobsen GR, et al: Laparoscopic adjustable gastric banding for the treatment of adolescent morbid obesity in the United States: A safe alternative to gastric bypass. J Pediatr Surg 40:86-91, 2005

12. Ponce J, Dixon JB: Laparoscopic adjustable gastric banding. Surg Obes Relat Dis 1:310-316, 2005

13. Ponce J, Paynter S, Fromm R: Laparoscopic adjustable gastric banding: 1,014 consecutive cases. J Am Coll Surg 201:529-535, 2005

14. Spivak H, Hewitt MF, Onn A, Half EE: Weight loss and improvement of obesity-related illness in 500 U.S. patients following laparoscopic adjustable gastric banding procedure. Am J Surg 189:27-32, 2005

32
Laparoscopic Repair of Inguinal Hernias

Felix Schier

The role of laparoscopic repair of inguinal hernias is not fully established. The approach is criticized for transforming a routine extraperitoneal procedure into a transperitoneal, technologically more complex operation that has been shown to result in a higher recurrence rate. In contrast, the advocates of the laparoscopic approach stress the reduced invasiveness, the absent manipulation of the chordal structures, the more correct diagnosis regarding associated direct and femoral hernias. Moreover, the contralateral internal ring can be visualized and repaired if patent. Finally, supporters cite the improved cosmesis.

This chapter describes a technique for closure of the internal inguinal ring with a nonabsorbable intraperitoneal suture without mesh and without incising the peritoneum. There are several variations to this technique. In general, the alternative techniques try to avoid intracorporeal suturing and knotting by introducing a thread through the abdominal wall, turning the thread around the internal inguinal ring, pulling it out, and knotting it outside the abdominal cavity. The results with these alternative techniques seem to be at least as good as with the approach described here.

INDICATIONS FOR WORKUP, AND PREOPERATIVE PREPARATION

The indications for laparoscopic inguinal hernia repair are the same as for the inguinal approach.

Older children are requested to empty their bladder preoperatively. A urinary catheter is not inserted. A full bladder does not hinder a laparoscopic hernia repair. However, in girls, a full bladder may obstruct the view of the internal genitalia. In these rare cases, a needle can be introduced through the abdominal wall and into the bladder for decompression. Until the repair is finished, the bladder should be mostly empty. The ovaries are inspected and the needle is withdrawn. No enema is ever given preoperatively.

OPERATIVE TECHNIQUE

The patient is placed in the supine position on the operating room table, and general endotracheal anesthesia is administered. A pad is not placed under the pelvis, as this maneuver would advance the great vessels unnecessarily close to the tip of the sharp trocars as they are introduced. The abdomen and scrotum are then prepared and draped. The surgeon stands on the side of the table opposite the side of the hernia being repaired (Fig. 32-1A). An intraumbilical 3-mm incision is made, and a Veress needle is gently introduced. Diagnostic laparoscopy is then performed.

The Veress needle is then replaced by a 3- or 5-mm laparoscope. Although 0-degree telescopes are adequate, 30-degree scopes provide better exposure of the internal inguinal ring. Two additional 2-mm cannulas are inserted at the level of the umbilicus, lateral to the rectus muscles (see Fig. 32-1B).

The internal inguinal rings are readily seen. A 4-0 nonabsorbable monofilamentous suture is shortened to

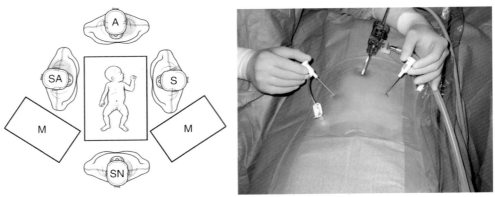

Figure 32-1.   For a laparoscopic hernia repair, the surgeon stands opposite the side on which the repair is being performed. **A,** A laparoscopic right inguinal hernia repair is being performed and the surgeon is to the patient's left. The surgical assistant/camera holder (SA) stands opposite the surgeon. The monitors are placed on either side of the foot end of the operating table with the scrub nurse (SN) between them at the end of the operating table. A, anesthesiologist. **B,** A 5-mm laparoscope is usually introduced through the umbilicus, although a 3-mm telescope can be used in some instances. Two additional 2-mm cannulas have been inserted just below the level of the umbilicus, lateral to the rectus muscles.

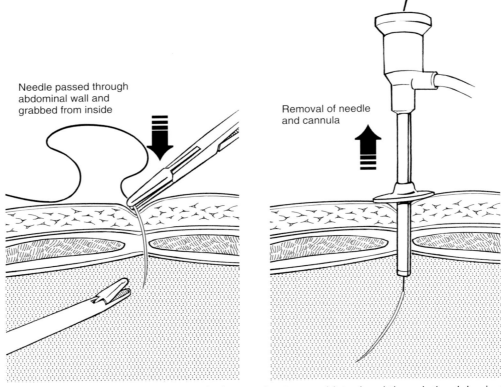

Needle passed through
abdominal wall and
grabbed from inside

Removal of needle
and cannula

Figure 32-2.   A 4-0 nonabsorbable monofilament suture is shortened to 7 cm and introduced through the abdominal wall near the internal inguinal ring using a traditional needle holder. This needle is secured in the abdominal cavity by a 2- or 3-mm laparoscopic needle driver. After suture ligation of the patent processus vaginalis, the needle is withdrawn through one of the 2-mm cannulas.

7 cm (3 in.) and inserted through the abdominal wall next to the internal inguinal ring using a traditional needle driver (Fig. 32-2). This needle is secured in the abdominal cavity by a 2- or 3-mm laparoscopic needle driver. A second laparoscopic needle driver is introduced through the other port and is used to align the needle. The internal inguinal ring is closed with several stitches placed in an N shape (Fig. 32-3).

On the anterior aspect of the internal inguinal ring, slightly more tissue is included, not only the peritoneum but also some underlying musculature. On the lower part, however, less tissue is included because of the close proximity of the nerves, testicular vessels, and vas deferens. It seems important to place the most medial stitches as close as possible to the epigastric vessels and the vas deferens (Fig. 32-4).

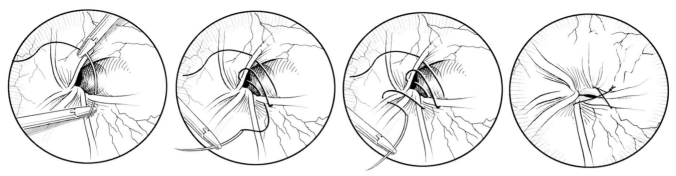

Figure 32-3.   A second laparoscopic needle driver is introduced through the other port and is used to align the needle. The internal ring is closed with several stitches placed in the shape of an N. On the anterior aspect of the internal ring, slightly more tissue is included. On the inferior part, however, less tissue is included because of the close proximity of the nerves, testicular vessels, and vas deferens. The most medial suture should be placed as close as possible to the epigastric vessels and the vas deferens.

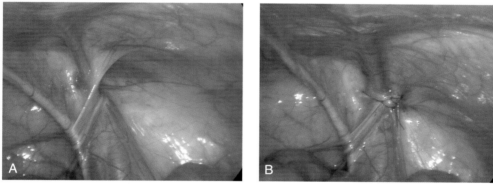

Figure 32-4.   **A,** Closure of an indirect right inguinal hernia. **B,** After laparoscopic hernia repair, the patent processus vaginalis is closed.

Almost all recurrences appear medial to the suture, close to the epigastric vessels. Rarely is a recurrent hernia noted laterally. Thus, in our experience, the inclusion of additional tissue medial to the epigastric vessels reduces the recurrence rate. Technically, the easiest repairs are in young infants. However, in newborns, there might be bowel distension, representing not a true obstacle to laparoscopic hernia repair but a visual restriction. In children older than 10 years, it might be difficult to secure the knot because of increased mechanical tension. It is helpful to reduce the intra-abdominal pressure and to exert digital pressure externally onto the internal inguinal ring to help close the internal ring. In most cases, a single N-shaped suture suffices. However, if there is doubt about whether the internal ring is completely closed, a second suture can be used.

In direct or femoral hernias (which seem to be much more frequently found during laparoscopy than in open surgery), we have experienced recurrences when only the peritoneum was closed by a single suture. Incising the peritoneum, exposing and suturing the underlying tissue, again with 4-0 nonabsorbable monofilamentous sutures, has reduced these recurrences. In these cases, the peritoneum is approximated as a second layer.

After hernia repair, the sutures are removed together with the 2-mm ports. Steri-Strips (3M, St. Paul, MN) are used to approximate the skin edges. The abdomen is desufflated through the umbilical cannula. The umbilical fascia is then closed with one 3-0 polyglactin suture. The umbilical skin is closed with Steri-Strips. Sterile dressings are then applied.

The patient is awakened and is usually ready for discharge several hours after the operation. A dressing change is suggested at the family doctor's office 4 days later. There are no restrictions in physical activity, including sports, or diet.

PEARLS

1. In a very small child, insert the cannulas more cephalad toward the chest. Suturing is easier when the ports are not on top of the internal inguinal ring.
2. The surgeon should change sides when performing bilateral hernias repairs. The surgeon should stand on the left side of the patient for a right inguinal hernia repair and on the right side of the patient for a left repair.
3. Polypropylene suture is acceptable. Deklene (Teleflex Medical, Mansfield, MA) is better. Deklene is not as rigid as polypropylene, and it keeps its shape almost

as well. Braided sutures tend to stick to the abdominal wall.

4. Cutting needles can be secured more firmly in needle drivers. Round needles tend to slip.

5. Suturing with two needle drivers is easier than with a needle driver and a forceps. Use a ratcheted needle driver for the dominant hand and a nonratcheted needle holder for the nondominant hand (ratchets are easier to release with the dominant hand).

PITFALLS

1. The medial aspect of the internal inguinal canal is the most crucial. Most recurrences occur at this site. Be sure that enough tissue is included into the suture at this area. The most important cause of recurrences is fear of injury to the epigastric vessels and the vas. Do not leave an opening here.

RESULTS

In our institution, 824 patients (75% boys), from 4 weeks to 14 years old (median, 1.4 years), have undergone laparoscopic inguinal hernia repair. The operating time has ranged from 6 to 42 minutes (median, 15 minutes). Indirect hernias were found in 93% of the patients, and direct hernias in 2.2%.

Femoral hernias were seen in 1% of the patients. Interestingly, 3% had no hernia. The follow-up has been from 1 month to 8 years (median, 4 years). Recurrences have developed in 3.5% of these patients. A second recurrence developed in 0.1%. Testicular atrophy has occurred in 0.1% of the boys. In 15% of the patients, a contralateral patent processus vaginalis was seen and repaired. An umbilical wound infection occurred in 0.1% of these children.

SELECTED REFERENCES

1. Schier F, Danzer E, Bondartschuk M: Incidence of contralateral patent processus vaginalis in children with inguinal hernia. J Pediatr Surg 36:1561-1563, 2001
2. Shalaby R, Desoky A: Needlescopic inguinal hernia repair in children. Pediatr Surg Int 18:153-156, 2002
3. Becmeur F, Philippe P, Lemandat-Schultz A, et al: A continuous series of 96 laparoscopic inguinal hernia repairs in children by a new technique. Surg Endosc 18:1738-1741, 2004
4. Patkowski D, Czernik J, Chrzan R, et al: Percutaneous internal ring suturing: A simple minimally invasive technique for inguinal hernia repair in children. J Laparoendosc Adv Surg Tech 16:513-517, 2006
5. Schier F: Laparoscopic inguinal hernia repair: A prospective personal series of 542 children. J Pediatr Surg 41:1081-1084, 2006

33
Principles of Pediatric Robotic Surgery

John J. Meehan

Robotic surgery is a new technology that may help expand the variety of procedures that can be accomplished in children using a minimally invasive approach. An enormous variety of cases have already been accomplished with robotic technology in children, and the list continues to grow. However, literature reports detailing the advantages of this approach have lagged behind this rapidly evolving field by a number of years, leaving the pediatric surgeon very little in the way of up-to-date information. In this chapter, we will review the history of robotic surgery, discuss the advantages and limitations of the current technology, and describe the relevant clinical applications of robotics in children.

HISTORY OF ROBOTICS

Most surgeons now perform a wide variety of basic minimally invasive procedures. However, complex procedures can still be quite difficult. Limitations in current laparoscopic equipment include loss of haptic feedback (force and tactile), loss of hand–eye coordination, and loss of dexterity. Depth perception is compromised as well, because laparoscopic surgery is performed using a single camera lens, creating a two-dimensional surgical image of a three-dimensional surgical field. Additionally, as the laparoscopic instruments pivot about the cannula site, the motion of the surgeon's hand translates to the opposite movement in the patient. This is known as the fulcrum effect. Another limitation is the restricted degrees of motion with standard laparoscopic instruments. Most current laparoscopic instruments have four degrees of motion, whereas the human wrist and hand have seven degrees of freedom of movement. Finally, physiologic tremors in the surgeon's hand are transmitted through the length of rigid instruments. Robotic surgery addresses most of these limitations.

The term *robot* was first introduced in the script for the play "R.U.R.: Rossum's Universal Robots" by Karel Capek in 1921. In its original Czech translation, *robota* means "drudgery" or "servitude." In the play, the robots were manufactured servants that closely resembled humans. The term has since been adopted for many forms of automated characters in movies, plays, and television. In reality, the term robot has been used to describe a multitude of automated devices, which are present in just about every form of industry. It was only a matter of time before the technology would enter the medical field.

One of the first robotic systems used in medicine was the Puma 560, a device first used in 1985 by Kwoh to perform neurosurgical biopsies (Fig. 33-1A). Three years later, Davies used the Puma 560 to perform a transurethral resection of the prostate. In 1988, PROBOT was introduced to perform prostatic surgery in England. In 1992, Integrated Surgical Systems unveiled the ROBODOC, a device used to mill out precise fittings in the femur for hip replacement surgery (see Fig. 33-1B).

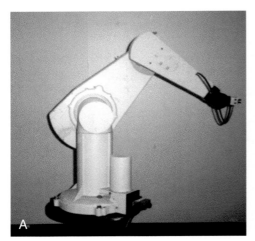
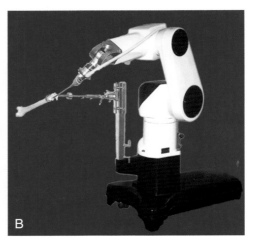

Figure 33-1.   A, The Puma 560 was one of the first robotic systems designed. **B,** The ROBODOC was used to mill out precise fittings in the femur for hip replacement surgery.

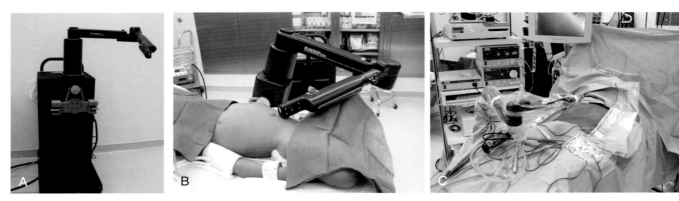

Figure 33-2.   A, The AESOP robotic camera holder on its cart. **B,** The AESOP positioned for a laparoscopic fundoplication in a young child. **C,** The AESOP positioned for a laparoscopic cholecystectomy. This device provides a steady camera view and can be voice activated. It is still being used in some centers to hold and manipulate the telescope or camera.

This was a significant advancement, and the ROBODOC became the first surgical robot to gain U.S. Food and Drug Administration (FDA) approval, bringing technology and robotics into mainstream medicine.

COMPUTER MOTION AND INTUITIVE SURGICAL

A group of researchers at the Department of Defense (DOD) teamed with scientists at Stanford's Research Institute (SRI). They were interested in finding a way to decrease wartime mortality by treating battlefield casualties from a remote operative station. This concept of "telepresence" would allow a surgeon to be in one location while potentially treating multiple casualties in a variety of sites. SRI developed the prototype for this concept, the Green Telepresence Surgery System. Although initially designed for open procedures, several of the engineers had the vision of bringing this technology into the realm of minimally invasive surgery.

Intuitive Surgical, Inc., (Sunnyvale, CA) was founded to test this concept. The DOD sold the licensed technology and intellectual property to this group, and this system was extensively redesigned into the da Vinci Surgical Robot.

As Intuitive worked on the da Vinci, another company, Computer Motion (CM), emerged. While Intuitive was working on the da Vinci, CM designed a camera system that responded to a surgeon's voice command. This became known as AESOP (Automated Endoscopic System for Optimal Positioning) (Fig. 33-2). Soon after Intuitive launched the da Vinci system in 1999, CM unveiled the Zeus system, and the competition between the two companies quickly accelerated. CM had a landmark event in robotics history in 2001. While seated at a console in New York, a surgeon performed the first transcontinental robotics procedure using the Zeus system by removing the gallbladder from a patient in Strasbourg, France. Meanwhile, the da Vinci was being used to help pioneer the minimally invasive prostatectomy.

Both systems enjoyed early success, but progress was hindered by legal battles between the two companies. Additionally, sales of the Zeus system became sluggish, and CM began having financial troubles. Eventually, the two companies agreed to drop their lawsuits and Intuitive purchased CM in 2003. Although this merger certainly saved funds that would have been wasted on legal expenses, it left the medical field with a sole provider of surgical robotics. With Intuitive now focusing on the da Vinci, the Zeus system was abandoned. A few of these systems are still in existence, but most have been relegated to laboratory use. Meanwhile, the da Vinci has flourished and its use has grown exponentially.

THE DA VINCI SYSTEM

The da Vinci robotic surgical system is a computer-enhanced telemanipulator currently approved by the FDA for adult and pediatric minimally invasive surgery. The system is composed of three main components: a master surgeon's console, a surgical cart, and a vision cart. The system provides the surgeon with stereoscopic vision, provides motion scaling and tremor reduction, and features instruments capable of seven degrees of motion, including grip, compared with the four degrees of motion provided by standard laparoscopic instruments.

MASTER SURGEON'S CONSOLE

The surgeon sits at the ergonomically designed surgeon's console up to thirty feet away from the operating table (Fig. 33-3). The console is attached to the surgical cart via electric cables, which transmit information between the master surgeon's console and the surgical cart ("robot") with virtually no delay. At the console, the surgeon receives video input from the operative field by placing his or her head into the high-resolution stereoscopic viewer. The viewer, consisting of two separate medical grade cathode ray tube monitors (one for each eye), precisely projects images viewed by the dual channel endoscope. The surgeon is then provided with a ten-fold, magnified, three-dimensional image of the operative field. The stereoscopic viewer is positioned at the console to project the three-dimensional image of the surgical field directly atop the surgeon's hands. This provides a more natural correspondence of hand–eye coordination and movement, thereby giving the surgeon a sensation of immersion within the operating field. Finally, the sides of the viewer contain infrared sensors that detect the presence of the surgeon's head, allowing manipulation of the robotic arms only when the surgeon's head is within the viewer.

In addition to receiving video input, the surgeon controls the three robotic arms of the surgical cart (the "robot") from the master surgeon's console. This is

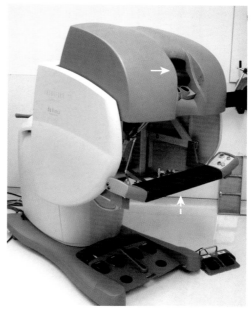

Figure 33-3. The da Vinci surgeon's console. The surgeon's head is placed into the high-resolution stereoscopic viewer (*solid arrow*) to receive video input from the operative field. The forearms are placed on the shelf (*dotted arrow*), under which are the master grips through which the surgeon's fingers are placed.

accomplished using dual master controls patterned after Castro-style needle drivers (Fig. 33-4A). By manipulating these master controls, the surgeon is able to control both the laparoscopic instruments, held by the two robotic operating arms, and the endoscope held by the third robotic arm. The surgeon's movements of the master grips are directly translated into corresponding movements of the tips of the articulating instruments. Similarly, wrist movements of the surgeon's hands are directly translated into wrist movements of the articulated instruments. The surgeon also receives gross force feedback via the master controls. However, fine, haptic sensation is unavailable to the surgeon.

The master surgeon's console also contains the remaining surgeon-system interface. Specifically, a series of pedals allows the surgeon not only to manipulate the camera but also to control camera focus and activate electrocautery (see Fig. 33-4B). To manipulate the endoscope, the surgeon depresses and holds down the camera control pedal. When this pedal is depressed, the master grips are disengaged from the instruments and instead control the movement of the endoscope. Similarly, the surgeon is able to rotate the camera as well as change the depth of the scope by simply manipulating the master grips. The clutch pedal allows the surgeon to disengage the master grips from the surgical cart, allowing repositioning of the master grips into a more comfortable configuration without moving the instruments or the endoscope.

Two control panels (the user interface panel and the user switch panel) are positioned aside the surgeon's

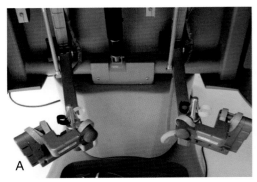
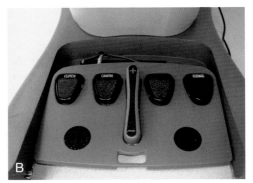

Figure 33-4. **A,** The dual master controls patterned after Castro-style needle drivers. The surgeon places fingers through the black and white finger grips. **B,** The foot pedals that allow the surgeon to manipulate the camera, control the camera focus, and activate electrocautery.

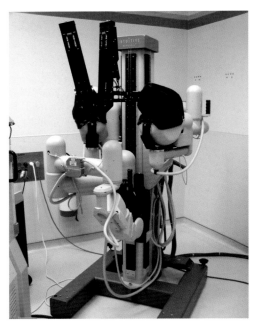

Figure 33-5. The patient-side surgical cart or "robot." The cart consists of motor-driven, cable-activated robotic arms mounted on a movable chassis.

hands. These controls are used to choose and calibrate either the 30-degree or the 0-degree endoscope, and they allow the surgeon to adjust motion scaling, select camera angle (up or down), allow changing between three-dimensional and two-dimensional viewing, place the system on and off standby, or completely disengage the system.

SURGICAL CART

The second component of the da Vinci system is the patient-side surgical cart, or "robot" (Fig. 33-5). In essence, this cart consists of motor-driven, cable-activated, robotic arms mounted on a movable chassis. The two robotic operating arms correspond to the surgeon's right and left hands. The third, central, robotic

arm holds and manipulates the dual-channel endoscope. A fourth arm, available as an upgrade to the older model or standard on the da Vinci model S, enables the surgeon to control three intracorporeal instruments simultaneously. The robotic arms are covered with sterile drapes before the robotics portion of the operation. After port placement, the surgical cart is wheeled into position adjacent to the operating table. This position is variable and depends on the particular operation being performed. The robotic arms are then attached or "docked" to pre-placed, unique cannulas.

The robotic arms are constructed to move around a "remote center." In traditional laparoscopic surgery, the fulcrum point of the patient's body serves as the "natural center" around which the laparoscopic instruments move. In contrast, the remote center of a robotic arm is determined by the setup joint position. In this manner, the fulcrum point around which the instruments and cannulas move does not vary during the operation, remaining steady despite possible changes in insufflation that may alter the position of the patient's abdominal wall.

Whereas the camera arm uses simple, mechanical adaptors to hold the endoscope in place, the robotic operating arms use unique sterile adaptors that serve as both an electrical and mechanical interface between the robotic arms and the articulating instruments. These reusable adaptors feature four notched wheels that correspond to matching wheels on both the sterile instruments and the robotic arms. By manipulating these wheels, the robotic arms transmit mechanical forces to the instruments, allowing the instruments' unique wristed movements and grip. Within the instruments themselves, the notched wheels are attached to a series of tungsten cables that travel the length of the instruments down to the tips. These cables precisely transmit the mechanical forces produced by the robotic arms to the tips of the surgical instruments. The sterile adapters also feature an electrical interface that allows the robotic arms to communicate with the individual instruments. Specifically, each instrument contains a microchip that tells the robotic arm which particular instrument is being attached and records the number of times that instrument has been used.

The da Vinci system features an array of surgical instrument tip configurations. These include a variety of fully articulating graspers, forceps, blades, and needle drivers. Additionally, the system features a variety of energy-delivering instruments, including monopolar hook and spatula cautery, bipolar forceps, and ultrasonic forceps. Both 5-mm- and 8-mm-diameter instruments are available.

VISION CART

The final component of the da Vinci system is the vision cart (Fig. 33-6). This is a movable tower that houses the dual light sources and camera equipment. It houses an insufflation device as well as a standard laparoscopic monitor for use by the assistant, who is positioned by the patient. To achieve stereoscopic vision, the system uses a unique dual-channel endoscope that attaches to two separate cameras. These cameras then attach to the two separate camera control units on the vision cart that allow for color balancing and gain adjustment. The cart also contains the equipment necessary to process the camera signals that provide the three-dimensional image at the surgeon's console.

The unique stereo endoscope is 12 mm in diameter and houses two separate 5-mm telescopes. The telescope is available in 0-degree and 30-degree versions. A 5-mm camera is also available, but is a single-channel

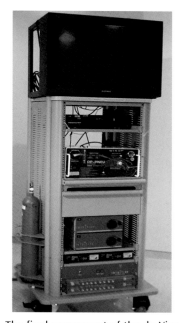

Figure 33-6. The final component of the da Vinci system is the vision cart, which is a movable tower that has the dual light sources and camera equipment. In addition, it also houses an insufflation device as well as a standard laparoscopic monitor for use by the assistant who is positioned at the patient's side.

telescope and thus does not provide a three-dimensional view of the operating field.

ROOM SETUP AND ANESTHESIA ISSUES

Among the challenges to the operating surgeon and robotic surgical (RS) team (beyond those of robot-specific hospital credentialing, and selection, training, and orchestration of the RS team) are the issues of room setup, anesthesia, and contingency management. An operating room should be designated as an RS suite, providing space to accommodate placement and mobility of the RS equipment (surgeon console, surgical cart, equipment cart).

For robotic operations, several patient-access issues related to anesthesia need to be addressed before draping the patient. First, management of the airway and ventilation circuit needs to be planned to provide clear, unobstructed flow of the extension tubing from the ventilator. We have found that a 6-foot ventilator extension tube is adequate, although dead-space ventilation must be considered. Second, for most pediatric operations, the robot is docked above the patient, making it difficult to urgently access the patient's airway without a specific plan for undocking and providing the anesthesiologist with unobstructed access to the patient's head and airway. These contingency issues must be planned and rehearsed.

For an operation in which esophageal bougies are used, the bougies should be positioned within the distal esophagus or stomach before draping, and they should be easily maneuvered by the anesthesiologist during the operation. An ether screen drape may be positioned and adjusted accordingly to provide the anesthesiologist the necessary space to accomplish these tasks. Finally, all potential points of contact between the patient and the robot once docked, outside the operative field, must be eliminated.

DA VINCI LIMITATIONS

The biggest obstacle to using the da Vinci robot is cost. In 2006, the cost of the standard da Vinci was $1.2 million, and the new da Vinci-S costs approximately $1.5 million. Added to this expense is an estimated $100,000 per year for a service contract for parts and repairs. Instrumentation is not included in this cost, and the 8-mm instruments have a life span of only 10 operations; the 5-mm instruments have a life span of 18 to 20 operations. A number of other issues make the da Vinci less than ideal. The standard da Vinci is limited to single-quadrant or two-quadrant surgery. In other words, it is great for looking at a focused area of the abdomen, but it loses its flexibility as the surgeon tries to move to other quadrants of the abdomen. This is because the instrument arms and camera arm have a limited range of motion. The range of motion of the

Table 33-1 Components of the da Vinci-S Surgical System: Dimensions

	Surgeon Console	Surgical Cart (Robot)	Vision Cart
Height (in./cm)	66/168	69/175	60/152
Width (in./cm)	36/91	36/91	22/56
Depth (in./cm)	62/158	50/127	27/69
Ground Clearance (in./cm)	2/5	1.9/4.8	7.5/19
Weight (lb/kg)	800/363	1200/544	200

new da Vinci-S has improved this limited range tremendously but not completely.

Before starting robotics, the biggest concern for most surgeons is the loss of haptic feedback. Currently, there is no haptic feedback with the da Vinci system. Although a system for haptic feedback is currently being engineered, it may be a number of years before this problem improves. Reliance must be on visual cues for a sense of how hard the surgeon is grasping or pulling on a structure. However, it is interesting that most robotics experts agree that this issue is far less concerning than they expected, as became apparent at the Society of American Gastrointestinal and Endoscopic Surgeons/Minimally Invasive Robotic Association (SAGES/MIRA) 2006 consensus meeting in New York City. Although it is still a concern, an overwhelming majority of these robotics experts found that haptic feedback is not as limiting as they had presumed it would be.

The size of the robot is also a limiting factor. Besides standing about 6 feet in height, the robot occupies a sizable footprint (Table 33-1). Access to the patient with such a large device hovering over the bed can seem troublesome. Instrument size can also be limiting, particularly in small children. Additionally, the instrument needs a certain amount of length outside the cannula so that it can articulate. Although the da Vinci has been used in neonates weighing as little as 2.2 kg, using it is a problem when the child is less than about 5 kg. Proper planning and flexibility in determining the best-suited cannula locations will help overcome these obstacles. Finally, the selection of instrument tips is considerably limited for small patients, particularly for the 5-mm instrument line.

CLINICAL APPLICATIONS OF PEDIATRIC ROBOTIC SURGERY

Numerous procedures have already been successfully performed using the robotic approach in children. Table 33-2 lists the pediatric procedures that have performed at the Children's Hospital of Iowa and the University of Iowa Hospitals and Clinics in Iowa City.

Table 33-2 Robotic Procedures That Have Been Performed at The Children's Hospital of Iowa

Abdominal Procedures

Cholecystectomy

Splenectomy

Adrenalectomy

Fundoplication

Esophagomyotomy

Pyloroplasty

Meckler's diverticulectomy

Small-bowel resection

Hemicolectomy

Total proctocolectomy with ileoanal pull-through

Treatment of rectal prolapse

Mesenteric lymphangioma

Ladd procedure

Choledochal cyst resection

Kasai portoenterostomy

Neuroblastoma resection

Duodenal atresia repair

Congenital diaphragmatic hernia repair

Thoracic Procedures

Intralobar sequestration resection

Resection of congenital cystic adenomatoid malformation

Anterior mediastinal mass resection

Posterior mediastinal mass resection

Bronchogenic cyst resection

Pulmonary lobectomy

Chest wall mass resection

Genitourinary and Pelvic Procedures

Extramucosal ureteral reimplant

Pyeloplasty

Ovarian cystectomy

Ovarian teratoma resection

Resection of a utricle

Essentially, any procedure can be done robotically. However, questions remain: Which are best performed open, which are best performed laparoscopically, and which are best performed robotically? The answers will almost certainly evolve as technology changes. Although the robot is ideally suited for complex operations, it is

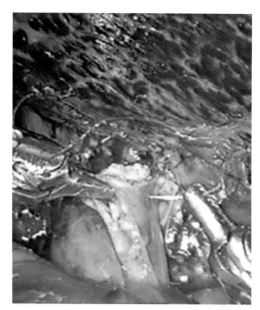

Figure 33-7. This view of the portal region during a Kasai procedure shows the excellent visualization with the 12-mm three-dimensional camera.

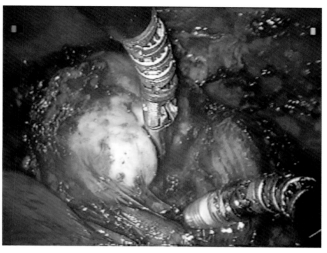

Figure 33-8. The articulating instruments allow easy dissection of thoracic masses.

probably best for a surgeon new to robotics to begin with simple procedures. Although there is clearly no benefit for using this robot for a cholecystectomy, it allows the surgeon to perform a basic minimally invasive procedure while learning the subtleties of the robot. Fundoplication and splenectomy are intermediate operations that will help expand the team's knowledge and experience with the system. The goal is not only to allow the surgeon to become familiar with the system but also for the support staff of assistants, scrub nurses, and circulators to learn this advanced technology.

Any operation that involves complex suturing or dissecting can be considered ideal for the da Vinci robot. An esophagomyotomy for surgical treatment of achalasia has already been shown to have better results in adults when done robotically than when the laparoscopic approach is used. In children, the Kasai portoenterostomy and resection of a choledochal cyst may be ideal procedures. The 12-mm three-dimensional camera gives superior visualization of the portal region during a Kasai procedure (Fig. 33-7). The robot is also ideally suited for procedures in the chest such as excision of esophageal masses or bronchogenic cysts. Another ideal thoracic operation for the robot is resection of solid intrathoracic tumors, particularly those in the mediastinum. The articulating instruments allow easy dissection of these masses, and circumnavigating the solid tumor within the rigid chest is remarkably easy with the articulating instruments (Fig. 33-8). Repair of duodenal atresia is another procedure that can seem significantly easier with the robot than with standard laparoscopic instruments. Although the view is two-dimensional, the 5-mm camera is preferred for this procedure, as the

12-mm camera is too big for the newborn. Procedures in the pelvis requiring suturing would also be ideal for the robot (e.g., extravesicular ureteral reimplant). Other genitourinary procedures including pyeloplasty and resection of a utricle are also ideally suited.

THE 2006 CONSENSUS MEETING ON ROBOTIC SURGERY

Organized by SAGES and MIRA, a consensus meeting on robotic surgery was held in the summer of 2006. The purpose of the meeting was to discuss a variety of important issues regarding robotic surgery, including clinical applications, credentialing, and research. The significant clinical applications for pediatric surgery have already been mentioned here. The credentialing subcommittee outlined several recommendations for training residents and staff surgeons alike, but it ultimately concluded that specific credentialing criteria should be dictated by each individual hospital. Finally, the research subcommittee defined the field of robotics and reiterated the need for further development of this advanced technology through a collaborative effort between physicians and industry. The meeting delegates also concluded that the three biggest limitations to robotic surgery were cost, training of new users, and lack of usable data in the literature resulting from the lag time between clinical experience and publication.

In conclusion, pediatric robotic surgery is a new technology that will very likely expand the scope of minimally invasive procedures that can be accomplished by many more surgeons. The movements of the robotic instruments closely simulate open surgery and return many of the positive aspects of open surgery back to the minimally invasive surgeon. The technology will continue to change, and pediatric surgeons should stay involved in this field to help drive our corporate colleagues to remember the needs of our smallest patients.

SELECTED REFERENCES

1. Kwoh YS, Hou J, Jonckheere EA, et al: A robot with improved absolute positioning accuracy for CT guided stereotactic brain surgery. IEEE Trans Biomed Eng 35:153-161, 1988
2. Mouret P: From the first laparoscopic cholecystectomy to the frontiers of laparoscopic surgery: The prospective futures. Dig Surg 8:124, 1991
3. Crothers IR, Gallagher AG, McClure N, et al: Experienced laparoscopic surgeons are automated to the "fulcrum effect": An ergonomic demonstration. Endoscopy 31:365-369, 1999
4. Davies B: A review of robotics in surgery. Proc Inst Mech Eng 214:129-140, 2000
5. Capek K: RUR: Rossum's Universal Robots. Dover, Reprint, 2001
6. Marescaux J, Leroy J, Rubino F, et al: Transcontinental robot-assisted remote telesurgery: Feasibility and potential applications. Ann Surg 235:487-492, 2002
7. Satava RM: Surgical robotics: The early chronicles: A personal historical perspective. Surg Laparosc Endosc Percutan Tech 12:6-16, 2002
8. Melvin WS, Dundon JM, Talamini M, et al: Computer-enhanced robotic telesurgery minimizes esophageal perforation during Heller myotomy. Surgery 138:553-558, 2005

34
Robotic Kasai Procedure

Sanjeev Dutta and Craig T. Albanese

The portoenterostomy reconstructive procedure, introduced by Morio Kasai in 1959, revolutionized the surgical management of biliary atresia and has become the standard of care for initial management of this disorder. Success of the procedure is indicated by resolution of the biliary obstruction, which depends on early diagnosis and operation, ideally before 8 weeks of age. This procedure has traditionally been performed through an open laparotomy, which also involves a cholangiogram to confirm the diagnosis, followed by Roux-en-Y portoenterostomy.

In recent years, surgeons with experience in advanced minimal-access techniques have successfully performed portoenterostomy using the laparoscopic approach. Compared with laparotomy, the laparoscopic approach has the potential advantages of improved visualization of the portal structures, decreased postoperative pain, and improved cosmesis. Potential disadvantages of the laparoscopic procedure are that the optics are only two-dimensional and the degrees of movement with laparoscopic instruments are limited compared with the robot.

The introduction of robotic surgical technology, with its potential for improved optical visualization and instrument dexterity, has added a new dimension to the minimal-access surgical approach to this disorder. Featuring wristed instrumentation with more degrees of freedom than standard laparoscopic instruments, stereoscopic visualization, nonreversed instrument control, tremor reduction, and motion scaling, robotic systems attempt to address many of the limitations of standard laparoscopic techniques.

INDICATIONS FOR WORKUP AND OPERATION

Biliary atresia is a neonatal condition characterized by progressive inflammatory obliteration of the extrahepatic biliary ductal structures, progressing to cirrhosis and liver failure if left untreated. Surgical management involves resection of the atretic bile duct with Roux-en-Y portoenterostomy to provide a biliary drainage conduit for the microscopic biliary radicles at the hilar plate. Despite this initial management, many children with biliary atresia progress to require liver transplantation.

The presence of conjugated hyperbilirubinemia in a jaundiced infant necessitates further evaluation. Investigations include ultrasonography, hepatobiliary scintigraphy, viral screen, alpha-1-antitrypsin (and other metabolic screens), and percutaneous liver biopsy. If hematologic, metabolic, genetic, and other nonsurgical causes are excluded, a diagnosis of biliary atresia must be entertained. Diagnostic confirmation is by intraoperative cholangiography, which can be performed as a preliminary procedure at the time of a planned portoenterostomy. In the case of minimal-access portoenterostomy, the cholangiogram is performed under telescopic guidance. For robotic portoenterostomy, we have performed the cholangiogram via a standard laparoscopic approach (described later), followed by introduction of the robotic platform once the diagnosis was confirmed.

Little preoperative preparation is necessary. Coagulation profiles should be corrected using fresh frozen plasma and vitamin K. Allowing only clear fluids for 12 hours before operation ensures minimal bowel residue. A single dose of prophylactic antibiotics to cover

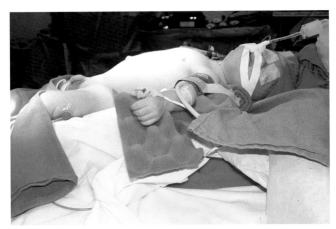

Figure 34-1. For a robotic Kasai procedure, the infant is elevated 4 inches off the operating table on blankets and foam padding to allow for the downward pitch of the back end of the robotic instruments.

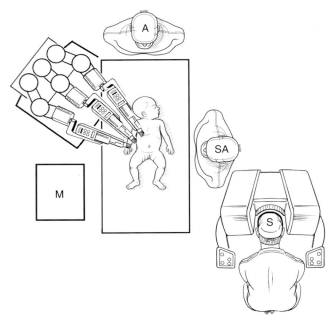

Figure 34-2. For a robotic Kasai operation, the infant is placed supine on the operating table. The robot is positioned over the infant's right shoulder. The surgeon's (S) console is located on the side of the room opposite the robot. The bedside surgeon (SA) is also located on the patient's left side. The monitor (M) is situated so all members of the operating team can have good visualization. A, anesthesiologist.

gram-negative and gram-positive organisms is administered in the operating room before the procedure.

OPERATIVE TECHNIQUE

The infant is elevated 4 inches off the operating table on blankets and foam to allow for the downward pitch of the back end of the robotic instruments (Fig. 34-1). The robot and operating personnel are positioned as seen in Figure 34-2. A 12-mm cannula is used instead of the usual 5-mm port in the umbilicus to accommodate the da Vinci (Intuitive Surgical, Sunnyvale, CA) stereoscope. Four (rather than three) additional ports are placed under direct laparoscopic visualization: two 5-mm robotic instrument ports on both sides of the umbilicus, one 3-mm left subcostal port for liver retraction, and one left lower quadrant 5-mm assistant's port (Fig. 34-3). This assistant's port is used for delivering and cutting sutures and for retracting, if necessary.

After cannula insertion, a cholangiogram is performed to confirm the diagnosis by transabdominal passage of a 22-gauge spinal needle directly into the gallbladder fundus, if present. After diagnostic confirmation, the da Vinci surgical cart is positioned directly at the head of the bed and docked to the operating ports. The 5-mm wristed robotic instruments are used. Two separate strategies can be used for the robotic procedure. In one approach, the surgical robot is used for the entire case, apart from the cholangiogram and construction of the Roux limb. Dissection of the atretic gallbladder is performed in top-down fashion using hook electrocautery and tissue forceps. This dissection is extended to the atretic cystic duct and the remains of the extrahepatic biliary tree to allow clear visualization of the portal structures—namely, the right and left hepatic arteries and bifurcation of the main portal vein. The atretic duct is transected distally at the superior border of the

duodenum. Careful attention is paid to dissection of the portal plate away from the portal vein confluence, including division of small portal branches, using hook electrocautery. The portal plate is then sharply excised, using the robotic Metzenbaum scissors through the left 5-mm port (Fig. 34-4). After excision, several cottonoid pledgets soaked in dilute epinephrine (1:200,000) are placed in the portal area to help control bleeding.

Once the portal plate is transected, the ligament of Treitz is identified telescopically and a length of small bowel is measured for Roux limb construction. Different-colored marking sutures are placed on either side of the planned site of bowel transection; one color denotes the future afferent limb, the other the efferent limb. The umbilical incision is then slightly enlarged (12 to 15 mm) and the small bowel exteriorized. A 10- to 15-cm Roux limb with jejunojejunostomy is created extracorporeally. The tip of the Roux limb is marked with a long suture to facilitate its intracorporeal identification and manipulation. The small bowel is returned to the abdomen and pneumoperitoneum is reestablished after tightening the umbilical fascia around the cannula with a suture. The Roux limb is brought antecolic to the portal plate. An enterotomy is made on the antimesenteric side of the limb with electrocautery, and the portoenterostomy is created using interrupted 4-0 Vicryl (Ethicon, Inc., Somerville, NJ) suture loaded on a TF needle (Fig. 34-5). Ports are removed and the fascia

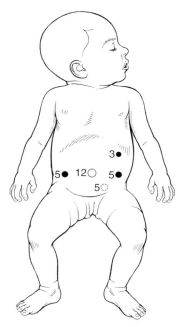

Figure 34-3. Port placement for a robotic Kasai. A 12-mm cannula is introduced in the umbilicus to accommodate the 12-mm, three-dimensional robotic telescope. Four additional ports are then introduced under direct visualization. Two 5-mm robotic ports (*solid circles*) are placed on either side of the umbilicus. A 5-mm port is placed in the infant's left lower abdomen for use by the bedside surgeon. A 3-mm cannula is introduced in the left subcostal region for liver retraction. The assistant utilizes the 5-mm port (*dotted circle*) in the left lower abdomen to deliver and cut sutures and to perform retraction, if necessary.

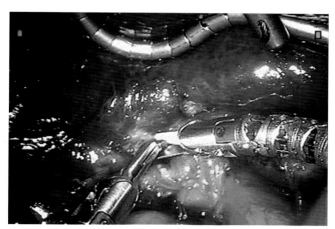

Figure 34-4. Transection of the portal plate using robotic Metzenbaum scissors, which have been introduced through the 5-mm port in the patient's left mid abdomen. Note the portal vein just below the scissors.

and skin incisions are closed with absorbable sutures after infiltration with 0.25% bupivacaine locally.

Certain aspects of the operation are easily performed laparoscopically, and perhaps use of the robot for these steps is overkill. The surgical robot is most useful in

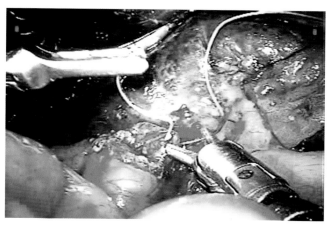

Figure 34-5. The anastomosis between the Roux limb and the portal plate is being performed with the robotic needle holder.

facilitating suturing. Therefore, as an alternative approach, the cholangiogram and portal dissection (excluding transection of the plate) can be performed without difficulty using conventional laparoscopy. With this approach, the ligament of Treitz is also identified laparoscopically and the small bowel marked with suture for subsequent orientation. Next, the enlarged umbilical incision is used to eviscerate the bowel and construct a Roux limb as previously described. Once the newly constructed Roux limb is returned to the abdomen, the robotic platform is brought in to transect the portal plate and perform the anastomosis. This approach avoids undocking and redocking the robot and can save considerable operative time.

POSTOPERATIVE CARE

Patients are admitted after the operation with a nasogastric tube in place. Diet is resumed when intestinal function recovers. Patients are discharged when a regular diet is tolerated and pain is controlled with oral medications. The infants are maintained on an intravenous antibiotic to prevent cholangitis until oral intake is resumed, and then oral prophylaxis is begun. They are discharged on oral antibiotic prophylaxis and fat-soluble vitamin supplementation, and they may also be prescribed cholestyramine and steroids if the surgeon chooses.

PEARLS

1. The Roux limb is most easily constructed extracorporeally through a slightly enlarged umbilical incision. Intracorporeal construction is cumbersome and time-consuming.
2. Dilute epinephrine-soaked cottonoid pledgets help to reduce oozing after hilar plate dissection, which improves visibility for subsequent portoenterostomy creation.

3. Excellent visualization of the portal confluence is achieved with the three-dimensional telescope, enabling complete dissection of the hilar plate to its posterior-most border.
4. The wrist action of the robotic Metzenbaum scissors allows an ideal angle for hilar transection.
5. The ergonomic arrangement of the robotic platform may reduce surgeon fatigue as compared with a standard laparoscopic approach, as this can sometimes be a long operation.

PITFALLS

1. The long arc of the 5-mm wristed instruments can be detrimental to mobility in the confined hilar space. Surgeons may choose to take advantage of the "tighter-wristed" 8-mm robotic instruments, but the drawback is that a larger incision is required.
2. The lack of haptic feedback with the robot can make suturing the portoenterostomy difficult. Adequate knot tying is discerned by visualizing formation of the knot as it is tied.
3. The lack of haptic feedback with robotic instruments also necessitates that great care be taken to avoid tearing through the parenchyma when passing the curved needle through the liver parenchyma.

RESULTS

There is too little experience with the robotic portoenterostomy to comment on outcomes. We have performed three procedures at our institution. At 3 to 18 months' follow-up, one patient has proceeded to liver transplantation. The long-term outcomes of robotic portoenterostomy will most likely mirror that of standard laparoscopy, which has been comparable to open approaches.

SELECTED REFERENCES

1. Grosfeld JL, Fitzgerald JF, Predaina R, et al: The efficacy of hepatoportoenterostomy in biliary atresia. Surgery 106:692-700, 1989
2. Schier F, Waldschmidt J: Experience with laparoscopy for the evaluation of cholestasis in newborns. Surg Endosc 4:13-14, 1990
3. Otte JB, de Ville de Goyet J, Reding R, et al: Sequential treatment of biliary atresia with Kasai portoenterostomy and liver transplantation: A review. Hepatology 20:41S-48, 1994
4. Esteves E, Clemente Neto E, Ottaiano Neto M, et al: Laparoscopic Kasai portoenterostomy for biliary atresia. Pediatr Surg Int 18:737-740, 2002
5. Lee H, Hirose S, Bratton B, et al: Initial experience with complex laparoscopic biliary surgery in children: Biliary atresia and choledochal cyst. J Pediatr Surg 39:804-807, 2004
6. Venigalla S, Gourley GR: Neonatal cholestasis. Semin Perinatol 28:348-355, 2004
7. Woo R, Le D, Krummel TM, Albanese C: Robot-assisted pediatric surgery. Am J Surg 188:27S-37, 2004
8. Martinez-Ferro M, Esteves E, Laje P: Laparoscopic treatment of biliary atresia and choledochal cyst. Semin Pediatr Surg 14:206-215, 2005
9. Dutta S, Albanese CT: Lessons learned during minimal access surgery for biliary atresia: Comparison of robotic and standard laparoscopic techniques. Pediatr Surg Int (in press)

35
Robotic Excision of Choledochal Cyst

James D. Geiger

Choledochal cyst is congenital dilation of the bile ducts. The estimated incidence in Western countries varies between 1 in 100,000 and 1 in 150,000 births. Its incidence is significantly higher in Asia, and it occurs more commonly in girls. The most widely used subdivision of choledochal cyst is the Todani classification. Type 1 cysts are the most frequently encountered and may be caused by an abnormal arrangement of the pancreatic and biliary ducts, also known as the *common channel*, which occurs in up to 92% of patients with choledochal cyst. If a choledochal cyst is not excised, a high incidence (20% to 30%) of cholangiocarcinoma has been reported, mainly after the second decade of life. Early diagnosis followed by cyst excision and Roux-en-Y reconstruction of the biliary tract is the treatment of choice, even in asymptomatic children.

INDICATIONS FOR WORKUP AND OPERATION

As a result of advances in diagnostic imaging, many asymptomatic choledochal cysts are diagnosed both prenatally and shortly after birth. Infants with a symptomatic choledochal cyst often present at 1 to 3 months of age with obstructive jaundice, acholic stools, and hepatomegaly, with a clinical picture indistinguishable from that of biliary atresia. Another group presents sometime after 2 years of age, usually with the more classic triad of abdominal pain, a palpable abdominal mass, and jaundice. A small subset of patients may present with pancreatitis.

The diagnostic evaluation of a choledochal cyst is centered on imaging studies. Ultrasonography is the best initial screening test. If a choledochal cyst is suspected, 99-technetium di-isopropyl-iminodiacetic acid (DISIDA) scintigraphy or magnetic resonance cholangiopancreatography will usually confirm the diagnosis and provide better anatomic details. Operative cholangiography should be performed to confirm the diagnosis and the anatomic information. Operative cholangiography can be performed either through the gallbladder or directly through the dilated bile duct.

OPERATIVE TECHNIQUE

The patient is placed supine on the operating table, and general endotracheal anesthesia is administered. Both arms are carefully padded and tucked. An orogastric tube is introduced to decompress the stomach, and a urinary catheter is inserted. The bed is usually angled to allow the da Vinci robot (Intuitive Surgical, Sunnyvale, CA) to be brought in at approximately a 45-degree angle over the patient's right shoulder (Fig. 35-1).

After prepping and draping, a 12-mm incision is made in a transverse direction in the inferior aspect of the umbilicus and the fascia is sharply incised. The Veress needle is inserted into the peritoneal cavity using a modified open technique. Utilizing the Step system (Covidien, Mansfield, MA), an expandable sheath is then inserted into the peritoneal cavity, and a 12-mm blunt tip cannula is introduced through the expandable sheath. (If the diagnosis is not certain by preoperative

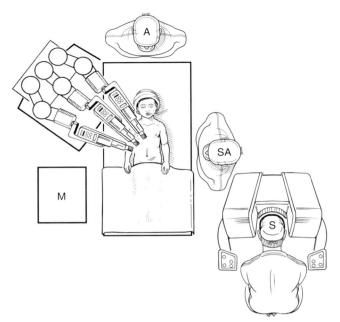

Figure 35-1.   For robotic excision of a choledochal cyst, the patient is placed supine on the operating table. The robot is positioned over the patient's right shoulder. The surgeon's (S) console is on the side of the room opposite the robot. The bedside surgeon (SA) is also located on the patient's left side. The monitor (M) is positioned so all members of the operating team can have good visualization. The scrub nurse can be positioned according to the surgeon's preference. A, anesthesiologist.

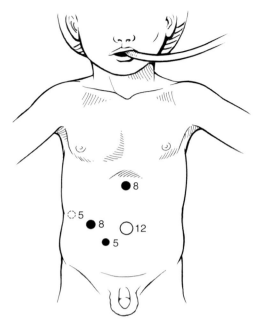

Figure 35-2.   Ports for robotic excision of a choledochal cyst. A 12-mm port is positioned in the umbilicus for use of a 12-mm, 30-degree angled three-dimensional telescope. Two 8-mm da Vinci cannulas are introduced, one in the mid-right upper abdomen and the other near the midline in the subxiphoid region. A 5-mm port is positioned in the right lower abdomen and is used as a retraction port by the bedside surgeon. An additional 5-mm port for liver retraction can be placed laterally near the right flank (*dotted circle*), if needed.

imaging, then a 5-mm port is inserted initially in the umbilicus for the intraoperative cholangiogram to confirm the diagnosis.) The peritoneal cavity is then insufflated with CO_2 to a pressure of 15 mm Hg. A 12-mm, 30-degree angled telescope is used throughout the procedure.

Two 8-mm da Vinci ports and a 5-mm accessory port are inserted (Fig. 35-2). A second 5-mm cannula can be inserted laterally in the right upper abdomen for additional liver retraction, if needed. (This has been needed in only one of our cases, when the falciform ligament was divided. The superior portion of the divided falciform ligament was secured and the liver was retracted cephalad. If exposure is still compromised, then another liver retractor, such as a fan retractor, can be introduced through this second 5-mm port.) We use the Step system for placing all cannulas. Before engaging the robot, the patient is placed in 30-degree reverse Trendelenburg position.

The surgeon begins the dissection by taking down the gallbladder in a retrograde fashion. Much of the initial dissection is accomplished with an atraumatic grasper in the surgeon's left hand and a hook cautery in the right hand. Additional retraction and exposure is provided with an atraumatic grasper placed through the accessory port. By taking down the gallbladder in a retrograde fashion, all of the short branches of the cystic artery are

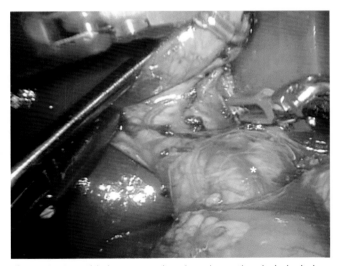

Figure 35-3.   This intraoperative view shows the choledochal cyst (*asterisk*) in the right upper abdomen. The gallbladder is being taken down from its liver bed.

ligated close to the gallbladder. Therefore, clipping or ligating the cystic artery separately is usually not necessary. The cystic duct is preserved and leads the surgeon down to the level of the choledochal cyst (Fig. 35-3). The portal dissection is then begun. The choledochal cyst must be carefully dissected, preserving the hepatic arteries as well as the portal vein lying posterior to it. When there is significant inflammation, the dissection, especially around the portal vein, can be quite treacherous. Sometimes, complete excision of the cyst is not possible, and then alternative reconstruction techniques can be accomplished by preserving the posterior wall of the cyst lying anterior to the portal vein. In the majority of cases, however, complete cyst excision is possible.

The cyst dissection in the porta hepatis is started on the inferior half of the cyst. Once the portal vein and hepatic vessels are separated from the cyst in its midportion, the dissection is carried inferiorly toward the pancreas (Fig. 35-4A). The cyst will eventually be found to taper rapidly to a small duct that often enters the pancreatic duct (see Fig. 35-4B). The common bile duct is then transected and suture ligated with careful attention to protect the pancreatic duct (Fig. 35-5). The cyst is then dissected cephalad until a transition from the abnormal cyst to normal-caliber hepatic ducts is identified. In some circumstances, the hepatic ducts may separately enter the large choledochal cyst and must be divided from it. The choledochal cyst and gallbladder are exteriorized through the umbilical port at the completion of the reconstruction. If the ducts were divided individually, a common confluence of the ducts is created by connecting the ducts with a few 4-0 Vicryl (Ethicon, Inc., Somerville, NJ) sutures placed along their medial walls (Fig. 35-6).

We prefer to complete the Roux-en-Y biliary reconstruction completely, using the da Vinci robot. Other groups have created the jejunostomy through an enlarged umbilical incision after performing the hepaticojejunostomy. We prefer a 20- to 30-cm Roux limb that is delivered to the porta hepatis in a retrocolic fashion. The jejunojejunostomy is either stapled or robotically sewn, depending on the size of the patient. All mesenteric defects are closed robotically. The hepaticojejunostomy is created with interrupted sutures using either 4-0 or 5-0 Vicryl or PDS (Ethicon Inc, Somerville, NJ) suture. As in our open technique, the back wall of the anastomosis is completed first, usually in an end-to-side fashion, with the entire back row of sutures placed before tying any of the sutures (Fig. 35-7A). The anterior anastomosis is accomplished with interrupted sutures, with the knots outside the anastomotic lumen (see Fig. 35-7B). A closed suction drain is situated in the porta hepatis and exteriorized through one of the port-site incisions. All of the other incisions are closed with absorbable suture. The skin incisions are approximated with Steri-Strips (3M, St. Paul, MN). The urinary cathe-

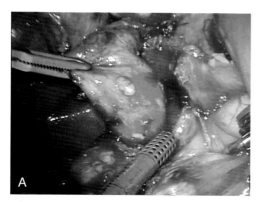
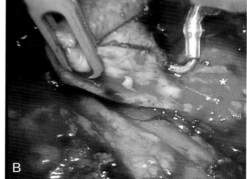

Figure 35-4. **A,** The cyst has been mobilized circumferentially and the dissection is proceeding down to the duodenum. **B,** The cyst tapers as it nears the pancreas (*asterisk*).

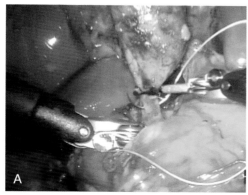
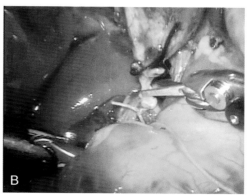

Figure 35-5. After ligating the cyst, the caudal aspect of the common bile duct is suture ligated (**A**) and then divided between the ligatures (**B**).

ter and orogastric tube are removed at the completion of the procedure.

POSTOPERATIVE CARE

The patients are admitted to a standard postoperative surgical unit and started on a diet as soon as there is evidence of return of bowel function. Some of our patients have started eating as early as 48 hours, but others have required a number of days for return of bowel function, most likely related to the return of function of the jejunojejunostomy. When ready for discharge, once-daily oral antibiotics and Ursodiol, usually three doses a day, are prescribed.

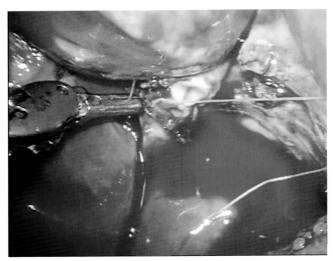

Figure 35-6.   Often, the right and left hepatic ducts are found to enter a large choledochal cyst, and they are divided separately from the cyst. It is helpful to create a common hepatic duct so that a single hepaticojejunostomy can be performed. Here, the two hepatic ducts are being sewn together to create a common hepatic duct.

PEARLS

1. Consider performing robotic cholecystectomies to gain experience with robotic port placement and robot positioning for operations in the right upper abdomen.
2. When undertaking a "new" procedure with the robot, it is good to have the company's clinical expert in attendance, as well as a second surgeon who is proficient in robotic operations.
3. Begin dissection of the cyst off the portal vein on the more inferior and lateral portion of the common bile duct.
4. Ligating the caudal end of the cyst facilitates the proximal dissection.
5. Divide the common hepatic duct sharply, and perform the hepaticojejunostomy the same way the open operation is done.

PITFALLS

1. Use of the 5-mm robotic instruments is advocated by some surgeons, but we find the working space to be larger than expected. Thus, we believe the 8-mm instruments allow more accurate dissection and suturing of the anastomosis.
2. Avoid placing the lateral da Vinci port posterior to the anterior axillary line.
3. Avoid positioning the da Vinci operative ports too close to the costal margins, especially if creation of the Roux limb will be accomplished robotically.

RESULTS

We have now completed five complex biliary operations using the da Vinci robotic device. This includes excision of four choledochal cysts in patients ranging from 3.5

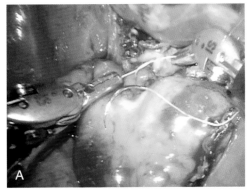
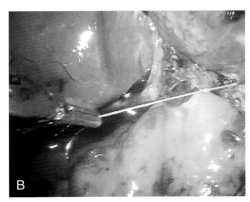

Figure 35-7.   The hepaticojejunostomy is being performed. **A,** The posterior wall of the hepaticojejunostomy anastomosis is being initiated. **B,** One of the lateral sutures between the hepatic duct and the Roux limb is being tied.

to 7 years old and the reconstruction of a complex biliary stricture in a 12-year-old. The Roux limb was fashioned in all patients robotically with the exception of one 3-year-old patient, whose jejunojejunostomy was completed extracorporeally through the umbilicus. The median follow-up has been 2.6 years, and all patients have had a normal bilirubin and no significant symptoms. One patient suffered an afferent limb obstruction 5 weeks postoperatively that was repaired by decompressing the limb, placing the bowel back into a good anatomic position, and reclosing the transverse colon mesenteric defect. There have been no other intraoperative or perioperative complications. The average length of postoperative hospitalization was 5.2 days.

Robotic excision of a choledochal cyst with Roux-en-Y hepaticojejunostomy is feasible and can lead to an excellent long-term outcome. The da Vinci robot provides excellent visualization and facilitates complex dissection and suturing. A larger experience and longer follow-up will be needed to determine if robotic excision of a choledochal cyst offers significant advantages to the patient.

SELECTED REFERENCES

1. Miyano T, Yamataka A, Kato Y, et al: Hepaticoenterostomy after excision of choledochal cyst in children: A 30-year experience with 180 cases. J Pediatr Surg 31:1417-1421, 1996
2. de Vries JS, de Vries S, Aronson DC, et al: Choledochal cysts: Age of presentation, symptoms, and late complications related to Todani's classification. J Pediatr Surg 37:1568-1573, 2002
3. Lee H, Hirose S, Bratton B, et al: Initial experience with complex laparoscopic biliary surgery in children: Biliary atresia and choledochal cyst. J Pediatr Surg 39:804-807, 2004
4. Yu ZL, Zhang LJ, Fu JZ, et al: Anomalous pancreaticobiliary junction: Image analysis and treatment principles. Hepatobiliary Pancreat Dis Int 3:136-139, 2004
5. Le DM, Woo RK, Sylvester K, et al: Laparoscopic resection of type 1 choledochal cysts in pediatric patients. Surg Endosc 20:249-251, 2006
6. Woo R, Le D, Albanese CT, et al: Robot-assisted laparoscopic resection of a type I choledochal cyst in a child. J Laparoendosc Adv Surg Tech 16:179-183, 2006

36
Robotic Fundoplication in Infants and Children

Michael S. Irish

Conventional, minimally invasive surgery for the treatment of pediatric gastroesophageal reflux disease (GERD) has become commonplace, if not the standard, in many pediatric surgical centers. Variations on minimally invasive techniques, instrumentation and outcomes from large series are well described in the literature, as are methods of diagnosis, indications for surgery, and outcomes. The use of robotic surgical systems has increased in the management of many pediatric surgical conditions, including surgical correction of GERD. One of the more commonly performed robotically assisted, minimally invasive (RMIS) procedures is the gastric fundoplication. Recently, the popularity of robotic fundoplication for this procedure has risen because of refinements in the technique and the development of smaller, more pediatrics-appropriate instruments. This chapter describes the use of a robotic surgical system (da Vinci, Intuitive Surgical, Sunnyvale, CA) for performing gastric fundoplication in infants and children. The preoperative investigation and indications for surgery do not vary from those described in Chapter 3 for the laparoscopic Nissen fundoplication. Presently, larger patient size is perhaps the only contraindication to robotic fundoplication. This limitation, as well as the advantages of RMIS for fundoplication, will be discussed in this chapter, along with outcomes of an initial series of patients treated with RMIS fundoplication.

OPERATIVE TECHNIQUE

All patients undergoing a robotic fundoplication are positioned supine, in reverse Trendelenburg, and elevated on foam pads (Fig. 36-1). Particularly for patients weighing less than 10 kg, this elevated position maximizes the vertical, extracorporeal range of motion of the robotic arms and avoids external collision of the arms with the table. A urinary catheter is inserted and the patient is prepared from the nipples to the pubis, and laterally to the posterior flank on either side. In smaller children, an appropriate-size rubber catheter serves nicely as an esophageal dilator and to decompress the stomach.

Although positioning of the ports for robotic fundoplication varies little from a laparoscopic fundoplication, there are subtle differences, particularly in the smaller patients. Extracorporeal range of motion of the robotic arms must be free of collision points. This requires careful planning because, unlike the laparoscopic technique in which a hand-held camera may be moved to another port, once the robotic port sites are chosen, they cannot be interchanged to compensate for a poorly placed port. External arm collisions occur with broad movements of the instruments placed through cannulas positioned too close to each other. We find that ports placed at least 7 to 8 cm (a hand-breadth) away from each other allow the best range of motion of the instruments. This distance is clearly not possible in an infant, in which case spacing the ports as far apart as possible in the illustrated array (Fig. 36-2) is desirable. Where cannula proximity is necessary in the smaller patients, limited intracorporeal range of motion of the instruments may need to be accepted. However, the degrees of motion of the instrument tip are generally preserved with this arrangement.

After the prepping and draping, cannula placement begins with insertion of an umbilical cannula for the telescope. An intraumbilical, vertical incision is preferred, followed by incision of the umbilical fascia. Pneumoperitoneum appropriate for the patient's size is established, and a hand-held, 5-mm laparoscope is inserted to initially explore the abdomen and to directly visualize placement of the subsequent ports. If a gastrostomy (GT) is needed, it is helpful to mark its anticipated location before insufflation. A 5-mm port is then placed there, through which the viscera can be manipulated for placement of subsequent cannulas. Next, liver retraction is addressed, and there are several alternatives to accom-

plish adequate liver retraction. An endoscopic Kittner (Aspen Surgical, Caledonia, MI), placed through a sub-xiphoid, 3-mm stab incision and held stationery by a table-mounted cannula sleeve stabilizer (Wolf, Vernon Hills, IL) provides excellent elevation and cephalad retraction of the left lobe of the liver, particularly in patients smaller than 10 kg (Fig. 36-3). A cannula need not be used here, as the Kittner will remain stationary. In a similar technique, an in-line, atraumatic, locking grasper can be inserted through a right flank incision,

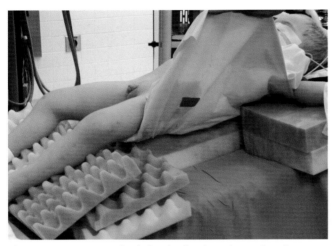

Figure 36-1. For a robotic fundoplication, the patient is elevated off the operating table on foam pads. For small patients, this elevated position maximizes the range of motion of the robotic arms and avoids external collision of the arms with the table.

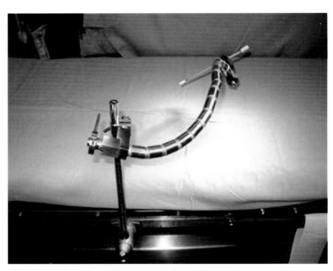

Figure 36-3. The table-mounted stabilizer allows excellent elevation and cephalad retraction of the left lobe of the liver. As seen here, a Kittner can be used to provide liver retraction.

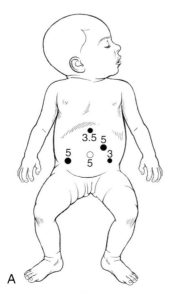
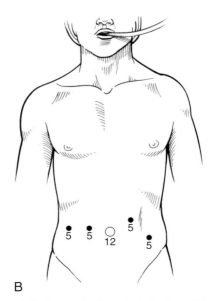

A   B

Figure 36-2. Port placement for a robotic fundoplication. **A,** For an infant, the site for exteriorization of the gastrostomy is the 5-mm left epigastric port. **B,** For an adolescent, a 12-mm port is placed through the umbilicus for utilization of the three-dimesional telescope. The other ports are 5 mm in size. Again, the 5-mm left epigastric port is used for the gastrostomy. It is important to position these ports as far apart from each other as possible, to allow the best range of motion of the instruments.

positioned beneath the liver, and secured to the diaphragm, thereby elevating the liver off the esophagus. Alternatively, any number of expanding or coiling retractors may also serve to gain adequate exposure, depending on the patient's size. Finally, with the four-arm robotic system, the third working arm may be used for exposure and liver retraction.

Placement of the right and left working ports or a fourth arm working port depends on the size of the patient. Although it is not always possible, placing the working ports 2 to 3 cm in front of the horizontal plane of the camera port allows visualized instrument exchanges. The 5-mm, "left arm" working port is placed in the right abdomen. In patients weighing less than 10 kg, this port is best placed in the right lower quadrant, and more cephalad in larger patients. This cannula is positioned to provide direct, in-line access to the esophageal hiatus, unobstructed by the liver. In a larger patient, where a fourth arm may be readily used as both a liver retractor and a working instrument, a 5-mm cannula is situated farther in the right flank for this purpose.

The 5-mm, "right arm" port may be inserted through the GT site or in the patient's left lower quadrant. It is advantageous, in smaller children and infants, to use the GT site as the right-arm working port and to place a 3-mm assistant's port in the right lower quadrant. The function of these ports may be interchanged (Fig. 36-4A).

After placement of the ports, liver retractor, and esophageal dilator, the surgical cart is docked (see Fig. 36-4B). The cart is brought in from the head of the table, centered on the camera port, and locked in a position that allows the arms to be lowered and locked on the cannulas. Once docked, the operating surgeon scrubs out and moves to the surgeon's console.

The operation begins with division of the short gastric vessels. This part of the procedure is performed with the surgeon distracting the stomach with an atraumatic grasping instrument in the left hand and dividing the short gastric vessels with either hook cautery or the robotic Harmonic Scalpel (Ethicon Endosurgery, Inc., Cincinnati, OH) in the right. Alternatively, division of the short gastric vessels may be performed with a hand-held Ligasure (Covidien, Mansfield, MA) before docking the robot. This short gastric dissection is carried to the left crus of the diaphragm. Using the blunt-tipped atraumatic grasping instruments, and with the help of an assistant distracting the stomach in either a left or right caudal direction, the phreno-esophageal ligament is divided using hook cautery from the right crus, across the anterior portion of the gastroesophageal junction, ending at the previously dissected plane at the left crus. Once this has been completed, an atraumatic grasping instrument is inserted through the right working port, and blunt dissection is carried out to open the retro-esophageal window from the right to left crus. If a large hiatal hernia is present, or if additional intra-abdominal esophageal length is needed, further dissection can be performed. Because of the maneuverability of the camera and articulating instruments, this dissection is facilitated and the surgeon has direct access to several centimeters in the lower mediastinum.

Crural reapproximation is completed with interrupted 2-0 or 3-0, braided, permanent suture on an RB or SH needle. The suture may be passed in a number of ways. In infants and small children, the suture may be introduced transcutaneously below the xiphoid. If a 5-mm assistant's port is used, the suture may be passed by the bedside assistant through this port with a 3-mm laparoscopic instrument. The length of suture is between 3 and 5 cm, depending on the size of the patient and the crural defect (Fig. 36-5). If additional exposure to the retroesophageal space is needed, a $^1/_4$-inch Penrose drain can be used to encircle the esophagus, and this is secured with an endoclip. The esophagus can then be elevated and retracted by the assistant to optimize exposure.

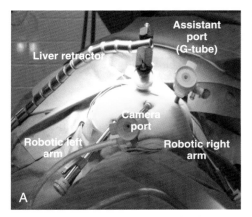
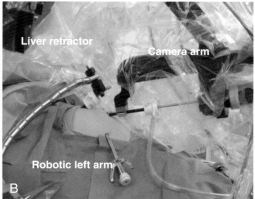

Figure 36-4.   Port placement for a robotic fundoplication. **A,** The ports are placed before docking the robot. **B,** The robot has been locked into a position that allows the arms to be lowered and locked onto the cannulas. Once the robot is docked, the operating surgeon scrubs out and moves to the surgeon's console.

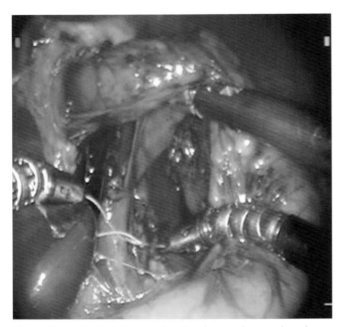

Figure 36-5. Crural reapproximation in a patient undergoing a robotic fundoplication.

A 360-degree fundoplication is then performed and inspected for any torsion, tension, or constriction. The wrap is secured with interrupted nonabsorbable sutures. Three sutures are placed incorporating the anterior wall of the esophagus. A 1.5- to 2.0-cm fundoplication is created for infants and small children, whereas a 2.0- to 2.5-cm wrap is preferred in larger children and adolescents.

GASTROSTOMY TUBE PLACEMENT

Robotic placement of a gastrostomy is possible, and we used it in three patients, but it is awkward and time consuming. Therefore, it is preferable to complete the fundoplication, undock the robot, and reinsert the hand-held laparoscopic instruments. The gastrostomy is then accomplished using the laparoscopic technique described in Chapter 6.

PEARLS AND PITFALLS

For Pearls and Pitfalls of laparoscopic Nissen fundoplication, please see Chapter 3, as they pertain to the procedure in general. The following Pearls and Pitfalls apply to *robotically assisted* fundoplication.

1. When beginning robotically assisted surgery it is advisable to do the following:
   (a) Begin with basic procedures (cholecystectomy, fundoplication) in healthy patients, preferably adolescents.
   (b) Direct the operating room setup, and communicate the logistics of the procedure (patient positioning, anesthesia positioning, and access, choice of instruments, and camera) to the operating room (OR) staff and anesthesiologist.
   (c) Rehearse urgent, open conversion protocol(s) with the OR staff, assistant, and anesthesiologist.
   (d) Plan subsequent cases with a dedicated robotics OR team
2. Carefully plan port positions to avoid external collisions of robotic arms (see text).
3. Use a standard endoscope rather than the robotic endoscope for intracorporeal guidance in placement of cannulas.
4. Remain scrubbed during the docking procedure until robotic arms are secured and instruments passed.
5. The assistant should be familiar with both robotic and laparoscopic instruments and technique, and should be capable of undocking the robot.
6. If an esophageal dilator is used, place it in the desired position before docking the robot.
7. When suturing, avoid grasping the suture excessively, as this will weaken the suture and may lead to breakage.
8. Use an assistant's port to avoid unnecessary robotic instrument exchanges. Have the assistant pass, cut, and retrieve suture material.
9. If a gastrostomy is also needed, it can be performed robotically, but it is more quickly accomplished using standard laparoscopic technique.

RESULTS

From October 2002 to July of 2006, 98 patients underwent RMIS at Blank Children's Hospital in Des Moines, Iowa. Sixteen children (seven girls, nine boys) with a mean age of 8.5 years (range, 1.2 months to 17 years) and a mean weight of 44.4 kg (range, 6.8 to 82 kg) underwent robotically assisted, laparoscopic Nissen fundoplication. Fourteen patients also needed a gastrostomy and one patient underwent pyloroplasty. The indications for surgery were gastroesophageal reflux in all cases, with the presence of a hiatal hernia in nine, esophageal stricture in one, failure to thrive in five, and delayed gastric emptying in one. All procedures were completed successfully with the da Vinci system without the need for conversion. Blood loss was negligible in all cases. The mean postoperative length of hospitalization for all patients was 4.2 days (range, 1 to 16 days). Postoperative complications included dysphagia in three of our earliest patients. One had spontaneous resolution and two required dilation. Additional complications included a superficial wound infection around the gastrostomy in one patient. A recurrent hiatal hernia with recurrent reflux developed in two patients, both requiring reoperation 18 and 36 months after their original surgery.

In this series, robotic fundoplication is shown to be feasible and safe in patients as small as 6.8 kg. Other centers have reported the use of this system for fundoplication in smaller patients. Advantages of this technology include the increased range of motion of robotic instruments, imparting the ability to perform delicate and precise procedures in small spaces. Currently, the use of a 5-mm camera sacrifices the advantage of three-dimensional vision available to the surgeon with the larger 12-mm camera. Finally, limited tactile feedback continues to be a disadvantage compared with open surgery. We do not directly attribute any of our complications to the robotic technique.

SELECTED REFERENCES

1. Holcomb GW III: Laparoscopy. In Ziegler MM, Azizkhan RG, Weber TR (eds): Operative Pediatric Surgery. New York, McGraw-Hill, pp 507-510, 2003

2. Luebbe BN, Woo R, Wolf SA, et al: Robotically-assisted minimally invasive surgery in children. Pediatr Endosurg Innov Tech 7:385-402, 2003

3. Jesch NK, Schmidt AI, Strassburg A, et al: Laparoscopic fundoplication in neurologically impaired children with percutaneous endoscopic gastrostomy. Eur J Pediatr Surg 14:89-92, 2004

4. Knight CG, Lorincz A, Gidell KM, et al: Computer-assisted robot-enhanced laparoscopic fundoplication in children. J Pediatr Surg 39:864-866, 2004

5. Diaz DM, Gibbons TE, Heiss K, et al: Antireflux surgery outcomes in pediatric gastroesophageal reflux disease. Am J Gastroenterol 100:1844-1852, 2005

6. Rothenberg SS: The first decade's experience with laparoscopic Nissen fundoplication in infants and children. J Pediatr Surg 40:142-146, 2005

7. Esposito C, Montupet P, van Der Zee D, et al: Long-term outcome of laparoscopic Nissen, Toupet, and Thal antireflux procedures for neurologically normal children with gastroesophageal reflux disease. Surg Endosc 20:855-858, 2006

37
Retroperitoneoscopic Nephrectomy

Jean-Stephane Valla

The lateral position for retroperitoneal access has been used for more than 10 years in adults and children. This access has been shown to be reliable for a large number of operations, particularly total ureteronephrectomy, pyeloplasty, and pyelotomy. The lateral position is familiar to the urologist, and it provides more complete access to the distal ureter. If an urgent open conversion is needed, the lateral position offers the best exposure to control injury to the great vessels. Thus, our usual approach is to perform nephrectomy retroperitoneally unless there are specific reasons to perform it transperitoneally.

However, despite the advantages of the retroperitoneal approach, the lateral approach is more often associated with perforation of the peritoneum and with reduction of space and visibility. Therefore, special attention must be paid to reduce exposure problems.

INDICATIONS FOR WORKUP AND OPERATION

The preoperative evaluation for total nephrectomy is the same whether the kidney is removed with the open or the minimally invasive technique. The complete absence of function on a renal scan is a good indication; if residual function is still present but less than 10% to 15%, the options are renal salvage or removal. Other factors, such as the presence of infection or hypertension, may help decide which option is best.

The usual indications for nephrectomy include a kidney destroyed by an obstructive or refluxing uropathy, a multicystic dysplastic kidney, or a pretransplant nephrectomy. There is no absolute contraindication to retroperitoneoscopic nephrectomy except renal malignancy. Relative contraindications include multiple prior renal surgeries, uncontrolled infection, and coagulopathy.

OPERATIVE TECHNIQUE

Children are prepared for surgery as usual without bowel preparation. General anesthesia with muscular relaxation and monitoring of end-tidal CO_2 is necessary. Nitrous oxide is generally contraindicated to help reduce bowel distension. A nasogastric tube is introduced for the same purpose. A bladder catheter is inserted to quantify diuresis. Preoperative antibiotics should be administered if the kidney has developed an infection.

The patient is placed in a lateral kidney position with lumbar hyperflexion to enlarge the space between the last rib and the iliac crest. The surgeon and assistant face the back of the patient (Fig. 37-1). The video column stands on the other side; the cables are fixed to the

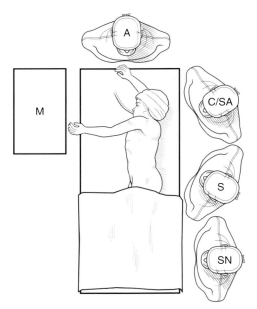

Figure 37-1.   Personnel for a left retroperitoneoscopic nephrectomy. The patient is placed in the true lateral position. The surgeon (S) stands at the patient's back with the surgical assistant/camera holder (C/SA) on the right. The monitor (M) is positioned in line with the operating instruments and opposite the surgeon. The scrub nurse (SN) is positioned to the surgeon's left. A, anesthesiologist.

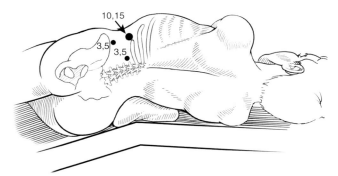

Figure 37-2.   For a left retroperitoneoscopic nephrectomy, the patient is placed in the lateral kidney position with lumbar hyperflexion to enlarge the space between the 12th rib and the iliac crest. A telescope is introduced through the initial skin incision (10 to 15 mm), made just below the tip of the 12th rib in the posterior axillary line (*solid arrow*). The primary working port (3 or 5 mm) is introduced in the costospinal angle at the junction of the lateral border of the erector spinae muscle with the underside of the 12th rib. The inferior port (3 or 5 mm) is inserted just above the iliac crest. It must not be placed too close to the iliac crest, because the bony crest could restrict the movement of the instruments placed through this site.

superior part of the operative field. If a total ureterectomy is needed at the same time, the position of the surgeon and the assistant, and the position of the video column, may change during the procedure, so the installation must be planned accordingly.

We favor an open technique for initial retroperitoneal access. This is a key point of the technique because the majority of complications deal with retroperitoneal access and the development of a working field. After sterile preparation and draping, anatomic landmarks are palpated (11th and 12th ribs, iliac crest, sacrospinalis muscle) and the surgeon mentally localizes the lateral peritoneal reflection. To avoid a frustrating gas leak, the size of the incision for the first cannula must be chosen carefully and depends on the size of the patient (0 to 18 years), the thickness of the abdominal wall (thin or obese child), the kidney disease (e.g., small or huge kidney, presence of perinephritis adhesion). Also, consideration must be given to the extraction of the specimen—for example, enlargement of the subcostal hole or inguinal incision to remove the entire ureter with the specimen. A 10-mm scope in a small child requires more working space and could compete with the operating instruments. The choice of which telescope to use must be adapted to each case. For example, when removing a dysplastic multicystic kidney in a normal child less than 2 years of age, a 5-mm telescope and two 3-mm cannulas for the operating instruments seems a good option. On the other hand, to remove a large hydrone-

phrotic infected kidney in an obese teenager, the only way to obtain primary access is by quite a large (15- to 20-mm) skin incision and the use of a large cannula with balloon.

The initial skin incision (8- to 15-mm long) is made just below the tip of the 12th rib at the posterior axillary line, in the area where the muscular wall is the thinnest (Fig. 37-2). A muscle-splitting dissection is used to gain access into the retroperitoneal space. Dissecting forceps, S-retractors, and Metzenbaum scissors are usually used to bluntly spread the external and internal oblique muscles. After piercing the white transversalis fascia with the tip of the scissors, the dissection is stopped when the yellow perirenal fat becomes visible. Two 2-0 stay sutures are placed on each side of the muscular layers. In the case of a large (15-mm) incision, it is sometimes possible to recognize the Gerota's fascia and incise it to begin CO_2 insufflation directly in the perirenal space. Most often, however, Gerota's fascia is not visible, so the working space is created in the retroperitoneal space and Gerota's fascia is opened in the following step.

To create an adequate working field, a small gauze is introduced in the retroperitoneal space and manipulated carefully to create the space. The surgeon must keep the dissection close to the posterior muscular wall to avoid peritoneal perforation. Next, the primary blunt port (5 to 10 mm, disposable or reusable) is introduced and secured to create a seal for the retropneumoperitoneum. CO_2 insufflation is started (8 to 10 mm in infants, 12 to 15 mm in children) and a 0- or 30-degree telescope is inserted. The working space, already created by the gauze, is progressively enlarged by moving the tip of the telescope, used as a palpator to free retroperitoneal fibrous tissues, behind the kidney. This allows visualization of the anatomic landmarks: the quadratus lumborum, psoas muscles, and posterior part of the kidney. A sufficient operating space is achieved by pushing away peritoneum and intra-abdominal organs and by dissecting the lateral peritoneal reflection at least to the anterior axillary line.

Next, two additional ports (3 or 5 mm) are placed under direct vision: the posterior port is introduced first, in the costospinal angle, at the junction of the lateral border of the erector spinae muscle with the underside of the 12th rib. Before placing the inferior port just above the iliac crest, an instrument (palpator for 3-mm port, endopeanut for 5-mm port) is inserted through the posterior port and is used to gently sweep medially the lateral peritoneal reflection in the lower part of the field so the third inferior cannula can be introduced safely. This inferior cannula must not be placed too close to the iliac crest, because the bony crest could restrict movement of instruments placed through this cannula. This port placement allows a triangulation of ports to maximize exposure and minimize instrument conflict in a small working space (see Fig. 37-2).

VASCULAR CONTROL

At this time, landmarks should be clearly visualized, especially the posterior part of the kidney, great vessels, and ureter. With the help of two atraumatic instruments (palpator, grasper, or peanut), Gerota's fascia is opened (if not already open) along the posterior part of kidney.

Anterior dissection should be limited at the beginning of the dissection to prevent peritoneal injury and to keep the kidney from flipping ventrally. On the other hand, if the anterior peritoneal adherences are kept intact, the kidney is automatically retracted anteriorly by the insufflation pressure and pushed to the top of the field, which yields good posterior access to the hilum (Fig. 37-3). If this spontaneous retraction is not sufficient, a third operating device, usually 3 mm, can be introduced in the midaxillary line for retraction of the kidney in the upper part of the field.

Dissection with a hook cautery or scissors cleans the artery and vein. They appear vertically oriented. The main renal vessels must be dissected in the inferior part of the field, where there is only one artery and one vein, and not too close to the kidney hilum where the vessels divide into several branches. The vessels do not need to be ligated and divided at their origin with the aorta and vena cava, but a sufficiently wide area of exposure (at least 1 cm) is necessary to allow safe control on each side of the intended site of division.

If the search for renal vessels proves difficult, the ureter may serve as a landmark. The ureter is easy to find

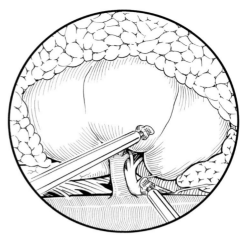

Figure 37-3. With the retroperitoneal approach, the kidney is automatically retracted anteriorly by the insufflation pressure and pushed to the top of the operating field, which yields good access to the hilum. The artery and vein are oriented vertically. If it is difficult to identify the artery and vein, it is usually easy to find the ureter in the retroperitoneal space, which can be dissected up to the pelvis where the vessels are found.

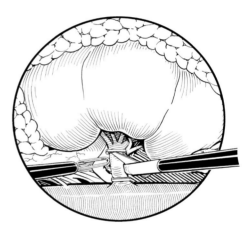

Figure 37-4. The artery is usually controlled first. Here, clips have been placed on the artery and it is being divided. In small patients, the artery can be ligated or divided with the harmonic scalpel or cautery.

in the retroperitoneal space, and its dissection up to the kidney leads to the renal vessels.

The artery is controlled first (Fig. 37-4). Many different means of hemostasis can be used, according to the anatomic situation and the vessel's diameter. Monopolar or bipolar coagulation with the hook can be used with smaller vessels. The ultrasonic scalpel or Ligasure (Covidien, Mansfield, MA) can be used for control of mid-size vessels and extracorporeal or intracorporeal ligatures or endoscopic clips can be used for large vessels.

After vascular control, dissection using electrocautery or the ultrasonic scalpel continues from cephalad to caudad around the kidney. Polar vessels can be encoun-

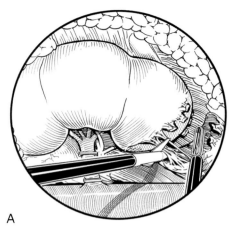
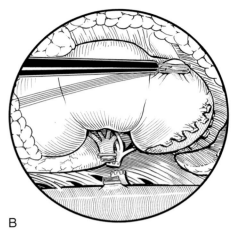

A   B

Figure 37-5.   After vascular control, dissection using electrocautery or the ultrasonic scalpel continues around the kidney. **A,** The kidney and adrenal gland can usually be separated through an avascular plane. **B,** The kidney has been completely freed.

tered at this time, and smaller vessels can usually be ligated with cautery. Larger vessels may require the ultrasonic scalpel. The kidney and adrenal gland can usually be separated using an avascular plane (Fig. 37-5A). Finally, the anterior part of the kidney is completely freed and the kidney is totally mobilized (see Fig. 37-5B).

URETERAL MANAGEMENT

In the case of a nonrefluxing or atrophic ureter, the ureterectomy can be limited to the lumbar part, and a ligature is not necessary prior to dividing it. On the other hand, in case of a refluxing or dilated ureter, a total ureterectomy is necessary to avoid postoperative complications related to the stump.

In children less than 5 or 6 years, it is possible to remove the lower part of the ureter by retroperitoneoscopy (Fig. 37-6). After changing the team position, the ureteral dissection is carried out down to the bladder, taking care not to injure the peritoneum (which is very adherent to the ureter), or the gonadal vessels. The smaller the child, the easier it is to reach the bladder. In boys, the vas is seen crossing the ureter and marks the inferior level of resection. The ureter can be ligated with a pre-tied ligature or an extracorporeal tie.

In children older than 5 or 6, particularly in girls with an ectopic ureter, it is preferable to remove the lower part of the ureter in an open manner through a low inguinal incision. This short incision allows ligation of the ureter close to the bladder or vagina. Moreover, the kidney and ureter can be extracted through this incision.

SPECIMEN REMOVAL

The benign nature of most pediatric renal diseases allows removal without concern for spillage. Endo-

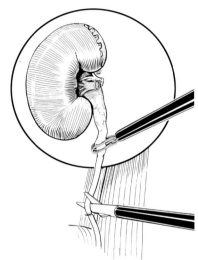

Figure 37-6.   In younger children, it is possible to remove the lower part of the ureter through the retroperitoneal approach. The ureter is dissected down to the bladder, taking care to avoid injuring the peritoneum or the gonadal vessels. Here, the distal ureter has been ligated with a ligature.

scopic retrieval bags are difficult to manipulate in the retroperitoneal space and are unnecessary most of the time. The difficulty of specimen extraction varies and depends on its size. In the case of a multicystic dysplastic kidney, extraction is very easy after puncture of all the cysts. In the same manner, in the case of a small kidney or a kidney with very thin cortex, extraction can be performed without morcellation. Large specimens can be removed after enlargement of the 10-mm hole, with or without the use of an endobag and morcellation. If a low incision (inguinal or Pfannenstiel) is needed for another purpose, the kidney can be removed through it.

After extraction, the port and telescope are reintroduced to check for hemostasis (at low insufflation pressure), particularly near the hilum. If needed, a drain is introduced through the inferior cannula. The ports are removed under direct vision. The closure of the fascia is easy because of the two stay sutures placed at the beginning of the procedure. Port sites are injected with bupivacaine and lidocaine. The skin is closed with subcuticular sutures or adhesive strips.

POSTOPERATIVE CARE

If drainage is needed, the drain is removed on postoperative day 1 or 2. An ultrasound is performed at 1 week and again at 1 month postoperatively to check the lumbar area.

PEARLS AND PITFALLS

1. *Dense perirenal adhesions* resulting from previous nephrostomy, repeated perinephritis, or xanthogranulomatous pyelonephritis were considered as a contraindication for retroperitoneoscopic nephrectomy at the beginning of our experience. Now, we attempt a retroperitoneoscopic approach on these patients and are successful most of the time.
2. In case of nephrectomy for *horseshoe or ectopic sigmoid kidney*, aberrant vascular anatomy is common and a careful dissection and clamping before vessel division is mandatory. The ultrasonic scalpel is advantageous for cutting between healthy and destroyed parenchyma.
3. Destroyed kidneys with *giant hydronephrosis* are usually soft with low pressure. A careful open approach allows one to avoid entering the renal cortex or pelvis during the first port placement. After the posterior part is dissected, the renal pelvis is decompressed with an aspirating needle under visualization, which greatly improves exposure and creates a large working space.
4. Creation of the working space in the retroperitoneum can be accomplished with conventional instruments or with an inflatable balloon. The balloon technique seems superfluous in children, because the pediatric retroperitoneum differs significantly from the adult retroperitoneum in generally having less fat and fewer adhesions. The most common complication is peritoneal tear, particularly in smaller children, in whom the peritoneum is thinner and less layered with fat. An accidental perforation induces pneumoperitoneum and reduces the retroperitoneal working space and visibility. In smaller children, the peritoneum is permeable, and intraperitoneal insufflation can occur after prolonged operative time, even without a visible tear.
5. The peritoneum is particularly vulnerable at the beginning of the procedure, when creating the retroperitoneal working space, and at the end of the procedure, when dissecting the anterior part of the kidney and the lower part of the ureter. If peritoneal insufflation occurs at the beginning of the procedure, there are several potential solutions: the most elegant, but also the most difficult, is to close the perforation with a purse-string 5-0 suture. The most simple is to desufflate the pneumoperitoneum continuously using a Veress needle. An unexpected peritoneal perforation has never been the sole reason for conversion in our experience.

RESULTS

From 1993 to 2006, 100 total nephrectomies were performed in our department for the following indications: multicystic dysplastic kidney (29 cases, two of which had crossed ectopia), kidney destroyed by reflux (35 cases), kidney destroyed by obstructive uropathy (28 cases with three cases of horseshoe kidney), small kidney with hypertension (three cases), small "invisible" kidney with incontinence (four cases), and xanthogranulomatous pyelonephritis (one case). There were no conversions, no major complications, and no significant blood loss (no transfusion). Intraoperatively, there were 25 cases of peritoneal perforation. In no case did peritoneal perforation induce a conversion. There were four cases of mild subcutaneous emphysema but no incidence of pneumomediastinum or pneumothorax. The mean operative time in these 100 patients was 95 minutes. Three mild postoperative complications occurred: one paralytic ileus, one wound infection, and one hematoma in the operative area. These complications disappeared in 1 week without reoperation. In 32 cases, a small suction drain was left for 24 hours. Pain medication was minimal, and no patient needed pharmacologic medication for relief after 48 hours. One day after surgery, solid food was offered. All children returned to normal unrestricted activities within 6 days. Clinical and ultrasonic checkups were performed 1 week and 1 month after surgery. The follow-up range was 6 months to 13 years (mean, 5.8 years).

SELECTED REFERENCES

1. El Ghoneimi A, Valla JS, Steyaert H, et al: Laparoscopic renal surgery via a retroperitoneal approach in children. J Urol 160:1138-1141, 1998
2. Diemunsch P, Becmeur F, Meyer P: Retroperitoneoscopy versus laparoscopy in piglets: Ventilatory and thermic repercussion. J Pediatr Surg 34:1514-1517, 1999
3. Hemal AK, Gupta NP, Wadhwa SN: Modified minimal cost retroperitoneoscopic nephrectomy, nephrectomy with isthmusectomy and nephroureterectomy in children: A pilot study. BJU Int 83:823-827, 1999
4. Valla JS: Videosurgery of the retroperitoneal space in children. In Bax NMA, Georgeson KE, Najmaldin A, Valla J-S

(eds): Endoscopic Surgery in Children. Berlin, Springer Verlag, pp 379-392, 1999

5. Capolicchio JP, Jednak R, Anidjar M, et al: A modified access technique for retroperitoneoscopic renal surgery in children. J Urol 170:204-206, 2003

6. Peters G: Complications of retroperitoneal laparoscopy in pediatric urology: Prevention, recognition and management. In Caione P, Kavoussi LR, Micali R (eds): Retroperitoneoscopy and Extraperitoneal Laparoscopy in Pediatric and Adult Urology. Milano, Springer Verlag, pp 203-210, 2003

7. Wakabayashi Y, Kataoka A, Johnin K, et al: Simple techniques for atraumatic peritoneal dissection from the abdominal wall and for preventing peritoneal injury during trocar placement under retroperitoneoscopy. J Urol 169:256-257, 2003

8. Borzi PA: A comparison of lateral and posterior retroperitoneoscopic approach for complete and partial nephroureterectomy in children. BJU Int 87:517-520, 2007

38
Robotic Pyeloplasty

Craig A. Peters

Laparoscopic pyeloplasty in children was first described in 1995, yet few surgeons have performed the procedure on a regular basis despite very satisfactory results by those who have. In all likelihood, this is because learning the delicate laparoscopic suturing is a significant challenge. However, the introduction of a robotic assist device, the da Vinci (Intuitive Surgical, Sunnyvale, CA), has diminished this obstacle. In many ways, pyeloplasty is an ideal procedure for the laparoscopic approach: the procedure itself (resecting a small segment of ureter and pelvis and reanastomosis) involves minimal tissue dissection, but accessing the renal pelvis, typically through a flank or dorsal incision, leads to a large portion of the morbidity. Therefore, we have converted to an entirely robotically assisted pyeloplasty for children and now rarely perform the conventional freehand laparoscopic procedure or an open pyeloplasty. This chapter describes our robotic approach and early outcomes (Table 38-1).

INDICATIONS FOR WORKUP AND OPERATION

The indications for a laparoscopic pyeloplasty are the same as for the open operation. Although vigorous debate continues about the indications for repair in asymptomatic children, the rationale is clear in many older children. Pain, infection, and impaired renal function are the absolute indications, and for those without symptoms, the operation choice is based on surgeon and parental preference. Before surgery, an understanding of the functional anatomy is necessary. A radionuclide renal scan can usually provide information about the level of function in the affected kidney. An ultrasound usually reveals the location of the obstruction but does not provide information about the ureter distal to the obstruction. Therefore, if the ureter has not been visualized in some manner, a retrograde pyelogram is performed at the time of repair to ensure that the distal ureter is normal. Although an abnormal distal ureter is rarely seen, it would be a major problem if this were not identified at the time of repair. A voiding cystourethrogram (VCUG) is optional and depends on patient age. Infants with hydronephrosis should have a screening VCUG performed, whereas older children without infection probably do not need this study.

Preoperatively, the patient is given a clear liquid diet the day before the operation, as well as a single suppository or oral laxative to clear the colon of bulky stool. Perioperative antibiotics are administered.

OPERATIVE TECHNIQUE

There are no anesthetic issues specific to pyeloplasty beyond those relevant to pediatric laparoscopy. Sufficient room for the robotic device is needed so that the patient can be accessed and instruments changed without interfering with the anesthesia team.

The patient is placed on a wedge to elevate the affected side about 30 degrees and is secured to the table with tape at the chest and upper legs (Fig. 38-1A). The table is rotated to both sides to ensure the patient is secure (see Fig. 38-1B). For port placement, the patient will be rotated with the affected side down to make the abdomen horizontal. For the operation, the patient will be rotated with the affected side up to provide about 60 degrees of elevation. This permits the colon to fall away

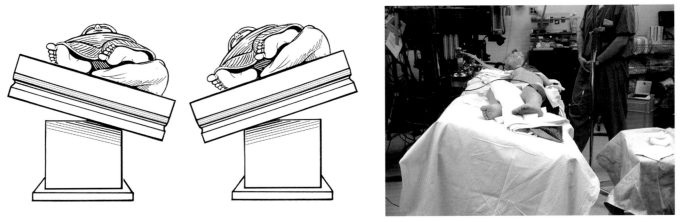

Figure 38-1. The patient is placed on a wedge to elevate the affected side about 30 degrees and is secured to the operating table with tape at the chest and upper legs. In the photograph, the patient is undergoing a left pyeloplasty. The table is rotated to both sides to ensure that the patient is secure.

Table 38-1 Demographic Data for a Series of >30 Patients Undergoing Open and Robotic Pyeloplasty

Parameter	Open	Robotic	*P* value
Age (mean)	6.6	6.9	.83
Operative time (min)	181	222	.012
Length of stay (days)	3.5	2.4	<.001
Postoperative narcotic equivalent	2.8	1.4	.001
Success rate	100%	97%	.16

From Lee RS, Retik AB, Borer JG, Peters CA: J Urol 175:683-687, 2006.

from the kidney. The robotic device is brought in from the side and over the patient's ipsilateral shoulder. The room should be laid out so that both the patient-side assistant surgeon and the scrub nurse can be opposite the robot (Fig. 38-2). Monitors are positioned to permit visualization by all members of the operating team at all times.

The most common arrangement of the cannulas is shown in Figure 38-3, with the endoscope (12 mm) positioned in the umbilicus. One working cannula (5 or 8 mm) is situated in the midline between the xiphoid and the umbilicus. The lower port is placed in the midclavicular line at the level of the anterior superior iliac spine. This cannula may be moved more medially for a small child or for a very large pelvis to prevent it from being too close to the working area and limiting its utility. The working upper epigastric port should not be in the midclavicular line, as it will be too close to the repair.

The umbilical cannula is inserted using an open technique by incising the umbilical skin and fascia in the midline and opening directly into the peritoneum. A 3-0 or 2-0 absorbable suture is placed around the fascia in a purse-string fashion, and it will be used for closure

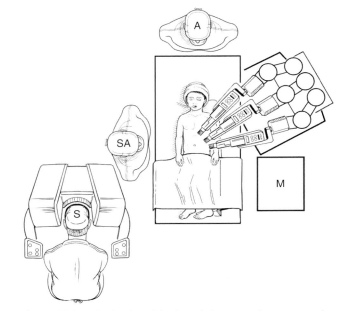

Figure 38-2. Optimal positioning of the operating personnel. The surgical assistant (SA) and the scrub nurse should be on the opposite side of the patient from the robot. The surgeon (S) is at the console. The monitor (M) is positioned to permit visualization by all members of the operating teams at all times. In this diagram, a left pyeloplasty is depicted. The robotic device is brought in from the side and over the patient's ipsilateral shoulder. A, anesthesiologist.

at completion. The two working ports are then introduced under vision after placing a box-stitch purse-string in the fascia. After the ports are inserted, the patient is tilted to the right and the robot is engaged. The robotic arms must be symmetrically arrayed about the camera, which should be directed toward the ureteropelvic junction (UPJ).

The procedure follows most of the same steps as the open and freehand laparoscopic operations. Two options are available for exposure: transmesenteric and

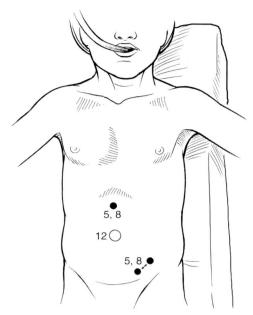

Figure 38-3.   The position of the cannulas. Here, a left pyeloplasty is being performed. The most common arrangement is shown, with a 12-mm telescope introduced through the umbilicus. A 5- or 8-mm working cannula is situated in the midline between the xiphoid and umbilicus. The lower cannula is placed in the midclavicular line at the level of the anterior superior iliac crest. This cannula may be positioned more medially in a smaller child or in a patient with a large pelvis, to prevent it from being too close to the working area and limiting its utility.

retrocolic. On the left side in smaller children, the dilated renal pelvis can usually be seen bulging through the mesentery medial to the colon. By incising the peritoneum over the UPJ and avoiding the mesenteric vessels, the UPJ can be exposed quickly. Alternatively, the colon can be reflected medially, exposing the kidney and pelvis. The UPJ is freed of surrounding tissue, as is the proximal ureter, avoiding devascularization. At this point, a hitch stitch is placed by inserting a 3-0 monofilament suture on an SH needle through the abdominal wall just below the ribs, and passing it through the upper renal pelvis away from the anticipated pyelotomy (Fig. 38-4). The suture is then passed back out the abdominal wall and secured with the correct tension, judged visually, to elevate the pelvis and UPJ. This stabilizes the pelvis for dissection and suturing. Also, it lifts the area of repair out of the pool of urine and blood that invariably develops.

The renal pelvis is incised first, and the cuff attached to the UPJ is used as a handle. This limits the amount of tissue handling and trauma during the procedure. The incision in the pelvis is made in an oblique angle running from the inferior aspect of the pelvis upward and medially. Unless the pelvis is massively enlarged, little effort is made to aggressively reduce its size. Some bleeding can be expected from the cut edge, and significant vessels may be spot cauterized.

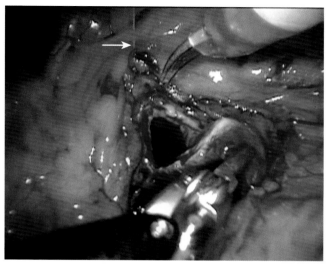

Figure 38-4.   A hitch stitch (*arrow*) is passed through the upper renal pelvis away from the anticipated pyelotomy to help elevate the pelvis and the UPJ. This stitch is introduced through the abdominal wall, and then passed through the pelvis and back out the abdominal wall.

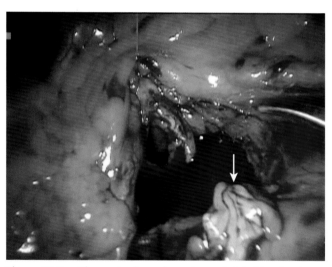

Figure 38-5.   The ureter (*arrow*) can be spatulated by simply cutting with scissors through the UPJ obstruction or by making a partial cut through the ureter just distal to the UPJ and then spatulating the ureter.

The ureter is then spatulated on its lateral aspect. Although it is unlikely to happen because of the large cuff of the renal pelvis, care is taken not to twist the ureter. The ureter can be spatulated by simply cutting through the UPJ obstruction with the scissors, or by making a partial cut through the ureter just distal to the UPJ and then spatulating the ureter (Fig. 38-5). The rest of the pelvis will be removed later. The ureteral spatulation should open up to a healthy, wide ureter. A small segment of a feeding tube can be inserted down the ureter if there is any question.

The pyeloplasty is begun by starting the anastomosis at the lower vertex of the ureteral spatulation. A running suture is usually used, although an interrupted suture technique can also be employed (Fig. 38-6). A monofilament absorbable suture is preferred, although these sutures usually have an annoying amount of memory. However, braided sutures are more traumatic on the tissues. The stitches are placed without pulling too tightly to purse-string the closure. Care is taken to avoid catching the other side wall of the ureter. It seems easier to pass the needle from the inside of the ureter to the outside, but the direction should be determined on a case-by-case basis. The anastomosis continues up to the level where the ureter was separated from the UPJ and pelvis.

At this point, the ureteral stent is inserted, if desired (Fig. 38-7A). We have found that placement of a double-J stent appears to enhance immediate postoperative recovery, avoids the need for a drain, and limits the risk of urinary extravasation. If a stent is not used, a perinephric drain is situated posteriorly at the end of the procedure. In younger children, the stent may be pre-

placed via cystoscopy with a dangling string for removal. Some older children will tolerate this as well for up to 2 weeks. The stent is usually removed cytoscopically in 4 weeks.

The stent is introduced by passing a 14-gauge angiocatheter through the abdominal wall below the costal margin and then inserting a guidewire through the angiocatheter. A stent of appropriate size for the patient is loaded onto the guidewire. After the guidewire is passed down the ureter, the stent is passed over the guidewire and down the ureter until the proximal curl of the stent is at the level of the pelvis. The wire is removed and the curl is positioned in the renal pelvis (see Fig. 38-7B). If there is any uncertainty about positioning, methylene blue dye may be instilled into the bladder and stent location confirmed by retrograde flow of the dye into the renal pelvis.

After the stent is in position, the front wall of the anastomosis is secured. The hitch stitch is then cut, and the pelvis allowed to drop back in position (Fig. 38-8). The peritoneum is closed over the anastomosis if the transmesenteric approach was used or the colon is allowed to fall back in normal position if the retrocolic approach was employed.

POSTOPERATIVE CARE

Postoperatively, a bladder catheter is left overnight. Patients are usually discharged the next day or occasionally the following day, depending on comfort and feeding. The stent is removed in 2 to 4 weeks with cystostomy, and an ultrasound is obtained 4 weeks later to assess hydronephrosis.

PEARLS AND PITFALLS

1. The critical elements for an efficient pyeloplasty include port placement and positioning, the transmesenteric exposure, and the hitch stitch.

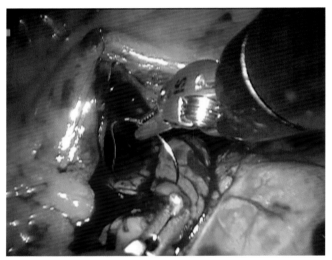

Figure 38-6. The pyeloplasty is initiated by starting the anastomosis at the lower vertex of the ureteral spatulation, as shown here. A running suture is usually used, although an interrupted suture technique can also be employed.

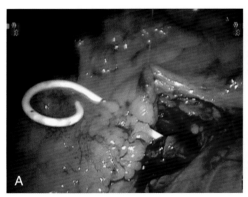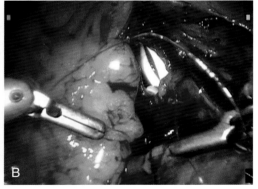

Figure 38-7. After creating the back wall of the anastomosis, the ureteral stent can be inserted, if desired. **A,** The stent is passed down the ureter until the proximal curl of the stent is at the level of the renal pelvis. **B,** After the stent is in position, the front wall of the anastomosis is secured.

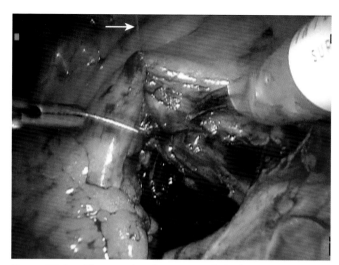

Figure 38-8. The completed anastomosis is shown before release of the hitch stitch (*arrow*). The peritoneum can be closed, if desired.

2. The guiding principle for port placement is to determine the approximate location of the UPJ and imagine a line between it and the umbilicus. An imaginary line between the two working ports should cross this at a right angle and be equidistant from the line of vision (Figure 38-3). This arrangement allows a symmetric array of the working instruments about the line of vision, which maximizes robotic efficiency and movement.
3. When appropriate, transmesenteric exposure is extremely efficient, as there is no need to mobilize the colon. Effective colonic mobilization requires a long line of dissection. Although very feasible, it does require some added operating time. Moreover, there is much more tissue trauma with the retrocolic approach than with the transmesenteric exposure.
4. The hitch stitch is an excellent means of stabilizing the working tissues and maintaining adequate exposure. Care should be taken to place the stitch high enough in the pelvis to avoid interfering with the pyelotomy. Also, the tension on the stitch needs to be monitored as it is being elevated to avoid tearing the renal pelvis.

RESULTS

We recently published a series of robotic pyeloplasties performed in over 30 children and compared them with an open contemporaneous and age-matched group of patients undergoing open pyeloplasty (Lee at al. 2006). There was one operative failure in the robotic group for a patient with a retrocolic pyeloplasty (the only one in the group). This patient had presented with severe pain. Apparently, the crossing vessel was not detected and the obstruction persisted. He then underwent correction using a transperitoneal pyeloplasty approach with good success. Compared with open pyeloplasty, the robotic approach was not significantly different in outcome or complications, but it did have shorter postoperative hospitalization and less postoperative analgesic requirements. Operative times were longer, but the last several cases had identical operating times.

SELECTED REFERENCES

1. Peters CA, Schlussel RN, Retik AB: Pediatric laparoscopic dismembered pyeloplasty. J Urol 153:1962-1965, 1995
2. Peters CA: Laparoscopy in pediatric urology: Challenge and opportunity. Semin Pediatr Surg 5:16-22, 1996
3. El-Ghoneimi A, Farhat W, Bolduc S, et al: Laparoscopic dismembered pyeloplasty by a retroperitoneal approach in children. BJU Int 92:104-108, 2003
4. Peters CA: Robotically assisted surgery in pediatric urology. Urol Clin North Am 31:743-752, 2004
5. Lee RS, Retik AB, Borer JG, Peters CA: Pediatric robot assisted laparoscopic dismembered pyeloplasty: Comparison with a cohort of open surgery. J Urol 175:683-687, 2006

39
Laparoscopic Varicocelectomy

Igor V. Poddoubnyi

A varicocele is a dilation of the pampiniform venous plexus and the internal spermatic vein. In the general population of healthy males, the overall incidence of varicocele is 10% to 15%. Approximately 30% to 50% of males with primary infertility have a varicocele. In fact, scrotal varicoceles are the most common cause of poor testicular sperm production and decreased semen quality. A varicocele is occasionally found in preadolescent boys. The incidence in older adolescents varies from 12% to 18%, with an average of 15%, an incidence similar to that in adult men. Accumulating evidence from animal and human studies has demonstrated that varicoceles are associated with a time-dependent decline in testicular function. Varicoceles may be a cause of progressive damage to the testes, resulting in further atrophy and impairment of seminal parameters.

INDICATIONS FOR WORKUP AND OPERATION

A varicocele is associated with a time-dependant arrest of growth in the testis in adolescent and adult males. Varicocelectomy is known to reverse this testicular growth arrest in adolescents. Surgical treatment is offered to the following:

- Adolescents with testicular growth retardation
- Adolescents with abnormal semen analysis
- Adolescents with symptoms: pain, heaviness, swelling

OPERATIVE TECHNIQUE

Laparoscopic varicocelectomy is performed under general anesthesia with muscle relaxation and controlled ventilation via endotracheal intubation or a laryngeal mask airway. Antibiotic prophylaxis is not administered routinely in these patients. A nasogastric tube is inserted and the stomach is kept deflated. The patient's urinary bladder is catheterized during the procedure.

The patient is placed on the operating table in the supine position. During the procedure, the patient is usually moved to a 10- to 15-degree Trendelenburg position with a slight tilt to the right. The operation is performed with the surgeon operating from the patient's right side. The assistant surgeon, situated on the left side of the patient, holds the camera. A scrub nurse with the instrument table is on the patient's right at the level of the lower limb (Fig. 39-1A). The laparoscopic tray with all necessary instruments and the monitor are on the patient's left at the level of the upper limb.

Three 6-mm cannulas are used in all cases. The first (with blunt tip) is introduced through the umbilicus using a modified open method. This port is used for insertion of a 5-mm 30-degree telescope. The two other 6-mm cannulas are inserted under visual control—one in a suprapubic position and the other in the left iliac area (see Fig. 39-1B). The following 5 mm instruments are usually used: straight atraumatic grasping forceps, curved atraumatic dissecting and grasping forceps, curved scissors, and needle holder.

With the patient in the supine position, the three 6-mm ports are inserted. The patient is moved to the Trendelenburg position with a slight tilt to the right. The spermatic vessels and vas deferens are identified entering the internal inguinal ring. In some cases (8% to 10%), minimal dissection and mobilization of the sigmoid colon is needed to provide optimal visualization of the vessels. A 1.5- to 2.0-cm peritoneal incision is made anterior to the spermatic vessels at a distance of 3 to 4 cm from the internal ring (Fig. 39-2). The entire spermatic vascular cord is freed from the underly-

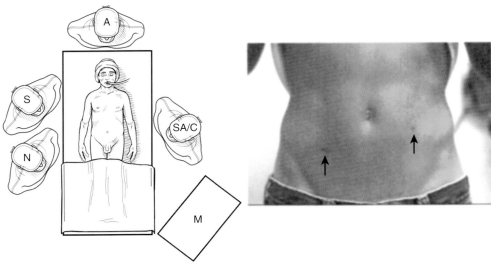

Figure 39-1. **A,** Personnel placement for a laparoscopic varicocelectomy. The patient is placed supine on the operating table and the bed rotated to a 10- to 15-degree Trendelenburg position with a slight tilt to the right. The surgeon (S) stands on the patient's right side and the assistant surgeon/camera hold (SA/C) on the patient's left. The scrub nurse (N) is to the right of the surgeon. The monitor (M) is positioned on the patient's left side at the level of the lower limb. **B,** For the operation, three 6-mm ports are used. The first is introduced through the umbilicus using a modified open method. After insertion of this cannula, a 5-mm 30-degree telescope is introduced through the cannula. Two additional cannulas (*arrows*) are used, one in the left lower abdomen and the other in the right lower abdomen.

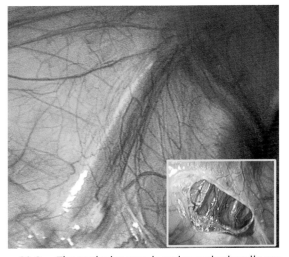

Figure 39-2. The testicular vessels and vascular bundle are viewed through the thin posterior peritoneum and are seen entering the inguinal canal. An incision is made in the peritoneum, exposing the vessels (*inset*).

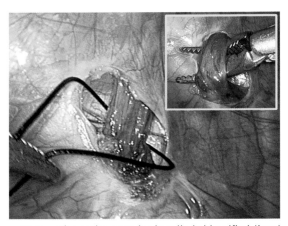

Figure 39-3. The entire vascular bundle is identified (*inset*), isolated, and encircled with a traction suture.

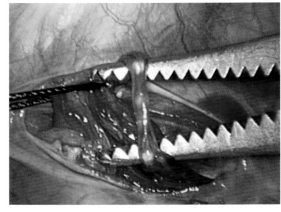

Figure 39-4. Usually, three to five lymphatics accompany the testicular vessels. These are identified and separated from the artery and veins. The lymphatic vessels are preserved to prevent the development of a postoperative hydrocele.

ing psoas muscle and a traction ligature (usually non-absorbable braided material) is placed under the bundle (Fig. 39-3). With careful observation, blunt dissection is used to separate the artery, veins, and lymphatic vessels. Three to five lymphatic vessels are usually seen and are thoroughly isolated from the other elements of the bundle (Fig. 39-4). Excellent intraoperative illumination and magnification facilitates visualization, identification, and dissection of these very thin lymphatic structures. With the exception of the dissected lymphatic vessels, all other elements of the vascular bundle are ligated with two nonabsorbable ligatures (Fig. 39-5). A

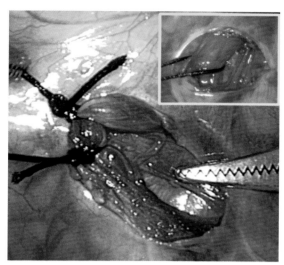

Figure 39-5. With the lymphatic vessels separated (*inset*), the vascular bundle is encircled with two nonabsorbable sutures and ligated.

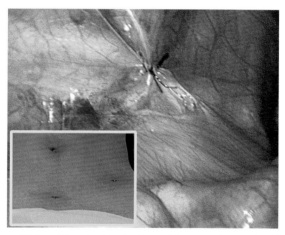

Figure 39-6. After double ligation of the vascular cord (with sparing of the lymphatic vessels), the peritoneal defect is closed. The incisions in this patient are seen in the *inset*.

thorough examination of the retroperitoneal inguinal region is performed, and all additional thin veins going through the internal ring are dissected and coagulated. The peritoneal defect is closed with an absorbable 5-0 suture (Fig. 39-6). The peritoneal cavity is inspected for any concomitant pathology. The instruments and laparoscope are withdrawn and the incisions are closed with intracutaneous absorbable sutures.

PEARLS AND PITFALLS

An analysis of about 2000 different laparoscopic procedures performed for varicocele in children during the past 12 years has helped us to develop the method that we consider optimal for these patients. The main objectives are to make the method simple and safe and to

avoid the common complications typical for varicocele surgery: persistence and recurrence (especially characteristic for artery-saving methods), hydrocele formation (typical for Palomo-type simple ligation of the whole vascular bundle), and orchitis (we came across this problem in the group of patients where indigocarmine was injected under the tunica albuginea for tinting and identification of the lymphatic vessels). The following pearls and features of our method help avoid these problems and minimize the complication rate:

1. Visualize the internal inguinal region to see all retroperitoneal vascular structures that pass through the internal ring. To prevent persistence and recurrence of the varicocele, all of these vessels have to be ligated (main vascular cord) or coagulated (additional veins). In 52 of our cases, we could see that the main bundle consisted of two parts separated from one another. The distance between the two parts of the cord varied from 1 to 4 cm. In 11 cases, one of the halves was seen to be medial to the external iliac artery and vein. This unusual anatomy could be the reason for recurrence.
2. Do not dissect separately every vein branch that is to be divided, because a thin vein can easily be missed and not ligated. We prefer to ligate the whole vascular bundle with the exception of the isolated structures (lymphatic vessels) that we want to preserve.
3. Do not preserve the artery, because artery-saving methods are complicated by significant recurrence. Moreover, postoperative Doppler examinations have shown no significant difference in testicular flow between patients undergoing the artery-saving technique when compared to patients who have had the entire vascular bundle ligated.
4. Consider dissection and preservation of the lymphatic vessels necessary to prevent hydrocele formation. No additional tinting of the lymphatic vessels (which can provoke orchitis) is needed. Intraoperative magnification makes it possible to visualize and dissect carefully these four to five lymphatic vessels. Also, temporary compression of the vascular cord with the use of the traction ligature facilitates this dissection and makes these vessels fill, which leads to easy identification.
5. Use the traction ligature as it facilitates all stages of dissection and inspection, especially of the lymphatic vessels. Double ligation of the vascular cord without cutting is a safe and reliable method that eliminates the possibility of postoperative bleeding.

RESULTS

More than 1000 pediatric patients aged 6 to 16 years underwent the described procedure from 1996 to 2005. The results of the treatment in this group were excellent.

There were no significant intraoperative or postoperative complications, conversions, or recurrences. The average operating time was 20.64 ± 3.24 minutes. The average hospital stay was about 24 hours.

SELECTED REFERENCES

1. Lyon RP, Marshall S, Scott MP: Varicocele in childhood and adolescence: Implication in adulthood infertility? Urology 19:641-644, 1982
2. Buch JP, Cromie WJ: Evaluation and treatment of the pre-adolescent varicocele. Urol Clin North Am 12:3-12, 1985
3. Reitelman C, Burbige KA, Sawczuk IS, et al: Diagnosis and surgical correction of the pediatric varicocele. J Urol 138:1038-1040, 1987
4. Kass EJ, Marcol B: Results of varicocele surgery in adolescents: A comparison of techniques. J Urol 148:694-696, 1992
5. Meacham RB, Townsend RR, Rademacher D, et al: The incidence of varicoceles in the general population when evaluated by physical examination, gray scale sonography and color Doppler sonography. J Urol 151:1535-1538, 1994
6. Jarow JP, Coburn M, Sigman M: Incidence of varicoceles in men with primary and secondary infertility. Urology 47:73-76, 1996
7. Esposito C, Monguzzi G, Gonzalez-Sabin MA, et al: Results and complications of laparoscopic surgery for pediatric varicocele. J Pediatr Surg 36:767-769, 2001
8. Varlet F, Becmeur F, Groupe d'Etudes en Coeliochirurgie: Infantile laparoscopic treatment of varicoceles in children: Multicentric prospective study of 90 cases. Eur J Pediatr Surg 11:399-403, 2001
9. Riccabona M, Oswald J, Koen M, et al: Optimizing the operative treatment of boys with varicocele: Sequential comparison of 4 techniques. J Urol 169:666-668, 2003

PART TWO

THORACOSCOPY

40
Principles of Thoracoscopy

Steven S. Rothenberg

Although thoracoscopy was first described in the early 1900s, it has undergone an exponential increase in popularity and growth over the past decade. In the 1970s and 1980s, the first significant experience in children was reported by Brad Rodgers. In these reports, equipment modified for pediatric patients was used to perform lung biopsies, evaluate various intrathoracic lesions, and perform limited pleural debridement in patients with empyema. However, even though there was increasing recognition of the morbidity associated with a standard thoracotomy, especially in small infants and children, there was little acceptance or adoption of these techniques until the early 1990s. Then began a dramatic revolution in the technology associated with laparoscopic surgery in adults, and the advances allowed this approach to be useful in children. The development of high-resolution microchips and digital cameras, smaller instrumentation, and better optics has enabled pediatric surgeons to perform even the most complicated chest procedures thoracoscopically.

INDICATIONS FOR WORKUP AND OPERATION

Today there are many indications for the thoracoscopic approach in infants and children (Table 40-1), and the number continues to expand with advances and refinements in technology and technique. Thoracoscopy is now being used extensively for lung biopsy and wedge resection in patients with interstitial lung disease (ILD) and metastatic lesions. More extensive pulmonary resections including segmentectomy and lobectomy have also been performed for infectious diseases, cavitary lesions, bullous disease, sequestrations, lobar emphysema, congenital adenomatoid malformations, and neoplasms. Thoracoscopy is also extremely useful in the evaluation and treatment of mediastinal masses. It allows excellent access and visualization for biopsy and resection of mediastinal structures such as lymph nodes, thymic and thyroid lesions, cystic hygromas, foregut duplications, ganglioneuromas, and neuroblastomas. Other advanced intrathoracic procedures include decortication for empyema, ligation of patent ductus arteriosus, repair of congenital diaphragmatic defects, esophageal myotomy for achalasia, thoracic sympathectomy for hyperhidrosis, anterior spinal fusion for severe scoliosis, and, most recently, primary repair of esophageal atresia.

The preoperative workup varies with the procedure to be performed. Most intrathoracic lesions require routine radiographs as well as a computed tomographic (CT) scan or magnetic resonance imaging (MRI) scan. A thin-cut, high-resolution CT scan is especially helpful in evaluating patients with ILD or presumed infectious conditions, as it can identify the most affected areas and helps determine the optimal site for biopsy (Fig. 40-1). As intraoperative ultrasound imaging improves, this modality may provide a more sensitive way for the surgeon to detect lesions deep to the surface of the lung and compensate for the lack of tactile sensation. Unfortunately, in its current state, this technology is still unreliable. An MRI scan may be more useful in evaluating vascular lesions, such as a vascular ring, or masses that may arise from or encroach on the spinal canal. Preoperative imaging studies can also help determine patient position and initial port placement.

OPERATIVE TECHNIQUE

The operative technique varies depending on the procedure being performed, but some general principles apply. In general, it is helpful to have single-lung ventilation, and in some cases (e.g., lobectomy), it is mandatory. This can usually be achieved by a contralateral mainstem intubation (Fig. 40-2A). A bronchial blocker can be useful as well when positioned in the ipsilateral mainstem bronchus (Fig. 40-2B). At times, this technique does not lead to total collapse of the lung as there may be some overflow ventilation because the endotracheal tube is not totally occlusive. This problem is overcome by the routine use of a low-flow (1 L/min), low-pressure (4 mm Hg) CO_2 infusion during the procedure to help keep the lung compressed. If adequate visualization is still not achieved, then the pressure and flow can be gradually increased until adequate lung collapse is obtained. Pressures of 10 to 12 mm Hg are tolerated without significant respiratory or hemodynamic consequences in most cases.

When thoracoscopy was first conceptualized, cannulas without valves were thought to be appropriate. However, in children, because of the need for positive-pressure CO_2 insufflation to help deflate the lung, cannulas with valves should be used. For some operations, it is important to keep the valved cannulas in place throughout the operation. For others, such as for debridement of empyema, the cannulas can be removed once an adequate working space is achieved to allow insertion of regular instruments to help remove the inflammatory peel. Stab incisions can also be used for 3-mm instruments. This stab incision technique is ideal for introduction of an assisting or retracting instrument (Fig. 40-3).

Patient positioning is also critical. The patient should be positioned so that gravity assists with exposure of the desired area and allows the lung to fall away (Fig. 40-4). Therefore, for anterior mediastinal operations, the patient is placed almost supine. For posterior mediastinal procedures, the patient is almost prone. For empyema, routine parenchymal biopsy, and lung resection, a lateral decubitus position is optimal. The specific details of each procedure will be discussed in the following chapters.

In addition to patient positioning, cannula placement is also important. As a general statement, the cannulas should be positioned like the bases in a baseball diamond (Fig. 40-5). The telescope should be positioned at home base, the working sites at first and third bases, and the target organ at second base. If a single monitor is used, it should be at center field. On occasion, especially in small patients (such as an infant

Table 40-1	Indications for Thoracoscopy in Children
Lung biopsy
Lobectomy
Sequestration resection
Cyst excision
Decortication or debridement for empyema
Foregut duplication resection
Esophageal myotomy
Anterior spine fusion
Diaphragmatic hernia or plication
Ligation for patent ductus arteriosus
Thoracic duct ligation
Esophageal atresia repair
Aortopexy
Mediastinal mass excision
Thymectomy
Sympathectomy
Pericardial window

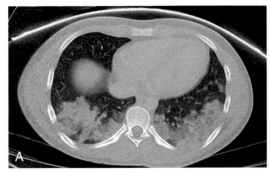
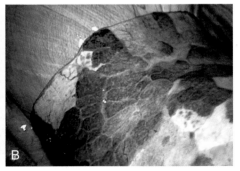

Figure 40-1. Preoperative imaging studies can be important when planning a thoracoscopic lung biopsy. A thin-cut, high-resolution CT scan is helpful in evaluating patients with interstitial lung disease or presumed infectious conditions. **A,** On a CT scan, parenchymal disease was presumed to be in the lower lobes. **B,** The operative view correlates with the CT scan. This patient had Wegener's granulomatosis.

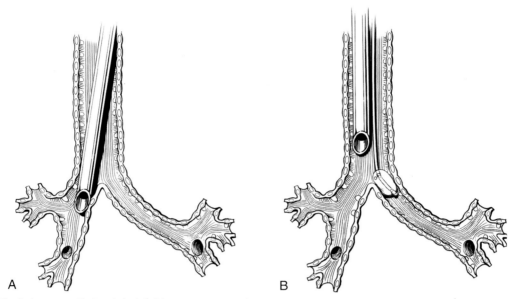

Figure 40-2. Single-lung ventilation is helpful in most cases and mandatory for some operations. In patients who are too young or too small for a double-lumen endotracheal tube, single-lung ventilation can be achieved with contralateral mainstem intubation. **A,** Right mainstem intubation is shown for a small child undergoing a left thoracoscopic procedure. **B,** A bronchial blocker can be useful as well with tracheal intubation and occlusion of the ipsilateral mainstem bronchus with the bronchial blocker. Tracheal intubation is depicted with the bronchial blocker passed into the left mainstem bronchus for a patient undergoing a left thoracoscopic operation.

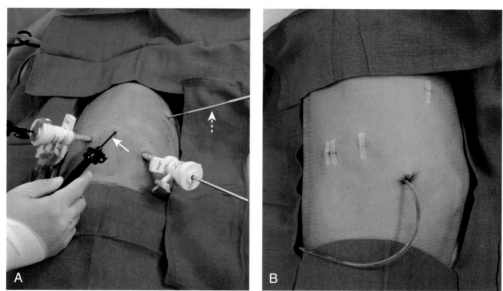

Figure 40-3. When cannulas are used for a thoracoscopic procedure in children, a valved cannula should be employed. **A,** Two 5-mm valved cannulas are seen. Additionally, it is often helpful to use the stab incision technique to insert an instrument to be used by the assistant (*solid arrow*), or a 3-mm retractor (*dotted arrow*). Escape of enough CO_2 to allow the lung to reexpand is rare. **B,** The incisions have been closed. In this patient, an esophageal duplication was extracted through the most lateral port. The silastic drain was removed soon after the operation.

undergoing esophageal atresia repair) and with 70-degree telescopes, it may be helpful to position the telescope at either first or third base and work through the home base and first or third base sites.

Finally, a chest drain or tube is not mandatory in all patients. If one is used, it can be exteriorized through one of the small working incisions, but it should be tunneled over the cephalad rib so as to create a tract that

will collapse once the drain or tube is removed (Fig. 40-6). This may help prevent the development of a post-pull pneumothorax.

POSTOPERATIVE CARE

The specifics of care vary depending on the procedure, but, in general, patients have less morbidity and recover

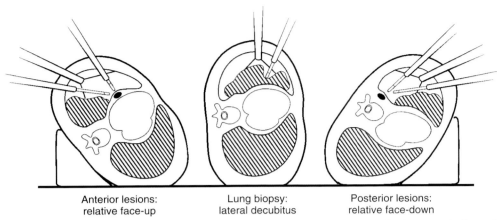

Anterior lesions: Lung biopsy: Posterior lesions:
relative face-up   lateral decubitus   relative face-down

Figure 40-4. The patient should be positioned so that gravity assists with exposure of the desired area and allows the lung to fall away. For an anterior lesion, the patient should be placed relatively face up. For a posterior lesion, the patient should be relatively face down so that the lung falls away. For lung biopsies or empyema operations, the lateral decubitus position is usually employed.

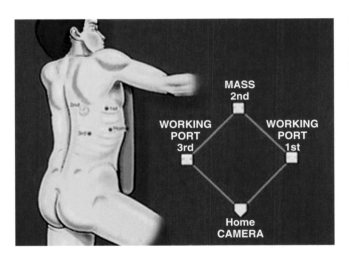

Figure 40-5. When trying to determine how to position the cannulas, think of a baseball diamond. The telescope should be at home base, with the working sites at first and third bases. The target organ is located at second base. A single monitor is usually used and is positioned in center field.

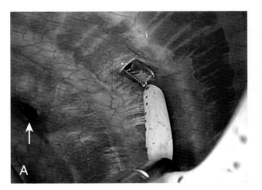
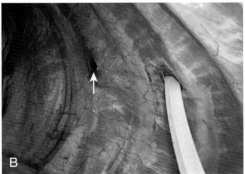

Figure 40-6. A chest tube is not mandatory for all thoracoscopic operations. However, if desired, a small silastic drain can be used rather than a stiff chest tube in most instances. **A,** A hemostat has been introduced externally through a stab incision but tunneled over the cephalad rib. It is shown entering the chest cavity one rib above the original stab incision. The original site of entry into the thoracic cavity is marked with an *arrow*. **B,** The drain is seen exiting the chest cavity cephalad to the original stab incision (*arrow*). With this technique, a postpull pneumothorax is not likely to develop as the drain is extracted through a subcutaneous tunnel rather than directly through the chest wall.

much more quickly from a thoracoscopic approach because of the lack of a long, painful thoracotomy incision. Unless there was significant injury to the lung or there is significant fluid to drain, a chest drain is not considered mandatory. The lung can be reexpanded on the operating table with a drain converted to water seal. If no leak is seen, the drain is removed before extubation. Most patients who are not being treated for associated conditions, infection, or lung disease are discharged within 24 hours.

PEARLS

1. Many patients develop oxygen desaturation with the initial collapse of the lung. However, most patients rebound within a few minutes. Be patient, and do not abandon the procedure.
2. Position the patient to assist completion of the operation thoracoscopically, not in anticipation of conversion. Do not create a self-fulfilling prophecy.
3. The surgeon and assistant should stand on the same side. Do not force your assistant to work backward.

PITFALLS

1. Relying on single-lung ventilation without planning to use CO_2 insufflation is a mistake, especially in smaller infants. Always use valved cannulas to prevent CO_2 escape.
2. Not having a clear plan of what is required, whether it is a simple biopsy or a complicated lobectomy, results in problems such as poor positioning of the patient, poor exposure, and a suboptimal outcome.

3. Discuss the planned operation, objectives, and issues with the anesthesiologist before the case. This may make the difference in your being able to complete the case thoracoscopically.
4. Use 3-mm instruments in an infant where it is difficult to use even 5-mm instruments.

SELECTED REFERENCES

1. Rodgers BM, Moazam F, Talbert JL: Thoracoscopy in children. Ann Surg 189:176-180, 1979
2. Rodgers BM: Pediatric thoracoscopy: Where have we come, what have we learned? Ann Thorac Surg 56:704-707, 1993
3. Rothenberg SS: Thoracoscopy in infants and children. Semin Pediatr Surg 3:277-288, 1994
4. Rothenberg SS, Wagener JS, Chang JHT, et al: The safety and efficacy of thoracoscopic lung biopsy for diagnosis and treatment in infants and children. J Pediatr Surg 31:100-104, 1996
5. Patrick DA, Rothenberg SS: Thoracoscopic resection of mediastinal masses in infants and children: An evaluation of technique and results. J Pediatr Surg 36:1165-1167, 2001
6. Rothenberg SS, Patrick DA, Bealer JF, et al: Evaluation of minimally invasive approaches to achalasia in children. J Pediatr Surg 36:808-810, 2001
7. Rothenberg SS: Thoracoscopic repair of tracheoesophageal fistula in newborns. J Pediatr Surg 37:869-872, 2002
8. Smith TJ, Rothenberg SS, Brooks M, et al: Thoracoscopic surgery in childhood cancer. J Pediatr Hematol Oncol 24:429-435, 2002
9. Rothenberg SS: Experience with thoracoscopic lobectomy in infants and children. J Pediatr Surg 38:102-104, 2003

41
Thoracoscopic Lung Biopsy

Michael P. La Quaglia and Steven S. Rothenberg

The need to obtain diagnostic lung tissue occurs often in infants and children. Disease processes such as interstitial lung disease (ILD), infectious lung disease, and metastatic lung lesions may require histologic examination for diagnosis and treatment. The ability to obtain these specimens thoracoscopically has greatly decreased the morbidity associated with open lung biopsy. Moreover, it may have changed the treatment algorithms to encourage earlier operative intervention to direct therapy.

INDICATIONS FOR WORKUP AND OPERATION

There is currently a wide variety of indications for thoracoscopic procedures in children, and the number continues to expand with advances and refinements in technology and technique. Thoracoscopy is being used extensively for lung biopsy and wedge resection in cases of ILD and metastatic lesions as well as for infectious diseases, cavitary lesions, and bullous disease. Thoracoscopy is most useful and applicable when lesions are peripheral and away from hilar structures. The surgeon should carefully document the number and location of suspicious parenchymal lesions. It is advisable to review the imaging study and localize abnormalities to a pulmonary segment.

The preoperative workup varies depending on the procedure to be performed. Most intrathoracic lesions require routine radiographs as well as a computed tomography (CT) or magnetic resonance (MRI) scan. A thin-cut (3- or 5-mm), high-resolution CT scan is especially helpful in evaluating patients with ILD as it can identify the areas most affected and assists in selection of a biopsy site because the external appearance of the lung is usually not helpful. CT-guided needle localization can also be used to direct biopsies for focal lesions that may lie deep in the lung parenchyma and, therefore, may not be visible on the surface of the lung at thoracoscopy. Needle localization is usually performed just before the thoracoscopy, with the radiologist marking the pleura overlying the lesion with a small blood patch or dye at the time of surgery (Fig. 41-1A). Alternatively, a small wire can be introduced into the lesion as well (Fig. 41-1B). As intraoperative ultrasound imaging improves, this modality may provide a more sensitive way for the surgeon to detect lesions deep to the surface of the lung and compensate for the lack of tactile sensation. Unfortunately, in its current state, this technology is still unreliable.

OPERATIVE TECHNIQUE

If possible, single-lung ventilation is advised to aid in collapsing the lung to be biopsied. This is usually accomplished by performing a mainstem intubation of the contralateral side (see Chapter 40). Alternatively, a 3 or 4 French Fogarty balloon catheter can be inserted through the vocal cords at the same time the patient is intubated with a single-lumen endotracheal tube. A fiberoptic bronchoscope is then passed through the endotracheal tube, and the blocker is guided into the ipsilateral mainstem bronchial orifice under direct vision (see Chapter 40). The surgeon should be present during this part of the procedure to assist the anesthesiologist with placement of the blocker and to confirm its correct positioning. The patient is positioned in a lateral decubitus position (Fig. 41-2). The chest is first

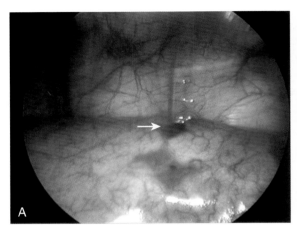
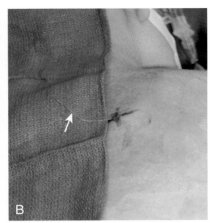

Figure 41-1. It is often necessary to mark lesions deep to the visceral pleural surface. A number of techniques are available. **A,** Thoracoscopic visualization of a small blood patch that has been placed over the lesion (*arrow*) by the radiologist. **B,** A small wire (*arrow*) has been introduced into the lesion by the radiologist and is seen exiting the patient's skin.

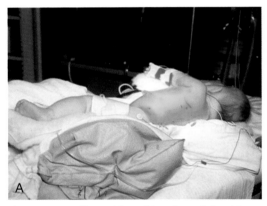
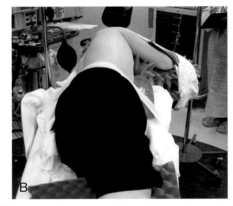

Figure 41-2. Patients are usually positioned in a lateral decubitus position for a thoracoscopic lung biopsy. A small child (**A**) and an adolescent (**B**) are positioned for a biopsy.

insufflated with CO_2 at a low flow (1 L/min) and low pressure (4 mm Hg) using a Veress needle in the midaxillary line in the 5th intercostal space. This helps collapse the lung and prevent inadvertent parenchymal injury with insertion of the first cannula. In all cases, valved ports should be used to allow continuation of the CO_2 insufflation to help keep the lung collapsed as there is often mild overflow ventilation from the contralateral lung.

Three ports are usually necessary and many lesions can be approached by placement of one port in the lower midaxillary line, one high in the axilla, and the final port in the parascapular line (Fig. 41-3). This may be modified depending on the location of the target lesion or lesions. The initial port is usually positioned in the midaxillary line to provide an initial survey of the entire lung surface. The other two cannulas are situated to facilitate resection of the desired tissue, usually one port anteriorly to grasp the desired tissue and the third site posteriorly in the largest interspace possible for

insertion of the endoscopic stapler. If necessary, the largest port can be removed and the stapler introduced directly through the chest wall (Fig. 41-4).

In patients over 15 kg, two 5-mm ports and one 12-mm port are used to allow access for the endoscopic stapler. The desired tissue is placed on stretch and the stapler is situated across the base of the desired specimen and fired (Fig. 41-5). Often, more than one application is necessary to complete the excision. If malignancy is not suspected, biopsy specimens are then exteriorized through the cannula or cannula site. In cases of presumed malignant lesions, the specimen can be exteriorized through the cannula. If too large, the specimen is placed into an endoscopic specimen bag and brought out through the cannula tract to prevent contamination of the port site (Fig. 41-6).

For infants, the telescope is inserted in the superior port and a grasping forceps is introduced in the anterior port. The tongue of lung tissue to be biopsied is grasped and elevated (Fig. 41-7A). Two endoloops are

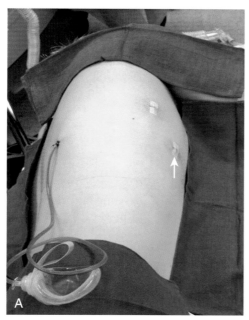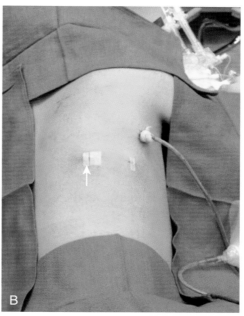

Figure 41-3. Three ports are usually necessary, and a triangular configuration generally works best. **A,** The stapler was introduced through the right inferior port (*arrow*). A 3-mm grasping forceps was introduced through the stab incision where the drain has been exteriorized, and the telescope and camera were inserted through the remaining port. This configuration was used for a posteriorly based lesion in the inferior aspect of the right upper lobe. **B,** The stapler was introduced through the posterior-most port (*arrow*). The drain was exteriorized through a stab incision through which a grasper was used to elevate the medial aspect of the right upper lobe. The telescope and camera were introduced through the remaining 5-mm port. In both of these patients, the stapler was introduced as far as possible from the lesion so that it could be opened in the small thoracic cavity.

Figure 41-4. In this patient, the largest port was removed and the stapler (*arrow*) was introduced directly through the chest wall. This technique can be useful when the thoracic cavity is small and will not allow the stapler to open with a cannula in place.

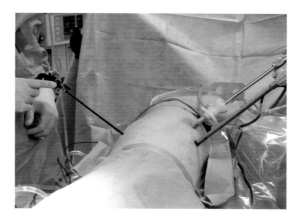

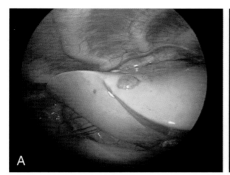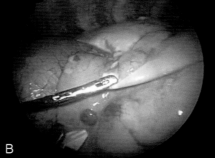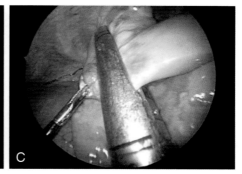

Figure 41-5. A 5-year-old with a Wilms tumor developed suspected metastatic lesions in the left upper lobe. **A,** The lesion is visualized on the inferior border of the left upper lobe. **B,** The edge of the left upper lobe is grasped to place the desired specimen on stretch. **C,** The stapler is then situated across the base of the lung containing the desired specimen, and fired. As in this case, more than one firing often is required to remove the desired lesion.

sequentially placed over the tissue, snaring the base of the specimen (Fig. 41-7B). The specimen is then resected distal to the loops using scissors (Fig. 41-7C).

After resection, a chest tube or drain is inserted through one of the port sites, and the other incisions are closed (Fig. 41-3). The patient is positioned supine and the endotracheal tube is withdrawn into the trachea. The collapsed lung is reexpanded, and the chest tube or drain is placed to water seal. If there is no evidence of an air leak (the finding in the majority of cases), the chest tube or drain can be removed and an occlusive dressing applied before extubating the patient. Removal of the chest tube before leaving the operating room eliminates a significant amount of postoperative pain.

POSTOPERATIVE CARE

Patients are admitted for observation after the operation. A chest radiograph is obtained in the recovery

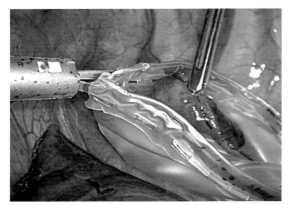

Figure 41-6. Placement of the specimen into an endoscopic retrieval bag should reduce or eliminate the possibility of port site contamination.

room. If a pneumothorax is not seen, the radiograph does not need to be repeated. Most patients require only one or two doses of an intravenous narcotic, and the majority are ready for discharge in 24 hours on oral analgesics. If a chest tube or drain is left, it should be removed as soon as the air leak resolves.

PEARLS

1. Both the surgeon and the assistant should be on the same side of the table so that no one is working opposite the telescope and camera.
2. If a discreet lesion (i.e., a metastatic lesion) is targeted, it may be helpful to place the patient in a modified decubitus position, either more prone or supine, so that gravity helps retract the lung to expose the desired area.
3. Whenever possible, biopsy along a lung edge so that a better tongue of tissue and a better seal are obtained (Figs. 41-5 and 41-7). The anterior segment of either the upper, middle, or lower lobe is ideal if there is diffuse disease.
4. Always obtain biopsies from two sites in patients with ILD so that there is tissue for comparison.
5. When using a stapler, it is generally better to use a tissue load rather than a vascular load.
6. Fibrin glue may be used as an extra sealant in patients with fibrotic lung tissue.
7. Use nonabsorbable pre-tied ligatures so that adequate tension can be used to cinch down on the noose and get a complete seal.

PITFALLS

1. Before the operation, discuss with the family the possibility that a lesion may not be seen. They should

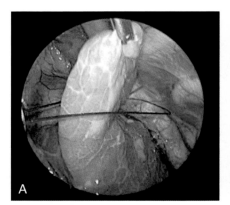 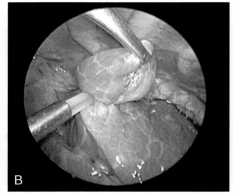 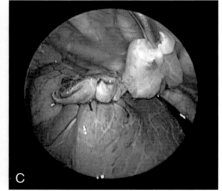

Figure 41-7. In infants in whom the thoracic cavity is not large enough to accept an endoscopic stapler, endoloops can be used to secure the lung at the base of the specimen. **A,** The tongue of lung tissue to be biopsied is grasped and elevated. An endoloop is positioned around the lung. **B,** The endoloop is closed around the base of the specimen. **C,** Usually, two endoloops are used. The specimen has been resected distal to the endoloops using scissors.

understand the circumstances under which conversion to an open thoracotomy might be needed.

2. Methylene blue, if not injected exactly in the parietal pleura, can result in diffuse staining, making identification of the site to be biopsied almost impossible.

3. Failure to use valved cannulas can result in an inability to adequately visualize the lesion because of incomplete lung collapse.

RESULTS

At Presbyterian St. Luke's Hospital in Denver, between January 2003 and December 2006, 280 patients underwent thoracoscopic lung biopsy, of which 279 operations were accomplished thoracoscopically. Ages ranged from 2 days to 18 years and weight from 2.1 to 117 kg. No patient was excluded on the basis of size or respiratory status. The endoscopic stapler was used in 185 cases and endoloops in 95 cases. A tissue diagnosis was obtained in 95% of cases. Chest tubes were left in only 10 patients after biopsy. Eight chest tubes were removed

in less than 24 hours. There was one delayed pneumothorax on day 3, which was successfully managed by needle aspiration. No other complications occurred.

SELECTED REFERENCES

1. Rothenberg SS, Wagner JS, Chang JHT, et al: The safety and efficiency of thoracoscopic lung biopsy for diagnosis and treatment in infants and children. J Pediatr Surg 31:100-104, 1996
2. Fan LL, Kozmetz CA, Rothenberg SS: The diagnostic value of transbronchial thoracoscopic and open lung biopsy in immunocompetent children with chronic interstitial lung disease. J Pediatr 131:565-569, 1997
3. Rothenberg SS: Thoracoscopic lung resection in children. J Pediatr Surg 35:271-275, 2000
4. Smith JJ, Rothenberg SS, Brooks M, et al: Thoracoscopic surgery in childhood cancer. J Pediatr Hemat Oncol 24:429-435, 2002
5. Partrick DA, Bensard DD, Teitelbaum DH, et al: Successful thoracoscopic lung biopsy in children utilizing preoperative CT-guided localization. J Pediatr Surg 37:970-973, 2002

42
Thoracoscopic Lobectomy

Steven S. Rothenberg

Thoracoscopy was first reported in the early 1900s. The first significant use in children was described in the late 1970s by Brad Rodgers, who used modified cystoscopy equipment for evaluation of intrathoracic lesions, small parenchymal biopsies, and limited pleural debridements. By the mid 1990s, thoracoscopic lung biopsy had become accepted as a superior technique for obtaining tissue in cases of interstitial lung disease or malignancy. Thoracoscopy has also become the preferred approach in the treatment of empyema and most mediastinal masses.

The thoracoscopic approach for lobectomy, because of the complex nature of the disease process and the surgical dissection, has not been as readily accepted. However, improvements in instrumentation and surgical technique over the past decade have made thoracoscopic lobectomy for congenital and acquired lung disease in children a viable option and in some cases is preferred.

INDICATIONS FOR WORKUP AND OPERATION

Indications for resection include both congenital and acquired disease. Congenital lesions include congenital cystic adenomatoid malformation, intralobar and extralobar sequestration, congenital lobar emphysema, and more rare causes of congenital airway obstruction that result in lung parenchymal injury. Acquired etiologies include severe bronchiectasis, right middle lobe syndrome, necrotizing pneumonia, and malignancy. In most cases, the preoperative evaluation consists of a routine chest radiograph and computerized tomographic scan. Occasionally, other studies such as a ventilation-perfusion scan may be needed to determine the degree of lung injury and whether a lobectomy is possible. Rarely, an aortogram or a magnetic resonance angiogram is necessary to identify a systemic vessel, as in the case of a sequestration or aberrant vascular supply. Bronchoscopy should be performed in cases where abnormal bronchial anatomy or obstruction is suspected.

OPERATIVE TECHNIQUE

The procedure varies slightly depending on the lobe being resected, but all procedures are performed with the patient in a lateral decubitus position. The room and personnel setup for a left lower lobectomy is shown in Figure 42-1. The surgeon and assistant stand at the patient's front with the monitor over the patient's back. In all cases, single-lung ventilation is desirable if at all possible, but a successful lobectomy can be performed using just CO_2 insufflation to collapse the lung. In larger patients, a double-lumen endotracheal tube is beneficial. In infants and smaller children, single-lung ventilation is obtained by mainstem intubation of the

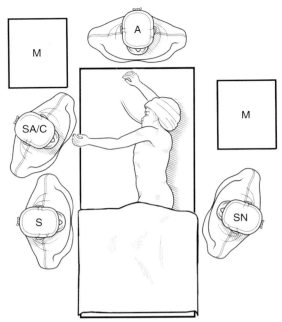

Figure 42-1.   The room and personnel setup for a left lower lobectomy. The surgeon (S) and surgical assistant/camera holder (SA/C) stand at the patient's front, with the monitor (M) over the patient's back. The scrub nurse (SN) can be positioned at the discretion of the surgeon. If the scrub nurse is positioned opposite the surgeon, as shown here, a second monitor may be helpful for viewing by the scrub nurse. A, anesthesiologist.

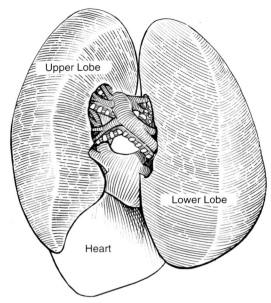

Figure 42-2.   The anatomy seen by the surgeon when the contents of the fissure between the left upper and lower lobes are exposed. The arteries are visualized first within the fissure, and the bronchial structures are behind the arteries. The pulmonary veins exit from the inferior portion of these lobes and drain into the heart.

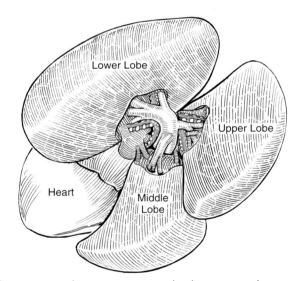

Figure 42-3.   The anatomy as seen by the surgeon when dissecting in the major and minor fissures of the right lung. The arteries are the first structures seen in the fissure, and the bronchial structures are behind the arteries. The pulmonary veins are inferior to the arteries and bronchial structures and drain into the heart.

contralateral side. A first- or second-generation cephalosporin is administered for prophylaxis in patients not already on antibiotics.

LOBAR ANATOMY

It is important to understand the anatomy of the structures in the various fissures. The anatomy of the fissure between the upper and lower lobes of the left lung is depicted in Figure 42-2. The anatomy of the structures in the major and minor fissures between the three lobes of the right lung is seen in Figure 42-3. When working anteriorly to posteriorly in the fissures, the surgeon encounters the arteries to the lobes first, followed by the bronchial structures. The lobar veins are not adjacent to the arteries and bronchi in the fissures but are seen more inferiorly in the mediastinum.

LOWER LOBECTOMY

The chest is initially insufflated through a Veress needle placed in the midaxillary line at the 5th or 6th interspace. CO_2 is insufflated at low flow and low pressure to help effect complete collapse of the lung. A flow of 1 L/min and a pressure of 4 to 6 mm Hg is maintained throughout the operation. Occasionally, it is necessary to use a higher pressure initially to facilitate complete collapse of the lung. Thus, it is important to use valved

ports so that a mild tension pneumothorax is maintained. We prefer the radially expandable ports as they prevent trauma to the intercostal vessels and nerves. After removal of the Veress needle, the first port (5 mm) is introduced at this site to determine the position of the major fissure and to evaluate the lung parenchyma. A 4-mm or 5-mm, 30-degree telescope is then inserted. This allows the surgeon to look directly down on the fissure and its contents. The location of the fissure dictates the positioning of the other ports. These working ports (3 mm or 5 mm), or instruments introduced without ports, are then inserted in the anterior axillary line between the 5th and the 8th or 9th interspaces (Fig. 42-4). The size of the cannulas depends on the size of the patient and the equipment to be used. If the endoscopic stapler is used, a 12-mm port is situated at the lower port site in the largest interspace possible that will align with the front edge of the fissure. This is usually

the 7th or 8th interspace. In smaller patients, the Ligasure (Covidien, Mansfield, MA) or endoscopic clips are used, and these require only a 5-mm cannula.

The first step in a lower lobectomy is mobilization of the inferior pulmonary ligament. During this mobilization, care is taken to look for a systemic vessel arising from the aorta in cases of sequestration (Fig. 42-5A). When found, the vessel is ligated and divided with either the Ligasure, clips, or ties (Fig. 42-5B). The inferior pulmonary vein is identified but not ligated at this point. Ligation of the vein before division of the pulmonary artery can lead to congestion in the lower lobe, which can then create space issues, especially in the smaller child and infant. After division of the inferior pulmonary ligament, the fissure is approached. If the fissure is incomplete, the Ligasure or stapler can be used to complete it. Gradually, moving anterior to posterior within the fissure, the pulmonary artery to the lower lobe is isolated (or the arteries, if more than one). Often, it is necessary to dissect into the parenchyma of the lower lobe to gain adequate exposure and length (Fig. 42-6). If possible, the artery is ligated at its main trunk to the lower lobe as it passes through the fissure. However, it is often easier to dissect the artery after the first or second bifurcation. This also provides a longer segment of artery to work with. The artery can be ligated and divided with the Ligasure in infants and with clips or the stapler in older children. The bronchus to the lower lobe lies directly behind the artery and can often be palpated before it is seen.

Once the artery is divided, the complete dissection of the vein is facilitated because of improved exposure. The vein is also ligated and divided in a variety of ways depending on the size of the vessel. Before ligating the vein, it is helpful to divide the pleura along the posterior border of the lobe to complete its mobilization (Fig. 42-7A). The inferior pulmonary vein is then ligated (Fig. 42-7B,C), and the bronchus to the lower lobe is isolated. The bronchus is divided with the endoscopic stapler in larger children (Fig. 42-8A) or cut sharply and

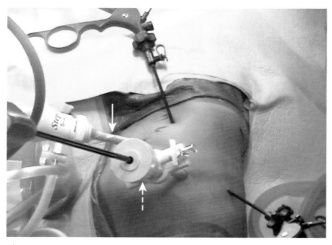

Figure 42-4. Port and instrument positions for a thoracoscopic left lower lobectomy. The initial port (*solid arrow*) is placed in the mid to anterior axillary line in the 5th or 6th interspace. After CO₂ insufflation and lung collapse, the 5-mm angled telescope is inserted. The location of the fissure dictates the positioning of the other ports. In this figure, a 5-mm port (*dotted arrow*) placed in the 9th intercostal space was subsequently exchanged for a 12-mm port for insertion of the stapler as well as extraction of the specimen. Instruments were placed directly through the skin for the other two working sites.

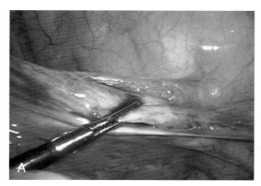
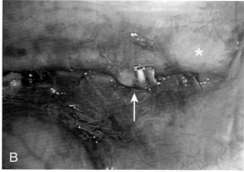

Figure 42-5. This patient was given a preliminary diagnosis of either a congenital cystic adenomatoid malformation or a sequestration. Thus, the initial step was to see if there was a systemic vessel emanating from the aorta, which would secure the diagnosis of sequestration. **A,** The vessel is seen to lie in the inferior pulmonary ligament. **B,** This systemic artery has been ligated with clips (*arrow*). The aorta (*asterisk*) is visualized cephalad to this aberrant systemic vessel.

closed with interrupted 3-0 PDS (Ethicon, Inc., Somerville, NJ) suture in smaller patients (Fig. 42-8B). In infants and patients less than 5 kg, it is possible to seal the bronchus with endoscopic clips. It is extremely important, especially in smaller patients, not to compromise the bronchus to the other lobes when dividing the lower lobe bronchus. For this reason, the stapler

should not be used in smaller patients as it may encroach on the upper or middle lobe bronchus. The specimen is then exteriorized either whole or piecemeal with a ring forceps, through the lower anterior axillary line port site, which is slightly enlarged if necessary (Fig. 42-9). If there is any concern about infection or malignancy, the specimen should be placed in an endoscopic bag. The endotracheal tube is then withdrawn into the trachea to ensure that the remaining lung inflates appropriately. A chest tube or drain is placed through the lower port site, and all incisions are closed in two layers with absorbable suture (Fig. 42-9).

RIGHT MIDDLE LOBE

The patient and personnel positioning is similar to that previously described for a lower lobectomy. However, the working ports are shifted slightly cephalad to allow good access to the minor fissure (Fig. 42-10). Dissection is started in the minor fissure going from front to back. The middle lobe arteries are encountered near the confluence of the minor and major fissures (Fig. 42-11). In some cases, it is helpful to complete the anterior portion of the major fissure to facilitate this dissection. The middle lobe vessels are isolated, usually at the bifurcation of the anterior and posterior segments, and are then sealed and divided as already described (Fig. 42-12). The lobe is retracted posteriorly, exposing the

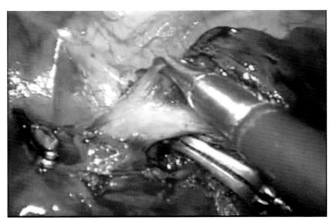

Figure 42-6. In this view, the main pulmonary artery to the left lower lobe has been identified and is being dissected prior to ligation. Ligation with either clips or the stapler is appropriate in older children. In infants and younger children, the Ligasure can often be used.

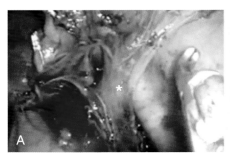 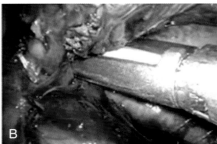 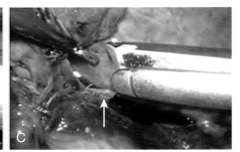

Figure 42-7. **A,** After the arterial supply to the left lower lobe has been ligated and divided, the vein (*asterisk*) is approached. **B,** A stapler is being applied across the pulmonary vein to the lower lobe. **C,** The vein (*arrow*) has been secured with the stapler.

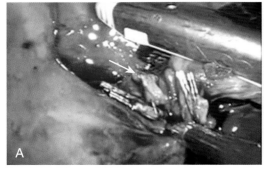 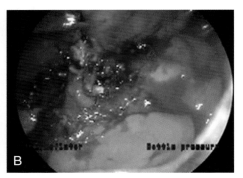

Figure 42-8. **A,** In an older patient, the bronchus is being divided with the stapler. Note the previously stapled pulmonary artery (*arrow*). **B,** In a smaller patient, the bronchus is being suture-ligated with interrupted 3-0 PDS sutures.

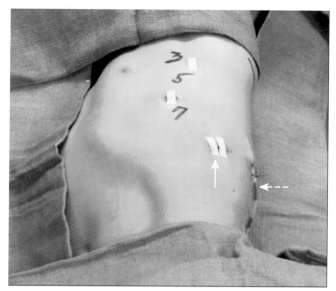

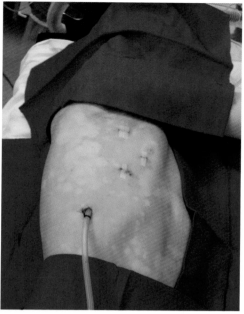

Figure 42-9.   The specimen can be exteriorized either whole or piecemeal through the lower anterior axillary line port (*solid arrow*), which can be slightly enlarged if necessary. A small Silastic chest drain (*dotted arrow*) was introduced through the more posteroinferior stab incision.

Figure 42-10.   The incisions for a thoracoscopic right middle lobectomy. These incisions are slightly more cephalad than those used for a lower lobectomy. Again, a small chest drain has been inserted through the most inferior stab incision.

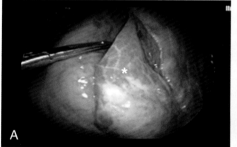
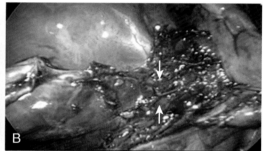

Figure 42-11.   **A,** The initial view of a collapsed middle lobe (*asterisk*) between healthy right upper and lower lobes. **B,** The fissure between the upper and middle and lower lobes has been dissected. The two arterial branches (*arrows*) to the middle lobe can be visualized at this point in the dissection.

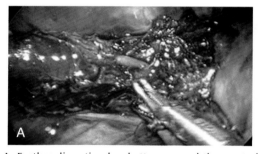
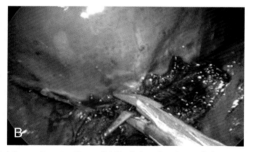

Figure 42-12.   **A,** Further dissection has better exposed these arterial branches to the middle lobe. **B,** One of these two arterial branches is being ligated with endoscopic clips.

middle pulmonary vein, which drains into the superior pulmonary vein (Fig. 42-13). The anterior pleura is divided sharply to facilitate this dissection.

Once the artery and vein are divided, the bronchus to the middle lobe is easily identified and usually enters the lobe near its apex (Fig. 42-14). In most cases, it is safest to divide the bronchus sharply and suture it closed rather than using a stapler. Even in larger children, the angle at which the endoscopic stapler must be placed can make it difficult to ensure that the upper and lower

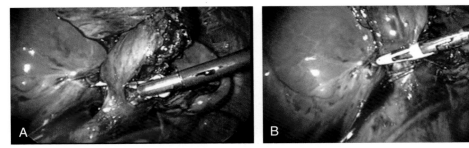

Figure 42-13. **A,** After ligation and division of the arterial vascular supply, the pulmonary vein to the middle lobe is exposed. **B,** Clips have been placed on the pulmonary vein as it enters the pericardium. The Ligasure is being used to seal the pulmonary vein proximal to these clips.

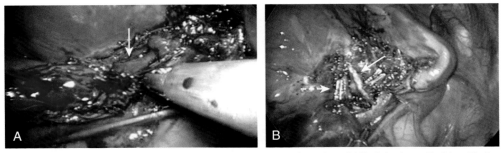

Figure 42-14. **A,** Once the artery and vein are divided, the bronchus (*arrow*) to the middle lobe is easily identified. **B,** The fissure after removal of the lobe. The staple line across the bronchus is marked with a *solid arrow*. The clips used for ligation of the pulmonary vein are marked with a *dotted arrow*. The clips that were used to ligate the arterial branches are just to the right of the bronchial staple line.

lobe bronchi are not compromised. Extraction of the specimen is like that of the lower lobe.

UPPER LOBECTOMY

The upper lobe is technically the most demanding segment to resect. This is primarily because it is necessary to peel the lobe off the main pulmonary artery, taking the branches to the upper lobe and preserving the main trunk as it passes to the more inferior lobes. However, the basic principles and approach are the same. Port placement varies slightly in that the ports are moved one or two interspaces cephalad and are positioned more anteriorly.

Dissection is begun by dividing the parietal pleura anteriorly, thereby exposing the superior pulmonary vein (Fig. 42-15). The vein is mobilized and sealed and divided usually at its first bifurcation. If it is a right upper lobectomy, care must be taken to preserve the middle lobe vein, which drains into the superior pulmonary vein almost immediately as it exits the pericardium. Once the vein is divided, the lobe is retracted posteriorly and inferiorly, exposing the main pulmonary artery as it transverses behind the upper lobe. The lung is gently teased off the artery until the segmental branches to the upper lobe are encountered (Fig. 42-16). These vessels are then dissected to give an adequate vascular length for safe ligation. If more length is necessary, then dissection should be carried into the paren-

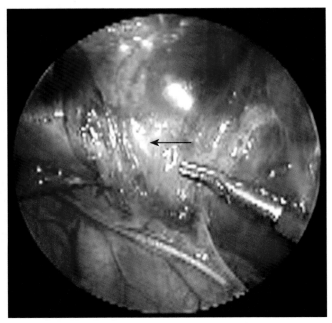

Figure 42-15. The initial step in a thoracoscopic upper lobectomy is division of the parietal pleura anteriorly, which exposes the superior pulmonary vein (*arrow*).

chyma of the upper lobe. The vessels are then sealed with the Ligasure, clips, or ties, depending on surgeon preference. Usually, three branches are encountered, the apical, posterior, and anterior segmental vessels. When the major fissure on the left is incomplete

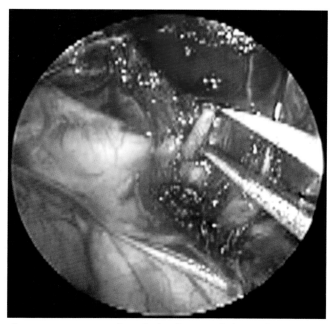

Figure 42-16. Once the vein has been sealed and divided, the segmental arterial branches of the upper lobe are encountered. In this view, the Ligasure is being used to dissect one of these branches and will be used to seal it before division.

anteriorly, it is helpful to complete it first as this will aid in exposure of the anterior or lingular branches. With the fissure completed posteriorly, the only remaining attachment is the upper lobe bronchus. By retracting the lung posteriorly and slightly superiorly, excellent exposure can be provided. The bronchus can then be divided and sutured closed, or clipped and divided. In larger patients, it can be divided with the endoscopic stapler. As with the other lobes, the lower port site is slightly enlarged, and the specimen is extracted piecemeal through this site. A chest tube or drain is inserted through the smallest incision, and the incisions are closed in layers with absorbable suture.

POSTOPERATIVE CARE

The chest tube or drain is placed to suction overnight, and a first-generation cephalosporin is administered for the first 24 hours. If no air leak is present in the morning, a chest radiograph is obtained with the tube or drain placed to water seal. If there is no pneumothorax, the tube or drain is removed. Intravenous narcotics are usually necessary only for the first night, and the patient is quickly transitioned to oral pain medication. Once the chest tube is removed and the patient is comfortable on oral analgesia, the patient can be discharged, with follow-up in 10 to 14 days.

PEARLS

1. Understanding the spatial relationships in the chest is the key to successful lobar resection. It is best to work from anterior to posterior in most cases, rather then flipping the lobe from one side to another. Flipping the lobe only results in additional operating time, repeated loss of exposure, and unnecessary manipulation of what may be inflamed and friable tissue.
2. Allow gravity to do the majority of the retracting. Rotate the operating table aggressively to improve exposure and obviate the need for adding another port for an additional instrument. However, if adequate exposure cannot be obtained, do not hesitate to insert an additional instrument, which can be done with the stab incision technique.
3. Maintain as dry a field as possible. Even a small amount of blood can obscure visualization significantly.
4. Whenever possible, divide the arterial branches first. This will decrease shunting within the lung, aiding the anesthesiologist. It will also diminish venous congestion within the lobe, which can make it more difficult to manipulate.

PITFALLS

1. Be sure to identify all segmental vessels. Failure to do so can result in avulsion of a vessel with uncontrollable bleeding, requiring conversion to an open thoracotomy. The most likely suspects are the apical branch to the lower lobes and the lingular branch to the left upper lobe.
2. Avoid mass ligations and divisions. Avoid the temptation to place a stapler across the major fissure without fully identifying all structures. You might get lucky but you can just as likely compromise arterial branches or bronchi to lung tissue you are not planning to resect.
3. Excessive manipulation of the lung tissue will result in slow bleeding, which may impair visualization. Use an atraumatic clamp on the lung and try to avoid repeated grabs and excessive tension.

RESULTS

From January 1994 through December 2005, 144 patients, from 2 days old to 18 years old and weighing 2.8 to 78 kg, underwent thoracoscopic lobectomy (Albanese and Rothenberg 2007; Rothenberg 2008). Of these operations, 112 were for sequestration or cystic adenomatoid malformation, 19 were for severe bronchiectasis, 10 were for congenital lobar emphysema, and 3 were for other lesions. Of the 144 procedures, 141 were completed thoracoscopically. There were 24 upper, 10 middle, and 110 lower lobectomies performed. The operative time ranged from 35 to 220 minutes (mean, 125 minutes). Chest tubes were inserted in 110 of the patients and remained for 0 to 3 days (mean, 1.2 days). The average hospital stay was 2.8 days. One intraoperative complication developed. Compromise to the left upper lobe bronchus occurred, which required a bronchoplasty. There was a 3% postoperative complication rate.

SELECTED REFERENCES

1. Rodgers BM, Moazam F, Talbert JL: Thoracoscopy in children. Ann Surg 189:176-189, 1979

2. Rothenberg SS: Thoracoscopic lung resection in children. J Pediatr Surg 35:271-275, 2000

3. Rothenberg SS: Experience with thoracoscopic lobectomy in infants and children. J Pediatr Surg 38:102-104, 2003

4. Albanese CT, Sydorak RM, Tsao K, et al: Thoracoscopic lobectomy for prenatally diagnosed lung lesions. J Pediatr Surg 38:553-555, 2003

5. De Lagausie P, Bonnard A, Berrebi D, et al: Video-assisted thoracoscopic surgery for pulmonary sequestration in children. Ann Thorac Surg 80:1266-1269, 2005

6. Cano I, Anton-Pacheco J, Garcia A, et al; Video-assisted thoracoscopic lobectomy in infants. Eur J Cardiothorac Surg 29:997-1000, 2006

7. Albanese CT, Rothenberg SS: Experience with 144 consecutive pediatric thoracoscopic lobectomies. J Laparoendosc Adv Surg Tech A 17:339-341, 2007

8. Rothenberg SS: First decade's experience with thoracoscopic lobectomy in infants and children. J Pediatr Surg 43:40-45, 2008

43
Thoracoscopic Congenital Diaphragmatic Hernia Repair

Mark L. Wulkan

This chapter discusses minimally invasive repair of a Bochdalek (posterolateral) congenital diaphragmatic hernia (CDH). The Bochdalek CDH develops in early gestation and is located in the posterolateral aspect of the diaphragm. It is associated with pulmonary hypoplasia and a significant incidence of respiratory failure. Patients with CDH typically have very immature lungs with decreased branching of both the arteries and the airways. The primary physiologic problem is pulmonary hypoplasia and respiratory failure, not the mass effect of abdominal viscera in the chest. The operative approach to CDH is typically transabdominal through a subcostal incision or, less commonly, through a low thoracotomy. The defect is closed primarily, if possible. If the defect cannot be closed, various synthetic materials as well as muscle flaps have been used. Both the laparoscopic and thoracoscopic approaches for CDH repair have been described. I prefer the thoracoscopic approach because of the ease of reduction of the abdominal viscera with CO_2 pneumothorax and the clear visualization of the defect.

INDICATIONS FOR WORKUP AND OPERATION

Congenital diaphragmatic hernia is often diagnosed prenatally. After the infant is born, a chest radiograph is confirmatory. Orogastric decompression and positive-pressure ventilation should be instituted once the diagnosis is suspected to prevent the abdominal viscera from expanding in the chest and causing a mass effect. The workup for infants with CDH typically consists of an echocardiogram to look for possible congenital heart disease and to quantify the degree of pulmonary hypertension. A baseline ultrasound of the head is also obtained in anticipation of possible extracorporeal life support (ECLS). In the past, CDH was thought to be a surgical emergency. It is now understood that the primary physiologic threat to the patient is not the mass effect of the abdominal viscera in the chest but the pulmonary hypoplasia. Thus, initiation of positive-pressure ventilation and nasogastric drainage at birth prevent further herniation and distention of the abdominal viscera.

We typically wait for the patient's respiratory status to stabilize before proceeding with operative repair. This is especially important for the minimally invasive approaches to CDH that use CO_2 insufflation. If the patient requires ECLS, thoracoscopic surgical repair is delayed until the patient is decannulated and on conventional respiratory support. Pervious ECLS is not a contraindication to thoracoscopic CDH repair. We have not attempted thoracoscopic CDH repair while the infant is on ECLS as this would be very difficult logistically, and unsafe because of the risk of bleeding.

OPERATIVE TECHNIQUE

Thoracoscopic repair of congenital diaphragmatic hernia is performed under general endotracheal anesthesia. A standard endotracheal tube is inserted. There is no need for bronchial blockers. There is usually plenty of room in the chest because of the pulmonary hypoplasia. Although not necessary, contralateral mainstem intubation can be used. Appropriate anesthetic monitors are placed, including an arterial line through which blood pressure and blood gases can be monitored.

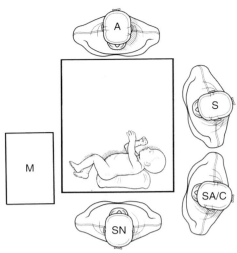

Figure 43-1.   The infant is positioned transversely at the end of the operating table with the left side elevated approximately 70 degrees. A wide preparation and drape is performed to allow access to the abdomen if conversion to a laparotomy is necessary. The operating surgeon (S) stands above the patient's head, with the monitor (M) placed just beyond the infant's feet. The surgical assistant/camera holder (SA/C) stands next to the surgeon. A, anesthesiologist; SN, scrub nurse.

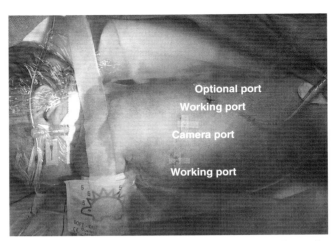

Figure 43-2.   The location of the ports for thoracoscopic repair of a left diaphragmatic hernia. In this case, a fourth port was used by the surgical assistant and was placed posterior to the working port used by the surgeon's left hand.

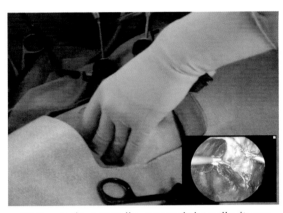

Figure 43-3.   As the suture line proceeds laterally, it may become more difficult to place the sutures. Suturing the lateral portion of the defect can be made easier by having an assistant put external pressure on the lateral chest wall to bring the tissues more in line with the instruments. *Inset:* The edge of the diaphragm is being grasped, and the suture has been introduced in the diaphragm a few centimeters from the edge.

The infant is positioned transversely at the end of the bed in a near-lateral decubitus position (at approximately 70 degrees) to allow access to the abdomen if conversion to a laparotomy is necessary. The operating surgeon stands above the patient's head with a monitor placed at the infant's feet (Fig. 43-1).

Initial Veress needle access is obtained through the 3rd or 4th intercostal space in the posterior axillary line. The chest is insufflated to 3 to 5 mm Hg using CO_2 at a flow rate of 1 L/min. Surprisingly, this is very well tolerated in this patient population. We have had neither problems with induction of clinically significant pulmonary hypertension nor any other hemodynamic perturbations. A 4-mm port is introduced at this site, and a 30-degree 4-mm telescope is inserted. Two additional 3- or 4-mm cannulas are inserted just inferior and to the right and left of the initial port site (Fig. 43-2). Occasionally, we forgo the use of cannulas and place the instruments directly through the chest wall. The right-handed instrument is positioned in the anterior axillary line, and the left-handed instrument is placed near the posterior axillary line. Typically, there is plenty of space in the chest because of the underdeveloped lung.

The abdominal viscera are gently reduced into the abdomen using blunt graspers, with care taken to cause no injury to the bowel or to any herniated viscera. The spleen is the last structure to be reduced. If there is a hernia sac, it can be used to help with the reduction of the viscera. Typically, I remove any hernia sac; however, this step may be optional if the sac is inverted on the abdominal side of the hernia. The defect is then closed

with interrupted sutures, starting medially and moving laterally. The needles are generally introduced through the chest wall for all stitches. This avoids dulling the needle by dragging it through a 3- or 4-mm port.

Early in our series, we used PDS (Ethicon, Inc., Somerville, NJ) suture with both extracorporeal and intracorporeal knot tying. Currently, we use silk or braided nylon as it is easier to tie intracorporeally. As the suture line extends laterally, it may become more difficult to place the sutures. Suturing of the lateral portion of the defect can be made easier by having an assistant put external pressure on the lateral chest wall to bring the tissues in-line with the instruments (Fig. 43-3). The lateral corner stitch may be brought around the rib, if necessary, as can be done with the open approach. Usually, this is done by making a nick in the skin where the needle is to be inserted into the chest cavity. The needle is then introduced extracorporeally through the chest wall and grasped intracorporeally. The suture is then driven back out the chest wall around a rib. The needle is not pulled all the way through the skin. When the back end of the needle is in the subcutaneous tissue, it is backed out the original hole (Fig. 43-4). An RB1 or SH needle works well for this suture.

If the closure of the diaphragm is under tension or is not possible, a prosthetic mesh can be introduced. I prefer an 8-ply Surgisis Gold (Cook, Inc., Bloomington, IL). GORE-TEX (WL Gore & Assoc., Flagstaff, AZ) and other biologic materials are also used in our institution, depending on the surgeon's preference. The easiest way to introduce the mesh into the chest cavity is to extend one of the graspers out through the opposite cannula site, grab the mesh, and pull the mesh into the chest

after it has been appropriately trimmed (Fig. 43-5). Interrupted sutures or continuous sutures can be placed between the rim of the diaphragmatic defect and the mesh. As there is usually no diaphragm laterally, the sutures are placed around the ribs. This may be done using the technique previously described (see Fig. 43-4). Once the defect is repaired, placement of a chest drain is optional. We tend not to leave chest drains routinely. The CO_2 insufflation is evacuated and the skin is closed.

PEARLS

1. Introduce the sutures into the chest directly using an external needle driver. This maintains the curve on the RB1 needle, which will facilitate suturing.

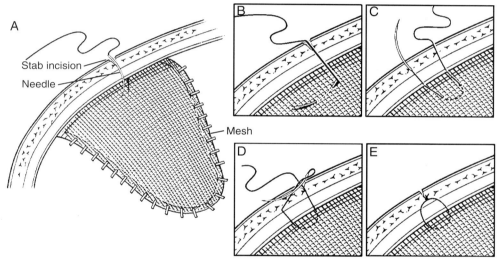

Figure 43-4. Suturing the lateral portion of the defect is the most difficult part of the thoracoscopic operation. **A,** The lateral corner stitches may be brought around the ribs to secure the diaphragmatic edge or mesh to the ribs. This is accomplished by making a small nick in the skin and introducing the needle into the thoracic cavity. **B,** Mesh has been used to close a portion of the diaphragmatic defect, so a horizontal mattress suture is placed through the mesh. **C,** The needle is then exteriorized through the chest wall, but the heel of the needle is left in the subcutaneous tissue. **D,** Next, the heel of the needle is backed out through the small nick in the skin. **E,** The suture is then tied in the subcutaneous tissue.

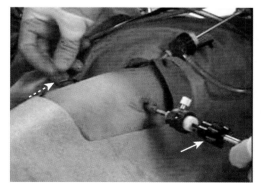
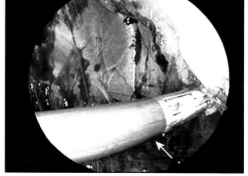

Figure 43-5. An easy way to introduce biologic mesh is to extend one of the graspers (*solid arrow*) out through the opposite cannula site (*dotted arrow*), secure the mesh, and then pull it into the chest after it has been appropriately trimmed.

2. To place the sutures laterally, it is often necessary to put external, manual pressure on the chest wall to bring the lateral edges into an ergonomic position for placement of the sutures (Fig. 43-3). These sutures may also be back-handed intracorporeally.

3. If the patient is having any hemodynamic problems at all, reduce the CO_2 inflating pressure, and then maintain CO_2 insufflation pressure at a lower level and flow.

PITFALLS

1. Make sure your ports are placed cephalad on the thoracic wall. If the cannulas are too low, it can be very difficult to suture.

2. Gently reduce the bowel and gently push the spleen through the defect. You may lift up the diaphragmatic leaf and place it over the spleen to help reduce it. Do not stab the spleen.

3. If there is total diaphragmatic agenesis, we usually convert to an open operation.

RESULTS

Four of the six surgeons at our institution are now performing thoracoscopic CDH repair, and 26 patients with CDH have undergone 28 attempted thoracoscopic repairs, with 20 successes (71%). Reasons for conversion were diaphragmatic agenesis (three), a large combination Bochdalek and hiatal hernia (one), misdiagnosis of a bilateral Morgagni hernia (one), strangulated colon within the hernia (one), inability to expose the posterior leaf (one), and hypercarbia (one). Three patients required ECMO preoperatively, and two of these were converted to an open repair. None had associated cardiac or other major congenital anomalies. Three patients had right-sided hernias, 22 had left-sided hernias, and one patient had bilateral Morgagni hernias. Of those repaired thoracoscopically, 10 were closed primarily, 5 were reinforced with a prosthetic material, and 5 were repaired with a prosthetic patch. Complications in patients who underwent successful thoracoscopic repair included one patient who died as a result of fungal sepsis, one death from postoperative respiratory failure and ECLS complications, one upper gastrointestinal bleed from gastritis, and two recurrences. These recurrences were both successfully repaired thoracoscopically. Complications in patients who were converted to an open procedure were as follows: chylothorax and superior vena caval thrombosis (one), and recurrent CDH (one).

SELECTED REFERENCES

1. van der Zee DC, Bax NM: Laparoscopic repair of congenital diaphragmatic hernia in a 6-month-old child. Surg Endosc 9:1001-1003, 1995
2. Holcomb GW 3rd, Ostlie DJ, Miller KA: Laparoscopic patch repair of diaphragmatic hernias with Surgisis. J Pediatr Surg 40:E1-5, 2005
3. Rozmiarek A, Weinsheimer R, Azzie G: Primary thoracoscopic repair of diaphragmatic hernia with pericostal sutures. J Laparoendosc Adv Surg Tech A 15:667-669, 2005
4. Yang EY, Allmendinger N, Johnson SM, et al: Neonatal thoracoscopic repair of congenital diaphragmatic hernia: Selection criteria for successful outcome. J Pediatr Surg 40:1369-1375, 2005

44
Thoracoscopic Decortication and Debridement for Empyema

Marjorie J. Arca and George W. Holcomb III

E mpyema thoracis is a collection of inflammatory fluid in the thoracic cavity. It usually arises as a complication of pneumonia, but it may also result from trauma, subdiaphragmatic infections, immunodeficient conditions, neoplastic processes, and other inflammatory states. Empyema formation annually occurs in 2% to 8% of children hospitalized for pneumonias. The progression of empyema is described in three stages: exudative, fibrinopurulent, and organizing. The exudative stage is characterized by sterile, thin fluid with minimal debris. The fibrinopurulent stage has thicker fluid, thick fibrin strands, loculations, and bacterial contamination. Finally, the pleural infection can progress to the organizing stage in which a thick fibrous peel can encase the lung, leading to compromised lung expansion.

Debridement refers to the removal of semisolid debris from the thoracic cavity. Decortication is the removal of the solid thick peel that may line either the parietal or the visceral pleura, or both. The goals of thoracoscopic debridement and decortication for empyema are to drain the infectious fluid from the pleural cavity and release the entrapped lung, to hasten resolution of symptoms, and to prevent pleural scarring.

INDICATIONS FOR WORKUP AND OPERATION

Since the introduction of routine vaccination for *Haemophilus influenzae*, the most common causative organisms for childhood pneumonias are *Streptococcus pneumoniae* and *Staphylococcus aureus*. Most patients have received a course of oral antibiotics before presentation. Symptoms range in severity. High spiking fevers, pleuritic chest pain, hypoxia, and a leukocytosis are suggestive of an empyema.

An algorithm for the diagnostic workup for a patient with parapneumonic fluid is outlined in Figure 44-1. The chest radiograph usually reveals haziness or opacification of a portion of the involved hemithorax. A lateral decubitus chest film may reveal layering of fluid. A chest ultrasound or a computed tomographic (CT) scan is a good diagnostic test to gauge the thickness of the fluid or to determine whether it is loculated (Fig. 44-2). Thin parapneumonic fluid collections with minimal fibrin debris (the exudative stage) may be drained simply with a chest tube. Patients with loculated fluid or fluid with thicker fibrin strands (the fibrinopurulent stage) are the best candidates for thoracoscopic drainage and debridement. Patients who fail to improve clinically in 48 to 72 hours with simple chest tube drainage should be considered for a thoracoscopic procedure. If the presence of a thick, solid peel encasing the lung is suggested on ultrasound or chest CT, the surgeon can start with thoracoscopy but must be prepared for an open decortication.

OPERATIVE TECHNIQUES

The procedure is performed under general anesthesia with endotracheal intubation. If possible, single-lung

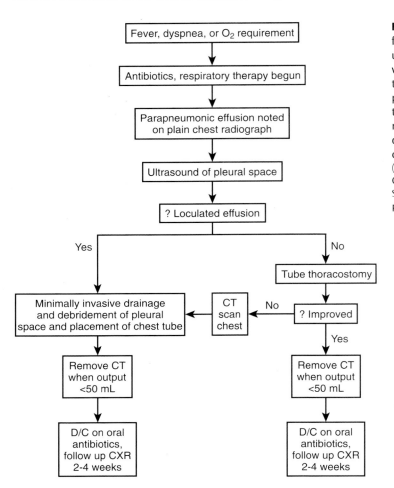

Figure 44-1. An algorithm for diagnostic evaluation for a patient with parapneumonic fluid. After either ultrasound or CT of the pleural space, it is determined whether the effusion is loculated. If it is loculated, thoracoscopic debridement and decortication is performed. If it is not loculated, then simple tube thoracostomy is preferred. However, if the patient does not improve with tube thoracostomy, thoracoscopic debridement and decortication is usually required. CXR, chest radiograph; D/C, discharge.
(Reprinted from Calkins CM, Holcomb GW III: Empyema. In Coran AG, Spitz L (eds): Operative Techniques in Pediatric Surgery. London, Edward Arnold, pp 187-195, 2006, with permission.)

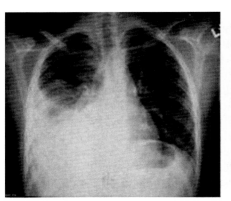
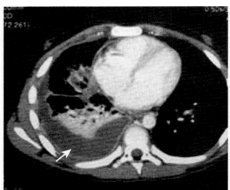
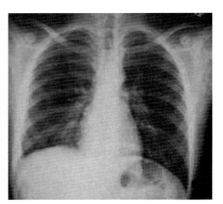

Figure 44-2. This 10-year-old was found to have a right parapneumonic infusion on chest radiograph (*left*). A CT scan was performed and revealed fluid (*arrow*) loculated in the right base (*center*). However, septations were also identified and the patient required thoracoscopic debridement and decortication. Six weeks after the operation, the chest radiograph (*right*) is completely clear.

ventilation using a double-lumen endotracheal tube is employed. The use of invasive monitoring devices such as an arterial line or central venous monitoring is left to the discretion of the anesthesiologist and usually depends on the severity of the patient's illness.

The patient is positioned in the lateral decubitus position with the affected side up. An axillary roll is placed (Fig. 44-3). A smaller child may need another roll at the waist to support the lower back. The larger child may need to be positioned where the iliac crest rests are level at the break in the operating table to open the intercostal spaces. Pressure points such as the proximal fibula, ankle, and foot must be protected with foam pads or lambskin. The arms are best bent at the elbow with the hands directed cephalad. The surgeon and assistant stand opposite one another, with the scrub nurse to the surgeon's right. Two video monitors are helpful as the operation is usually performed in all parts of

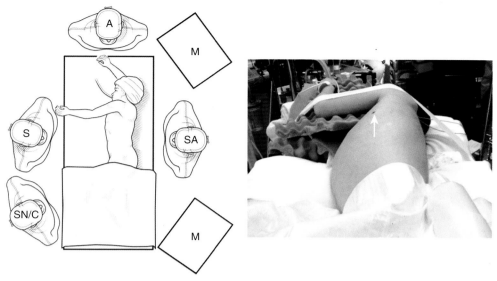

Figure 44-3. For a thoracoscopic debridement and decortication, the surgeon (S) and surgical assistant (SA) stand on either side of the patient. Usually, the scrub nurse holds the camera (SN/C). A monitor (M) is positioned at the head and at the foot of the operating table because the entire thoracic cavity is usually affected by the empyema. A, anesthesiologist. In the patient shown, an attempt was made at initial fibrinolytic therapy through a small chest drain. However, this was unsuccessful and the patient was taken to the operating room for a thoracoscopic debridement and decortication. Such patients are placed in a lateral decubitus position, as shown. Note the site where the chest drain was removed (*arrow*).

the thoracic cavity (Fig. 44-3). One monitor should be positioned at the foot of the operating table and one at the head of the table.

Almost all empyemas affect the caudal portion of the thoracic cavity. Initial access to the empyema can be gained through a 10-mm incision in the anterior axillary line at the level of the 4th or 5th intercostal space (Fig. 44-4). A 10-mm valved cannula with a blunt tip is then introduced through this incision and into the thoracic cavity. Valved cannulas are used initially to allow positive-pressure insufflation up to 6 mm Hg to help compress the lung and to create a working space within the rigid thoracic cage. Alternatively, if a chest tube was previously placed, this site can be used for insertion of the initial port. After removal of the chest tube, the 10-mm cannula is introduced through this established tract. After introduction of this initial cannula, a 10-mm angled telescope is introduced through the cannula and is used to further create a working space by sweeping the adhesions and lung away from the chest wall. Once the underlying lung has been freed and a working space created, a second 10-mm incision is made and a cannula is inserted into the same interspace in the posterior axillary line. The third incision and cannula are positioned in the midaxillary line in the 9th or 10th intercostal space (Fig. 44-4). This incision will be the site for exteriorization of the chest tube after completion of the thoracoscopic debridement and decortication. With this arrangement, a working triangle is formed.

Initially, an endoscopic suction device is used to evacuate the thoracic cavity of its liquid contents. The pleural fluid is sent for Gram stain and culture. The fibrinous

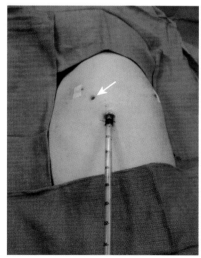

Figure 44-4. The triangular orientation of the ports for thoracoscopic debridement and decortication. A 10-mm incision is used at each site so that the ports can be removed and ring forceps introduced through the incisions and the thoracic wall to perform the debridement and decortication. The most inferior site is selected for exteriorization of the chest tube. The *arrow* indicates the site for previous exteriorization of a chest catheter, which was used with an attempt at fibrolytic therapy to resolve the empyema.

material is debrided from the visceral and parietal pleural surfaces using atraumatic blunt-tipped endoscopic forceps. Once the lung is collapsed and an adequate working space is achieved, the cannulas can be removed and curved ring forceps introduced directly

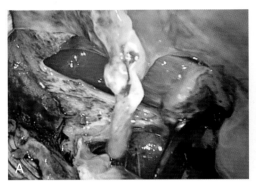
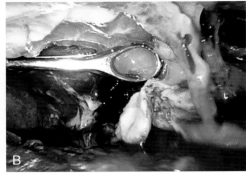

Figure 44-5. Typical appearance in a patient with empyema. **A,** Note the thick fibrinous exudate hanging from the parietal pleura. **B,** Ring forceps have been introduced through a 10-mm incision to allow extensive grasping of the purulent exudate. Note the collapsed lung at the bottom of the photograph.

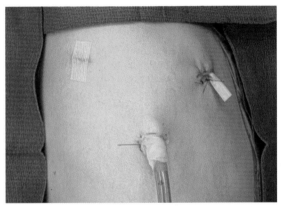

Figure 44-6. Exteriorization of the chest tube through the most inferior working site. The latex drain was left in one of the working incisions as this site was previously used for insertion of a chest tube. Closure of these sites is possible if drainage is accomplished with a small drain to help prevent postoperative infection at the site.

through the chest wall incisions to debride the pleural space (Fig. 44-5). Depending on which portion of the thoracic cavity is being debrided, the instruments and telescope are rotated between the three incisions to triangulate the area being addressed. The surgeon must be careful to avoid lung injury when performing the debridement. All pockets of fluid must be drained adequately. At the conclusion of the operation, the chest cavity is irrigated with warm saline.

A single chest tube (usually 20, 24, or 28 French) is inserted into the pleural space under thoracoscopic visualization (Fig. 44-6). Typically, the most inferior port site is used as the exit site, with the tube directed posteriorly within the chest cavity. The tube is inserted through this most inferior incision but is then tunneled over the cephalad rib to create a soft tissue tract and help prevent the development of a pneumothorax when the chest tube is removed. The incisions are closed in layers with absorbable suture. The chest tube is placed under −10 to −20 cm H_2O suction, depending on the size of the child.

POSTOPERATIVE CARE

The chest tube is maintained on suction until drainage is less than 50 mL in a 24-hour period and all air leaks have resolved. It is then placed to water seal. If the lung is completely expanded and there is no significant reaccumulation of pleural fluid on chest radiographs, then the chest tube is removed. Antibiotics are chosen to reflect the organisms cultured from the empyema fluid. Patients are discharged when they are afebrile and able to tolerate pain on oral medications. Typically, they receive at least a 14-day course of antibiotics. A follow-up visit and chest radiograph are recommended 3 to 4 weeks after discharge.

PEARLS AND PITFALLS

1. The use of either ultrasound or CT imaging before thoracoscopic debridement and decortication helps differentiate between lung consolidation and a large pleural effusion. These two processes can look similar on a chest radiograph.
2. Some authors recommend placing the incisions in the same horizontal plane so that they can be interconnected if a thoracotomy becomes necessary. However, conversion to a thoracotomy is rarely needed unless it is very late in the disease process.
3. The diaphragmatic surface of the lower lobe and the lung apex should be examined carefully for pleural peel and loculated fluid.
4. If small pieces of solid debris are intimately adherent to the lung and their removal would result in lung injury, it may be best to leave them alone.
5. A few small air leaks usually resolve postoperatively with the chest tube in place.
6. It is often helpful to see how well the lung insufflates under thoracoscopic visualization by having the anesthesiologist hand-ventilate to pressures of −30 mm Hg prior to closing.
7. Patients who have had a prolonged severe respiratory infection usually present in a suboptimal nutritional

state. It is imperative to feed these children adequately and in a timely fashion to facilitate healing and recovery.

RESULTS

A consensus panel of the American College of Chest Physicians has published guidelines regarding the management of empyema in adults. They recommended drainage for all complex parapneumonic effusions, stating that simple tube thoracostomy alone might be insufficient for managing empyemas. The panel listed fibrinolytics, video-assisted thoracoscopic decortication (VATS), and open thoracotomy as "acceptable" approaches for complex empyemas in adults, basing their recommendations on case reports and historically controlled comparisons.

In 2004, Gates published a systematic comparison of 44 retrospective studies published from 1987 to 2002 describing the management of complex empyemas in children. The studies were categorized by treatment modalities: chest tube alone, fibrinolytics, open thoracotomy, and VATS. There were 1369 patients available for analysis. Using a Kruskal-Wallis nonparametric test, Gates concluded that early VATS or thoracotomy led to a shorter length of stay than the two other treatment modalities.

From 2000 to 2006 at Children's Mercy Hospital, 47 patients underwent thoracoscopic debridement and decortication for surgical treatment of empyema. The mean age was 7.4 years. Twenty-five patients were male. Twenty-eight operations were on the right side and 19 were on the left. The mean time between admission and the thoracoscopic operation was 3 days (range, 0 to 10 days). The mean duration of postoperative chest tube drainage was 3.6 days (range, 2 to 6 days). The mean postoperative hospitalization was 4.76 days (range, 2 to 12 days). All patients recovered uneventfully. No patient required a second operation.

SELECTED REFERENCES

1. Colice GL, Curtis A, Deslauriers J, et al: Medical and surgical treatment of parapneumonic effusions. Chest 18:1158-1171, 2000
2. Tan TZ, Mason EO J, Wald ER, et al: Clinical characteristics of children with complicated pneumonia caused by Streptococcus pneumonia. Pediatrics 110:1-6, 2002
3. Gates RL, Caniano DA, Hayes JR, Arca MJ: Does VATS provide optimal treatment of empyema in children? A systematic review. J Pediatr Surg 39:381-386, 2004
4. Calkins CM, Holcomb GW III: Empyema. In Coran AG, Spitz L (eds): Operative Techniques in Pediatric Surgery. London, Edward Arnold, pp 187-195, 2006

45
Thoracoscopy for Treatment of Spontaneous Pneumothorax

Bradley M. Rodgers

The use of thoracoscopy for the treatment of patients with a spontaneous pneumothorax has gained general acceptance over the past decade. Thoracoscopy has an advantage over standard axillary thoracotomy in that it provides a view of the entire visceral pleura through significantly smaller incisions. Any of the procedures that have been described for achieving a pleurodesis for treatment of spontaneous pneumothorax through an open thoracotomy can be performed thoracoscopically.

INDICATIONS FOR WORKUP AND OPERATION

A spontaneous pneumothorax is generally categorized as primary (PSP) or secondary (SSP). Children with SSP have underlying pulmonary disease such as cystic fibrosis or asthma. Patients with PSP have no known underlying pulmonary disease, although approximately a third are found to have subpleural blebs (Fig. 45-1). Most patients with PSP or SSP experience some degree of respiratory distress and pain in the ipsilateral chest. The workup for patients with a suspected pneu-mothorax includes a careful history, particularly looking for the possibility of previous episodes that were unrecognized, as well as a history of underlying lung disease.

The diagnosis of a pneumothorax by physical examination in children is difficult because of the transmission of breath sounds from the contralateral lung. Particular attention should be paid to the position of the trachea in the suprasternal notch as it will shift to the contralateral side in patients with a tension pneumothorax. An upright posteroanterior chest radiograph confirms the presence of a pneumothorax (Fig. 45-2). A chest computed tomography (CT) scan may demonstrate subpleural blebs. Many patients with a spontaneous pneumothorax are symptomatic enough that a chest tube or catheter should be placed immediately. On the other hand, many patients with relatively small pneumothoraces will absorb the air, given some time. I prefer not to insert a chest tube in patients who are candidates for thoracoscopy and are stable from a respiratory standpoint to avoid stimulating pleural inflammation.

The traditional indications for pleurodesis in children with PSP are (1) a second pneumothorax on the ipsilateral side, (2) simultaneous bilateral pneumothoraces, (3) a continued air leak (>7 days), (4) an initial tension pneumothorax, and (5) difficulty in accessing medical care. Another indication in adult patients is a high-risk occupation (flying, diving). With the ease and success of thoracoscopic treatment of these patients, many surgeons are liberalizing the indications and offering pleurodesis to patients with significant respiratory difficulties created by an initial pneumothorax. Some surgeons have advocated a chest CT scan at the initial episode to look for evidence of subpleural blebs on the ipsilateral or contralateral side as an indication for pleurodesis. All children with SSP should be offered pleurodesis with the initial episode as ipsilateral recurrence is uniform and symptoms may be severe.

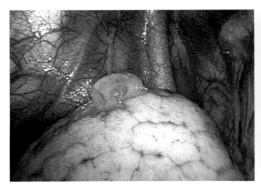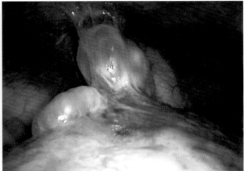

Figure 45-1.   Patients with primary spontaneous pneumothoraces generally do not have a known underlying pulmonary disease. However, subpleural blebs are found in at least one third of these patients.

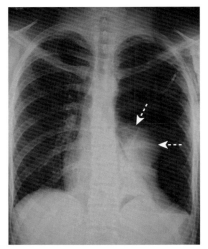

Figure 45-2.   An upright posteroanterior chest radiograph confirms the presence of a pneumothorax. In this chest radiograph, there is marked collapse of the left lung (*arrows*). The majority of the pleural cavity is filled with air.

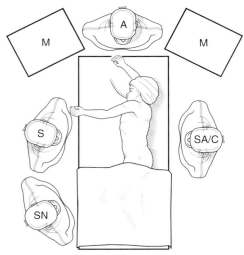

Figure 45-3.   Most patients with spontaneous pneumothorax have blebs in the upper lobes. These patients are placed in a full lateral position with careful padding. The surgeon (S) and surgical assistant/camera holder (SA/C) are positioned on opposite sides of the operating table. If two monitors (M) are used, they are positioned at the head of the table on either side of the anesthesiologist (A). The scrub nurse (SN) can be positioned at the surgeon's discretion, but is usually caudal to the surgeon.

OPERATIVE TECHNIQUES

The anesthetic considerations for thoracoscopic pleurodesis depend in large measure on the stability of the patient and the planned procedure. At one extreme, a quick, relatively painless talc pleurodesis may be performed under sedation along with an intercostal nerve block with the patient breathing spontaneously. On the other hand, a more involved procedure, such as an apical pleurectomy, is better performed under general anesthesia, perhaps with unilateral ventilation. In general, unilateral ventilation of the contralateral lung offers some advantages when performing a thoracoscopic pleurodesis, but it may make identification of subpleural blebs more difficult. We currently perform the majority of these procedures with the patient under general anesthesia with a double-lumen endotracheal tube. We supplement the general anesthesia with a local anesthetic at the cannula sites or with a formal rib block.

Patients in whom a talc pleurodesis is to be performed under local anesthesia are placed in the position of maximal respiratory comfort. All patients having general anesthesia are placed in a full lateral position with careful padding. The surgeon and surgical assistant/camera holder are positioned on opposite sides of the operating table, as these blebs are usually located at the apex of the lung. When two monitors are used, they are positioned on either side of the patient's head (Fig. 45-3).

We prefer to use the Step cannula system (US Surgical, Norwalk, CT) for thoracoscopy, believing that it reduces the trauma to the intercostal neurovascular bundle.

Three ports are usually required: a 12-mm port for the stapler, a 5-mm cannula for the camera, and a 3-mm port or stab incision for a grasping instrument (Fig. 45-4). If a chest tube was not previously required, a 5-mm Step cannula is initially introduced in the 5th intercostal space, midaxillary line, to avoid the latissimus and serratus anterior muscles. A 5-mm 0- or 30-degree telescope is then inserted. The visceropleural surface is carefully examined with the ipsilateral lung ventilated with low inspiratory pressure, looking for evidence of disruption of the visceral pleura as a cause for the pneumothorax. The ipsilateral lung is then collapsed with CO_2 insufflation and occlusion of the ipsilateral bronchus. A second 5-mm Step cannula is introduced in an adjacent interspace in either the anterior or posterior axillary line, and a dissecting instrument is used to bluntly dissect any loose adhesions between the lung and chest wall and to retract the lung to allow inspec-

tion of the entire visceral pleural surface. If a subpleural bleb is encountered, usually at the apex of the lung (Fig. 45-5A), a 12-mm cannula will be needed to accept the roticulating endoscopic stapler with a vascular cartridge. We prefer to position this cannula as low as practical on the chest wall and in the posterior axillary line to allow maximal space to open the stapler. The bleb is grasped with the dissecting forceps and the lung is resected with multiple firings of the stapler (Fig. 45-5B,C). The specimen is then extracted through the 12-mm port. We do not routinely use a specimen bag for this retrieval.

A pleurodesis is then performed. The majority of our patients are treated with a talc pleurodesis. The talc atomizer (Sclerosol Sterile Talc Powder, Bryan Corp., Woburn, MA) is inserted through the 5-mm cannula, and the entire visceral and parietal surfaces are dusted with 2 to 4 g talc, concentrating at the apex of the chest. When a mechanical pleurodesis is being performed, the working port must be a 10-mm cannula. Therefore, the 10-mm telescope is removed and a 5-mm scope is inserted through the 5-mm cannula. We prefer to wrap a piece of Marlex mesh (Davol, Inc., Cranston, RI) around the tip of a 5-mm dissecting forceps and to secure it with several ligatures (Fig. 45-6) for the

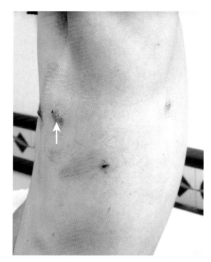

Figure 45-4. A triangular configuration for the ports is ideal. In the tall, lean patient shown, the stapler was introduced through the port in the anterior axillary line (*arrow*). A stab incision was placed just inferior to the scapula, and a grasper was introduced through it to elevate the bleb. The telescope was positioned through the most inferior port. The stapler was introduced through the medial port because that was where a relatively large chest tube had been placed previously at a different hospital.

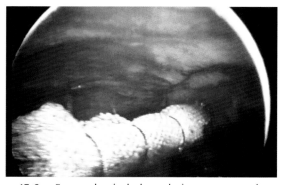

Figure 45-6. For mechanical pleurodesis, we wrap a piece of Marlex mesh around the tip of a 5-mm dissecting forceps and secure it with several ligatures. The Marlex allows a vigorous abrasion of the parietal pleural surface without accumulating fibrous tissue and losing its abrasive capacity.

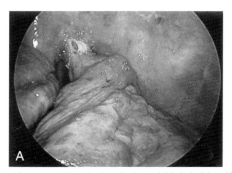
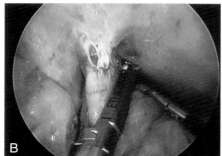
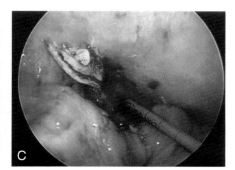

Figure 45-5. **A,** A subpleural bleb is identified in the apex of the lung, and air is seen emanating from rupture of the bleb. **B,** The bleb is grasped with a dissecting forceps, and a stapler is positioned across the tip of the lung to be resected. **C,** The bleb has been ligated and divided with the stapler.

mechanical pleurodesis. The Marlex allows a vigorous abrasion of the parietal pleural surface without accumulating fibrous tissue and losing its abrasive capacity. The pleura is abraded over as much of the surface as can be visualized with particular attention paid to the apex.

When an apical pleurectomy is anticipated, the cautery is used to score the pleura over the surface of the 4th rib posterolaterally, and the entire apical cap of parietal pleura is removed using blunt dissection. The pleura is incised sharply over the superior vena cava or great vessels to avoid cautery dissection in this region. This dissection is accomplished by inserting a second 5-mm Step cannula and using a 5-mm cotton-tip dissector. At the completion of all of these procedures, the working ports are removed. A 16 or 18 French chest tube or a soft drain is inserted through the posteroinferior incision under direct visualization and secured to the chest wall with the tip of the tube or drain positioned at the thoracic apex. The telescope and its cannula are then removed. The port sites are closed in layers using interrupted absorbable sutures in the thoracic wall musculature and subcutaneous tissues. The skin is closed with subcuticular absorbable sutures. The chest tube or drain is connected to underwater seal drainage, without suction. A chest radiograph is obtained in the recovery room. Suction is not applied to the chest tube or drain if the lung is fully expanded. If there remains a pneumothorax, 10 cm of suction is applied.

POSTOPERATIVE CARE

The chest tube or drain is placed to underwater drainage for 12 hours and is removed after the lung is fully expanded. Full expansion of the lung is confirmed with a chest radiograph after removing the tube or drain, and the patient is discharged to be followed up in 2 weeks with a repeat chest radiograph.

PEARLS

1. The use of a chest CT scan may demonstrate subpleural blebs, identifying a patient at high risk for recurrence.
2. All of the pleural adhesions must be taken down to visualize the entire pleural surface and ensure a complete pleurodesis.
3. Talc pleurodesis can be performed rapidly under four-rib intercostal block in children with SSP and significant respiratory insufficiency.

4. Eliminating suction on the chest tube postoperatively may minimize persistent air leaks.

PITFALLS

1. The use of unilateral pulmonary ventilation on the contralateral side offers some advantages in this patient population, but pleural leaks on the affected side may be difficult to discern.
2. You *must* visualize the entire visceral pleural surface.
3. When removing the ports, carefully inspect the cannula sites for signs of intercostal bleeding.

RESULTS

Since 1982, we have used thoracoscopy for the treatment of all pediatric patients with a spontaneous pneumothorax considered appropriate for pleurodesis. We have performed a total of 42 thoracoscopic procedures in 32 patients. Sixteen patients had PSP and 16 had SSP. Thirty-eight procedures were performed with talc pleurodesis, and four underwent pleural abrasion. In addition, two of the latter had an apical pleurectomy. There have been two partial recurrences, both in patients with SSP: one had undergone a pleural abrasion and the other a talc pleurodesis. Four complications have occurred. Three patients with cystic fibrosis had prolonged air leaks (7, 8, and 12 days) and one patient experienced an episode of bleeding from an intercostal vessel requiring repeat thoracoscopy for control. Follow-up has ranged from 6 months to 24 years.

SELECTED REFERENCES

1. Ozcan C, McGahren ED, Rodgers BM: Thoracoscopic treatment of spontaneous pneumothorax in children. J Pediatr Surg 38:1459-1464, 2003
2. Freixinet JL, Canalis E, Julia G, et al: Axillary thoracotomy versus videothoracoscopy for the treatment of primary spontaneous pneumothorax. Ann Thorac Surg 78:417-420, 2004
3. Choudhary AK, Sellars ME, Wallis C. et al: Primary spontaneous pneumothorax in children: The role of CT in guiding management. Clin Radiol 60:508-511, 2005
4. Sawada S, Watanabe Y, Moriyama S: Video-assisted thoracoscopic surgery for primary spontaneous pneumothorax: Evaluation of indications and long-term outcome compared with conservative treatment and open thoracotomy. Chest 127:2226-2230, 2005

46
Thoracoscopic Biopsy of a Mediastinal Mass

Danny C. Little and George W. Holcomb III

Management of mediastinal masses in children depends on obtaining tissue for diagnosis. Historically, several modalities have been available, including percutaneous fine-needle aspiration, cervical mediastinoscopy, mediastinotomy, thoracotomy, and sternotomy. In recent years, the indications for thoracoscopy have expanded in adult and pediatric patients. Initial reports focused on biopsying pulmonary masses and debriding empyemas. With improved video technology and finer instrumentation, thoracoscopy can now be used for evaluating mediastinal disorders.

Thoracoscopic biopsy of mediastinal masses is a safe and effective procedure in children. When the surgeon has sufficient experience with minimally invasive techniques and familiarity with the standard open techniques, morbidity should remain low and mortality very rare. Postoperative discomfort is minimal and the cosmetic results are excellent. Most children recover rapidly and can be discharged within 24 hours.

INDICATIONS FOR WORKUP AND OPERATION

Mediastinal masses are often identified incidentally. However, 40% of primary masses are malignant. They may be detected on routine chest radiographs, computed tomography scans, or magnetic resonance images (Fig. 46-1). Three-dimensional reformats may better assess the origin and extent of disease and thus enhance operative planning. The anatomic location of the mediastinal mass is often suggestive of the specific pathology. Posterior mediastinal calcifications may be seen in neuroblastoma whereas calcium deposits in the anterior mediastinum are seen with germ cell tumors.

Preoperatively, consideration should be given to the child's ability to tolerate single-lung ventilation. There is no single test to predict this, but clinical experience has shown that collapse of the ipsilateral lung is tolerated in most children. At the same time, a large anterior mediastinal mass must raise concern about overwhelming tracheal compression when general endotracheal anesthesia is administered, especially in the supine position.

OPERATIVE TECHNIQUE

General anesthesia is induced in the supine position. Anesthetic technique varies according to patient size, pulmonary status, and required exposure. Single-lung ventilation is preferred. This can be accomplished with a double-lumen endotracheal tube in older children. The smallest double-lumen endotracheal tube that is available currently is 27 French, which corresponds to a 6.0-internal-diameter single-lumen tube. In most instances, the patient needs to be older than 7 or 8 years. Selective intubation of the contralateral mainstem bronchus with a cuffed endotracheal tube is often successful. Moreover, pleural insufflation with 6 to 10 mm Hg of CO_2 may help deflate the lung. A Fogarty or Swan-Ganz catheter can be used as a bronchial blocker, and bronchoscopy can facilitate optimal placement.

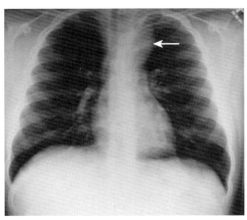
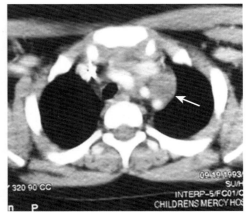

Figure 46-1.   In this patient, the chest radiograph reveals a left mediastinal mass (*arrow*). On the chest CT scan, the mass is identified by an *arrow*, and the vascular structures are seen to be medial and inferior to the mass.

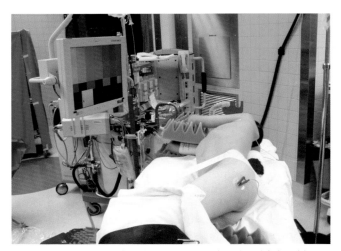

Figure 46-2.   The patient is placed in a right lateral decubitus position for a left middle mediastinal biopsy. The operating table may be gently flexed at the iliac crest to enlarge the intercostal spaces. A bean bag may be advantageous to support larger patients.

The importance of proper positioning cannot be overemphasized. The child is situated so as to allow the lung to fall away dependently after collapse, thus allowing maximal mediastinal visualization. Thus, apical lesions may be more easily viewed in a reversed Trendelenburg position. The opposite would be true for diaphragmatic lesions. The operating table may be gently flexed at the iliac crests to enlarge the intercostal spaces (Fig. 46-2). A bean bag may be required to support larger patients. Cushioning should be placed along joints and pressure points. The patient is prepped and draped as for a standard lateral thoracotomy. The surgeon and assistant stand at the patient's back with the monitor opposite them (Fig. 46-3A).

Preoperative antibiotics covering skin flora are recommended. Using an open technique, a 5-mm valved cannula is introduced in the 4th or 5th intercostal space in the midaxillary line. Insufflation may be added with

initial pressure of 4 to 6 mm Hg without deleterious effects. Additional 5-mm valved ports or stab incisions are placed between the anterior and posterior axillary lines. Optimal port placement is achieved when cannulas surround the pathology in a triangular configuration (Fig. 46-3B).

Straight and angulated telescopes of 0, 30, and 70 degrees should be readily available. If pleural adhesions are encountered, blunt dissection with the suction-irrigation device or blunt forceps may assist in the pleural dissection. The majority of the dissection can be accomplished bluntly with the occasional use of electrocautery or the ultrasonic shears. For the typical middle mediastinal mass, there is often uncertainty as to the location of the great vessels, and preoperative imaging is essential to understanding the relationship of the mass to the surrounding vessels. Usually, the mass is located lateral to the great vessels (or at least a portion of it is located lateral to these vessels) and can be biopsied without concern for massive bleeding. If there remains uncertainty, the planned biopsy site can be aspirated using a small needle to ensure it is not a vascular structure. It is often helpful to place a suture through the site from which the biopsy is to be taken; this allows manipulation of the site without tissue trauma to the resulting specimen. Therefore, we place a 2-0 silk suture in a figure-eight fashion through this biopsy site (Fig. 46-4A). Next, the area to be biopsied is outlined with either a hook cautery or a Maryland dissecting instrument connected to cautery (Fig. 46-4B). Once this area is outlined, scissors connected to cautery can be used to take the actual biopsy (Fig. 46-5A). The suture that was placed through the mass can be very helpful to manipulate the mass for appropriate exposure. Once the biopsy specimen has been removed, hemostasis can usually be controlled with the cautery. An endoscopic bag is quite helpful when exteriorizing the specimen to prevent tumor spillage and contamination of the pleural cavity (Fig. 46-5B). It is important to remember that numerous histologic studies may be needed to

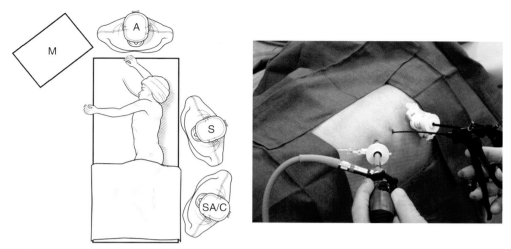

Figure 46-3.   For biopsy of a mediastinal mass, whether in the anterior, posterior, or middle mediastinum, the surgeon (S) and surgical assistant/camera holder (SA/C) stand at the patient's back, with the monitor (M) positioned opposite them. A, anesthesiologist. For biopsy of a middle mediastinal mass, as is being performed in the photograph, a 5-mm valved cannula is introduced in the 4th or 5th intercostal space in the midaxillary line. After insufflation, additional 5-mm valved ports or instruments introduced through stab incisions are placed between the anterior and posterior axillary lines to triangulate the lesion. An angled telescope is used.

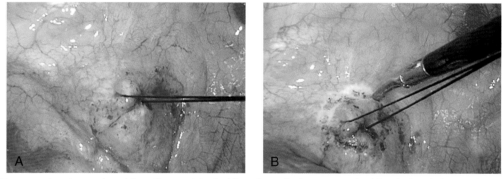

Figure 46-4.   **A,** A silk suture has been placed in a figure-eight fashion through the mass to be biopsied to help manipulate the specimen without traumatizing it. **B,** The biopsy site is being outlined with a Maryland dissecting instrument connected to cautery.

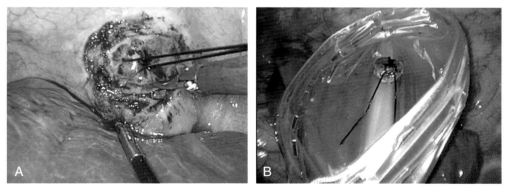

Figure 46-5.   **A,** Once the area is outlined, scissors connected to cautery can be used to take the biopsy. The suture, which has been placed through the mass, is very helpful for manipulation of the mass for adequate exposure. **B,** The biopsy is placed into an endoscopic retrieval bag.

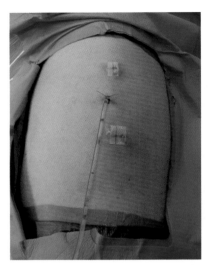

Figure 46-6. If desired by the surgeon, a small, fluted, closed suction drain can be introduced through one of the small incisions and directed toward the apex. Bulb suction is usually sufficient. Some surgeons do not place a drain for this operation.

determine the patient's diagnosis, so it is important to have an adequate volume of tissue for these studies.

The use of a chest drain is usually dictated by surgeon preference. A small fluted Blake drain (Johnson & Johnson, New Brunswick, NJ) can be placed through the most caudal 5-mm incision and directed towards the apex. Usually, bulb suction is sufficient (Fig. 46-6). An intercostal nerve block using 0.25% bupivacaine hydrochloride is used. The small incisions are closed in layers with absorbable suture.

POSTOPERATIVE CARE

The patients are admitted to the surgical floor after the operation and allowed to begin oral intake when desired. Postoperative analgesia is facilitated with intravenous ketorolac (0.5 mg/kg intravenously, up to 10 mg) and oral analgesics. The drain output and chest radiograph are reviewed the following day. Most children are ready for removal of the drain on the first postoperative day. Occasionally, a small pneumothorax is identified, which generally can be followed expectantly. Over 80% of our patients are ready for discharge within 48 hours.

PEARLS

1. Closely communicate with the anesthesiologist when using thoracic insufflation to avoid a hemodynamically significant tension pneumothorax.
2. Use valved cannulas if using insufflation.
3. Insert a 12-mm cannula if using the linear stapler.
4. Ensure meticulous hemostasis with the use of unipolar cautery, ultrasonic shears, or Ligasure (Covidien, Mansfield, MA) to provide a dry operative field and allow optimal visualization.
5. Properly identify the great vessels using endoscopic ultrasound, if needed.

6. Perform needle aspiration of the mass prior to dissection to rule out a vascular structure.
7. Use gravity as much as possible to allow the collapsed lung to fall away from the field of vision.
8. Closely communicate with the pathologist to ensure that the tissue sample is adequate. A frozen section evaluation may be necessary to ensure that diagnostic material was obtained.
9. Place a chest drain for any child with severe parenchymal disease and for those requiring aggressive support with high positive-pressure ventilation.

PITFALLS

1. Recognize that a bronchial blocker may become dislodged back into the trachea. This is especially critical if positioned within the relatively short right main bronchus.
2. Identify the phrenic nerve.
3. Watch for excessive thoracic pressures resulting in impaired ventilation and decreased venous return to the heart.
4. Recall that complete excision is not the goal. The goal is to obtain an adequate biopsy for histologic examination to further guide the patient's management.

SELECTED REFERENCES

1. Davis RD Jr, Oldham HN Jr, Sabiston DC Jr: The mediastinum. In Sabiston DC Jr, Spencer FC (eds): Surgery of the Chest. Philadelphia, Saunders, pp 498-5334, 1990
2. McGahren ED, Kern JA, Rodgers BM: Anesthetic techniques for pediatric thoracoscopy. Ann Thorac Surg 60:927-930, 1995
3. Yim APC: Video-assisted thoracoscopic management of anterior mediastinal masses. Surg Endosc 9:1184-1188, 1995
4. Rieger R, Schrenk P, Woisetschläger R, Wayand W: Video-thoracoscopy for the management of mediastinal mass lesions. Surg Endosc 10:715-717, 1996
5. Saenz NC, Conlon KC, Aronson DC, et al: The application of minimal access procedures in infants, children, and young adults with pediatric malignancies. J Laparoendosc Adv Surg Tech A 7:289-294, 1997
6. Sandoval C, Stringel G: Video-assisted thoracoscopy for the diagnosis of mediastinal masses in children. JSLS 1:131-133, 1997
7. Rothenberg SS: Thoracoscopy in infants and children. Semin Pediatr Surg 7:194-201, 1998
8. Partrick DA, Rothenberg SS: Thoracoscopic resection of mediastinal masses in infants and children: An evaluation of technique and results. J Pediatr Surg 36:1165-1167, 2001
9. Lobe TD: Thoracoscopy in pediatric surgery. In Ziegler MM, Azizkhan RG, Weber TR (eds): Operative Pediatric Surgery. New York, McGraw-Hill, pp 427-438, 2003

47

Thoracoscopic Excision of Foregut Duplications

Sanjeev Dutta and Craig T. Albanese

Duplications of the foregut represent abnormalities of ventral budding of the embryonic lung primordium, and they usually manifest as posterior mediastinal cystic lesions. They are typically adjacent and adherent to the esophagus or bronchial structures. Rarely, they are located in a subdiaphragmatic position. Esophageal lesions are identifiable histologically (and sometimes on radiographs) by their two distinct muscle layers, whereas bronchogenic lesions will have cartilaginous tissue in their walls. Either lesion may have ciliated respiratory epithelium. These lesions are usually discovered on imaging for respiratory symptoms or on a prenatally performed ultrasound. Bronchial cysts may be located centrally—for example, at a subcarinal location—or in the peripheral mediastinum. Esophageal duplications are adjacent to, or embedded in, the wall of the esophagus.

INDICATIONS FOR WORKUP AND OPERATION

Foregut duplications are benign, although rare cases of malignant transformation have been described in all age groups. Patients often present with a cough, wheeze, or respiratory distress, and can develop bronchitis or pneumonia. They can become infected, causing adhesion and fibrosis of the surrounding pleural tissue. Bronchial lesions can grow to cause airway obstruction, and children may present with pulmonary distension for this reason. Esophageal lesions can cause luminal obstruction, which is usually partial. Operative removal is indicated to prevent these sequelae as foregut cysts do not resolve spontaneously.

Computed tomographic (CT) scanning is recommended for lesions discovered on a chest radiograph or prenatal ultrasound. The CT scan helps delineate the exact location and size of the lesion, which dictates the side of the operative approach (Fig. 47-1). Although the majority of lesions can be excised using a thoracoscopic approach, some investigators recommend thoracotomy for bronchial cysts located at a subcarinal position deep in the mediastinum because obtaining a pleural window to access these lesions can be difficult. In addition, subcarinal lesions causing bronchial obstruction may be more amenable to thoracotomy when pulmonary distension on the side ipsilateral to the obstruction makes the lesion inaccessible. Moreover, the child may not tolerate creation of a pneumothorax for access on the contralateral side. Asymmetric subcarinal lesions are amenable to thoracoscopy as they can be teased from their subcarinal position by progressive dissection and traction.

For esophageal lesions deeply imbedded in the esophageal wall, some investigators also advise the judicious use of thoracoscopic resection because of the risk of esophageal perforation. This is a relative contraindication, depending on operator experience and comfort with the possible need to suture the esophageal wall. In general, experienced minimal-access surgeons are aptly skilled and comfortable performing esophageal repair, if needed. Finally, infectious complications can make these lesions difficult to resect because of dense adhesions and fibrosis around

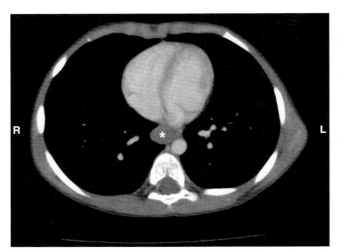

Figure 47-1.   This CT scan in an 8-year-old shows a foregut duplication cyst (*asterisk*) adjacent to the esophagus. The lesion measured 2 × 1.5 cm. This patient subsequently underwent right thoracoscopy with resection of the lesion.

the lesion and between the parietal and visceral pleura.

OPERATIVE TECHNIQUE

The technique of thoracoscopic resection of foregut cystic duplications has been described in detail (see references 5 through 8). General endotracheal anesthesia is used. The ipsilateral lung should be isolated and collapsed (Fig. 47-2). If intubation with a double-lumen endotracheal tube is not possible because of the patient's small size, selective ventilation can be achieved by using a Fogarty balloon catheter or bronchial blocker introduced into the ipsilateral mainstem bronchus. In infants, selective ventilation can be achieved by simply intubating one mainstem bronchus, either blindly or with the assistance of a small fiberoptic bronchoscope. Patients are positioned in a lateral decubitus position for middle mediastinal lesions or placed semiprone (20 to 30 degrees) for posterior mediastinal masses. They are secured with either a bean bag (Olympic Vac Pac, Olympic Medical, Seattle, WA), or with rolls and tape. All bony prominences and the contralateral axilla are padded.

The surgeon and assistant stand next to one another, on the patient's anterior side, with the monitor positioned at the patient's back (Fig. 47-3). A Step (Covidien, Mansfield, MA) sleeve over a Veress needle is introduced through a 5-mm incision placed in the axilla at the midaxillary line, and a 5-mm port is introduced through the expandable sleeve. Low-pressure insufflation (4 to 6 mm Hg) at a low flow rate (1 to 2 L/min) is used to aid in lung parenchymal compression, optimizing exposure and minimizing the need for

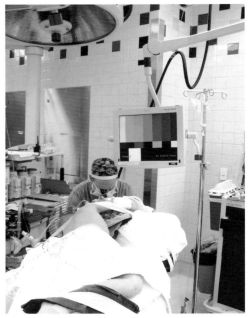

Figure 47-2.   The optimal positioning of the patient for excision of a posterior mediastinal mass is the semiprone position. In this child with a right thoracic duplication, a double-lumen endotracheal tube is being introduced. The anesthesiologist is using fiberoptic bronchoscopy through the double-lumen endotracheal tube to confirm its position.

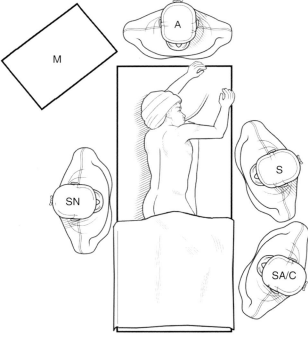

Figure 47-3.   This patient is undergoing right thoracoscopy for removal of an esophageal duplication cyst. The surgeon (S) and surgical assistant/camera holder (SA/C) stand at the patient's front. The monitor (M) is positioned over the patient's right shoulder to keep the target lesion in line between the surgeon and the monitor. The scrub nurse (SN) can be positioned according to the surgeon's preference. A, anesthesiologist.

mechanical lung retraction. Three or four additional ports (3- to 5-mm size) are inserted between the anterior and posterior axillary lines at various levels of the chest, depending on the location of the lesion (Fig. 47-4). A 5-mm, 30-degree angled telescope is used, and dissection instruments include monopolar hook diathermy, scissors, blunt graspers, and the ultrasonic dissector. For esophageal lesions, an esophageal bougie of appropriate size should be placed to aid identification, dissection, and resection.

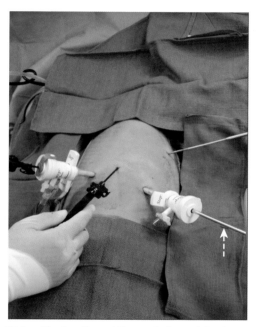

Figure 47-4. The location of the ports for a right thoracoscopy and resection of a duplication cyst. As is evident, two 5-mm ports and two stab incisions are used. The uppermost stab incision is used for insertion of a diamond-shaped retractor to help retract the lung away from the lesion. In this case, the 45-degree angle telescope (*arrow*) was placed through the lowest port. The surgeon worked through the two lateral ports.

RESECTION OF ESOPHAGEAL DUPLICATIONS

The pleura is excised over the lesion, with an intraesophageal bougie in place to help identify the esophagus. These lesions rarely grow to the size of bronchogenic cysts, so decompression before excision is not usually necessary. Lesions embedded in the wall of the esophagus are removed by blunt separation of the muscular fibers, followed by excision in a submucosal plane (Fig. 47-5). Inadvertent perforation of the esophagus requires closure with absorbable sutures. Alternatively, the cyst may share a long common wall with the esophagus. The surgeon may choose to resect the lesion while leaving the common wall intact as would be done in the excision of a bronchogenic cyst. However, stripping of the retained mucosal lining and diathermic obliteration of any small mucosal remnant is necessary to prevent recurrence. The esophageal bougie is removed, and a nasogastric tube is inserted if esophageal repair is performed. A chest tube is placed at the discretion of the surgeon, and the skin incisions are closed after local anesthetic infiltration (Fig. 47-6).

RESECTION OF BRONCHOGENIC CYSTS

The technique for excision of a bronchogenic cyst is very similar to that of an esophageal duplication. The surgeon works through two ports, with a grasping forceps in one hand and a dissection instrument in the other. The assistant guides the telescope and may use an additional port to assist with retraction, if desired or necessary. Excision of very large lesions may be facilitated by transthoracic needle decompression of the lesion. The mediastinal parietal pleura over the lesion is incised. Continuous traction is placed on the lesion while a combination of blunt and sharp (with diathermy) dissection is applied along its wall. Small vessels are cauterized.

The cyst may terminate in a narrow stalk communicating with the airway or may share a common wall. After complete resection of such a lesion, the resultant

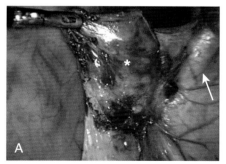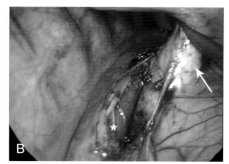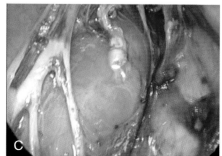

Figure 47-5.   Excision of an esophageal duplication cyst adjacent to the lower esophagus. **A,** The cyst (*asterisk*) is being retracted away from the posterior-lying esophagus. **B,** The esophagus is identified (*asterisk*) after the cyst has been excised. In **A** and **B,** the inferior pulmonary vein is marked with an arrow. **C,** The wall of the esophagus is inspected, as are branches of the vagus nerve as they course along the lateral wall of the esophagus. Histologic examination of the specimen revealed this to be an esophageal duplication cyst.

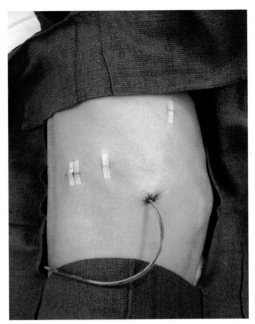

Figure 47-6.   Closure of the incisions after excision of a duplication cyst in the right chest. A soft, pliable chest drain was introduced through the most inferior port and removed the next morning. The patient was discharged the next afternoon.

airway defect is closed using an absorbable suture. If a common wall is left intact, the mucosal lining of the cyst should be stripped or obliterated. The resected lesion can be removed in several ways. If decompressed, it can be withdrawn intact through a port site or pulled out of the port piecemeal. Conversely, the lesion may be placed in an endoscopic bag and the bag exteriorized.

Possible communication with the tracheobronchial tree necessitates short-term chest tube drainage. A small tube or drain is brought through one of the cannula sites. A long-acting local anesthetic is infused at each port site (or as intercostal nerve blocks), and the skin of each incision is closed using intradermal absorbable sutures.

POSTOPERATIVE CARE

Patients are admitted after the operation, and the chest tube, if present, is removed on the first postoperative day if no air leak is evident. Patients are discharged (usually 1 or 2 days postoperatively) when the chest tube is removed and they are tolerating liquids and oral pain medication. When the esophagus was repaired, a water-soluble contrast esophagram is performed on postoperative day 5, and the diet is resumed thereafter.

PEARLS

1. A bougie in the esophagus helps to delineate this structure during dissection.

2. Decompression of large lesions may facilitate dissection.
3. Keeping the dissection intimate to the wall of the lesion avoids injury to other structures.
4. Before final removal of the telescope after resection of bronchogenic cysts, gentle pulmonary insufflation with saline in the thorax allows identification of any air leaks.

PITFALLS

1. A common wall shared by the lesion can lead to perforation of the airway or esophagus, necessitating repair. A thoracoscopic approach should be avoided if there is discomfort with this level of technical complexity.
2. If a common wall is being left intact, its mucosal lining should be completely stripped or obliterated to avoid recurrence.
3. Central mediastinal bronchogenic lesions may have communication with the airway, so a chest tube or drain should be placed to avoid a postoperative pneumothorax.

RESULTS

Michel and colleagues performed thoracoscopic resection of 15 bronchogenic cysts and two esophageal duplications over a 5-year period in patients ranging in age from 2 months to 6 years. The lesions ranged in diameter from 2 to 4 cm. An esophageal perforation was discovered in one patient on postoperative day 1, necessitating thoracotomy for repair and tube thoracostomy drainage. A second patient, in whom a bronchogenic cyst was adherent to the lung parenchyma, developed a postoperative pneumothorax after chest tube removal, requiring insertion of another tube. The remaining patients were discharged after a median hospital stay of 3 days, without evidence of recurrence over a 30-month median follow-up.

Merry and colleagues reported an experience with thoracoscopic resection of seven foregut duplications in children with a mean age of 27 months and a mean weight of 11.4 kg. Six lesions were bronchogenic cysts and one was an esophageal duplication. The median postoperative hospitalization was 2 days. One patient who underwent excision of a cyst and did not have a chest tube inserted at the initial operation developed a postoperative pneumothorax requiring placement of two chest drains. A second patient, who had a bronchogenic cyst excised leaving a common wall treated by laser ablation, was found to have a recurrent lesion 1 year later.

Partrick and Rothenberg reported excision of 12 foregut duplications in a series of 39 patients who underwent thoracoscopic resection of mediastinal masses over a 7-year period. They stressed prone positioning in these patients and did not use chest tubes. All patients resumed oral feeding the same day as surgery and were discharged in less than 48 hours.

SELECTED REFERENCES

1. Di Lorenzo M, Collin PP, Vaillancourt R, et al: Bronchogenic cysts. J Pediatr Surg 24:988-991, 1989
2. Bolton JW, Shahian DM: Asymptomatic bronchogenic cysts: What is the best management? Ann Thorac Surg 53:1134-1137, 1992
3. Harvell JD, Macho JR, Klein HZ: Isolated intra-abdominal esophageal cyst: Case report and review of the literature. Am J Surg Pathol 20:476-479, 1996
4. Shah RS, Varela PJ, Merry CM: Selective ventilation using a Fogarty balloon catheter as a bronchial blocker: An essential technique for pediatric thoracoscopic surgery. Pediatr Endosurg Innov Tech 1:147-150, 1997
5. Harmon CM, Coran AG: Congenital anomalies of esophagus. In O'Neill JA, Rowe MI, Grosfeld JL, et al (eds): Pediatric Surgery. St. Louis, Mosby-Year Book, pp 941-967, 1998
6. Michel JL, Revillon Y, Montupet P, et al: Thoracoscopic treatment of mediastinal cysts in children. J Pediatr Surg 33:1745-1748, 1998
7. Merry C, Spurbeck W, Lobe TE: Resection of foregut-derived duplications by minimal-access surgery. Pediatr Surg Int 15:224-226, 1999
8. Partrick DA, Rothenberg SS: Thoracoscopic resection of mediastinal masses in infants and children: An evaluation of technique and results. J Pediatr Surg 36:1165-1167, 2001

48
Thoracoscopic Repair of Esophageal Atresia and Tracheoesophageal Fistula

Steven S. Rothenberg

E sophageal atresia (EA), with or without a tracheo-esophageal fistula (TEF), is one of the more uncommon congenital anomalies, occurring in 1 in 5000 births. Traditionally, these patients have presented shortly after birth because of an inability to pass an orogastric tube, respiratory distress, or an inability to tolerate feeding. The condition may be associated with other major congenital anomalies (such as those seen in the VACTERL association, which may include vertebrae, imperforate anus, cardiac anomalies, tracheoesophageal fistula, renal anomalies, and limb anomalies), or it may be an isolated defect. Improvements in maternal–fetal ultrasound have resulted in a prenatal diagnosis in a number of cases. Patients with EA/TEF require relatively emergent surgical intervention to prevent aspiration of gastric acid and overdistention of the intestines. Those with pure atresia can be managed in a more leisurely fashion, as long as the infant's oral secretions are controlled by continuous or intermittent suction. In 2000, the first successful thoracoscopic repair of an EA/TEF in a newborn was reported (Rothenberg 2000). More recently, a six-institution review of over 100 cases was published (Holcomb et al. 2005). These papers have shown the safety and efficacy of thoracoscopic repair for this condition.

INDICATIONS FOR WORKUP AND OPERATION

All patients with EA/TEF can be considered for thoracoscopic repair. The decision to approach these patients thoracoscopically depends on a number of different factors, the most important being the stability of the infant and the experience of the surgeon and anesthesiologist with thoracoscopy in neonates. The infant first needs to undergo a thorough evaluation to determine if there are any other congenital anomalies. The most relevant is an echocardiogram to determine the anatomy and function of the heart, as well as the location of the aortic arch.

There are very few absolute contraindications to the thoracoscopic approach for this condition. Currently, these include severe hemodynamic instability requiring significant vasopressor support, and significant prematurity (<1500 g). Relative contraindications include significant congenital cardiac defects, smaller size (1500 to 2000 g), or significant abdominal distention. Congenital heart defects are not an absolute contraindication to the thoracoscopic approach, and repairs have been successfully completed in patients with atrial septal defects, ventricular septal defects, or tetralogy of Fallot. However, patients with severe cardiac anomalies may not be able to tolerate even the short periods of single-lung ventilation that are required to ligate the fistula or perform the anastomosis. It is also important to determine the side of the aortic arch as this determines the surgical approach. A right-sided arch implies that a left-sided approach is preferable. This can be done with minimal added difficulty. Imperforate anus or cloacal anomalies are not a contraindication, and a thoracoscopic EA/TEF repair can be combined with a laparoscopic evaluation and repair of these associated conditions. Other anomalies that may change the surgical approach include the association of intestinal atresias. A proximal bowel atresia may result in significant early gastric distention,

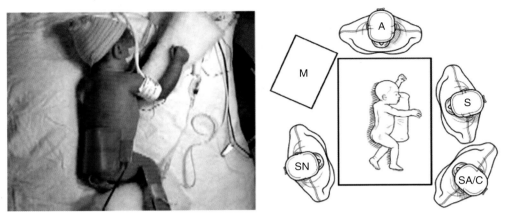

Figure 48-1. Optimal positioning of the newborn for a thoracoscopic repair of esophageal atresia and fistula is shown. The infant should be placed in a modified prone position to allow the lung to fall away from the posterior mediastinum. The diagram shows personnel placement for this operation. The surgeon (S) and surgical assistant/camera holder (SA/C) stand at the front of the patient with the monitor (M) over the infant's shoulder so that the area of dissection is in line between the telescope and camera and the monitor. The scrub nurse (SN) can be positioned depending on the surgeon's preference. A, anesthesiologist.

which may cause immediate problems. The surgeon must evaluate each situation separately and determine the most appropriate approach. Much of the decision will depend on the surgeon's and anesthesiologist's experience with thoracoscopy in neonates.

OPERATIVE TECHNIQUE

General endotracheal anesthesia is administered, but low peak pressures should be used until the fistula is ligated to prevent overdistention of the abdomen. A local anesthetic (0.25% bupivacaine) is inserted at the cannula sites. An attempt should be made to obtain a left mainstem intubation by blind manipulation of the endotracheal tube. However, if this cannot be achieved easily, the endotracheal tube should be left in the trachea just above the carina. Extra time should not be wasted trying to manipulate the tube down the left side as effective collapse of the right lung can be achieved with CO_2 insufflation alone. The decision to perform preoperative bronchoscopy is controversial. The surgeon can follow the guidelines used for open EA/TEF repair. A urinary catheter is also optional.

Once the endotracheal tube is secure, the patient is positioned in a modified prone position (Fig. 48-1). If there is a right-sided arch, then the left side is approached. This positioning gives the surgeon access to the area between the anterior and posterior axillary line for port placement while allowing gravity to pull the lung away from the posterior mediastinum. Generally, small towel rolls are sufficient to provide stabilization for positioning. A small bean bag may also be used. This positioning allows excellent visualization of the esophageal segments and fistula.

The surgeon and the assistant stand at the front of the infant and the monitor is placed at the infant's back (Fig. 48-1). This arrangement allows the surgeon and the assistant to work in line with the monitor. The assistant should also be able to see the monitor. The scrub nurse is situated on either side of the patient or at the front of the table, depending on the room layout. Because of the fine manipulations necessary during the operation, the surgeon and the assistant should position themselves in the most ergonomic and comfortable position.

Port placement is extremely important because of the small chest cavity and the delicate nature of the dissection and reconstruction. The procedure can be performed with three ports, but occasionally a fourth port is necessary for lung retraction (Fig. 48-2). Stab incisions can be used for insertion of 3-mm instruments. The initial cannula (3 to 5 mm) is introduced in the 5th intercostal space at approximately the posterior axillary line. This is the camera port, and it allows excellent visualization of the posterior mediastinum in the area of the two esophageal segments. A 30- or 45-degree telescope is useful to allow the surgeon to look down on the area of dissection. The two instrument ports are placed in the midaxillary line, one to two interspaces above and below the camera site. The upper, 5-mm port is for introduction of the clip applier and needle holder. The lower port is a 3-mm port. Ideally, these ports are situated so that the instrument tips approximate a right angle (90 degrees) at the level of the fistula. This positioning facilitates suturing in the small working space. A fourth cannula (3 mm) can be inserted lower in the thoracic cavity to help retract the lung. The operative principles are the same as those used for the open procedure.

Once the chest cavity has been insufflated and the lung collapsed, the surgeon should first identify the tracheoesophageal fistula. In most cases, the fistula enters the membranous portion of the trachea just above the carina. This level is usually demarcated by the azygos vein (Fig. 48-3). After the azygos is identified, it should be mobilized for a short segment using a curved dissector or scissors. The vein is then cauterized and divided. It is often easiest to divide the vein with a small hook cautery, although bipolar cautery or other sealing devices may also be used.

With the vein divided, the lower esophageal segment is identified and followed proximally to the trachea (Fig. 48-4A). Because of the magnification afforded by the

thoracoscopic approach, it is easy to visualize exactly where the fistula enters the back wall of the trachea. One or two 5-mm endoscopic clips can then be applied across the fistula (Fig. 48-4B). Care should be taken to identify and avoid injuring the vagus nerve. The fistula can then be safely divided distal to the clip with scissors. The distal esophageal segment may retract, making it difficult to visualize. Therefore, it may be preferable to wait until the upper pouch is dissected before completely dividing the fistula. The fistula may also be suture ligated, but this technique requires delicate suturing at a time when an air leak from the divided fistula may be causing increased respiratory compromise.

Attention is now turned to the thoracic inlet. The anesthesiologist exerts pressure on the naso-esophageal tube to help identify the upper pouch. The pleura overlying the upper pouch is incised sharply and the pouch is mobilized with blunt and sharp dissection. In some cases, it is helpful to place a stay suture in the tip of the

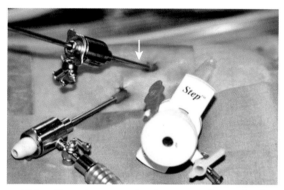

Figure 48-2. Port placement for thoracoscopic repair of esophageal atresia and fistula. The initial cannula (*arrow*) is introduced in the 5th intercostal space in the posterior axillary line. This camera port allows excellent visualization of the posterior mediastinum with a 30- or 45-degree angled telescope. The two instrument ports are then introduced in the midaxillary line one to two interspaces above and below the camera site. The upper port is 5 mm for introduction for the endoscopic clip applier and needle holder. The lower port is 3 mm in size. These ports should be situated so that when the instrument tips are introduced through them, they will approximate a 90-degree angle at the level of the fistula. A 3-mm instrument can be introduced in the lower thoracic cavity to help retract the lung if needed.

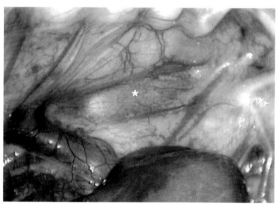

Figure 48-3. The initial view upon entering the chest in a patient with esophageal atresia and tracheoesophageal fistula. The tracheoesophageal fistula is located beneath the azygos vein, which will be divided. The upper esophageal pouch (*asterisk*) is seen clearly with a bougie in it. The collapsed lung is seen at the bottom of the photograph.

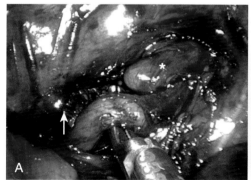

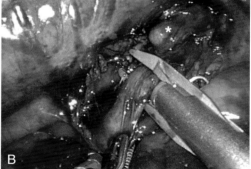

Figure 48-4. **A,** After ligation and division of the azygos vein (*arrow*), the tracheoesophageal fistula has been mobilized and is being encircled with an angled dissecting instrument. The upper esophageal pouch (*asterisk*) was immobilized before ligation and division of the fistula. **B,** The tracheoesophageal fistula is being ligated with a 5-mm endoscopic clip applier. Two clips are usually applied and the fistula is divided distal to the second clip. The upper esophageal pouch is marked with an *asterisk*.

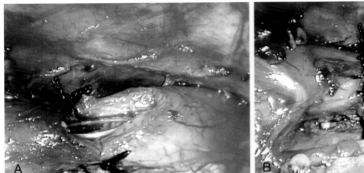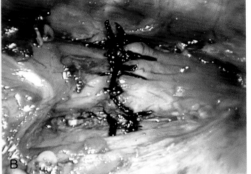

Figure 48-5. **A,** Esophageal anastomosis. The posterior suture line has been completed with interrupted sutures. A small silastic tube introduced through the nose is guided through the anastomosis and into the stomach. **B,** The completed anastomosis.

pouch to aid in applying traction. The plane between the esophagus and the trachea is usually seen well, and the two can usually be separated using sharp dissection. Mobilization of the upper pouch is extended into the thoracic inlet.

Once adequate mobilization is achieved, the distal tip of the pouch is resected. An adequate opening is needed to prevent later stricture formation.

With the two esophageal ends mobilized, the anastomosis is performed using a 4-0 or 5-0 suture on a small tapered needle. The sutures are placed one at a time in an interrupted fashion. The back wall is secured first (three to five sutures), with the knots being intraluminal. A small silastic tube is then passed under direct vision through the anastomosis into the stomach (Fig. 48-5A). The anterior wall is then completed with the nasogastric tube acting as a guide to prevent incorporation of the posterior wall and to ensure patency of the anastomosis (see Fig. 48-5B). Adequate bites of tissue are needed to prevent the sutures from tearing the esophagus. Also, it is imperative to incorporate the mucosa in every stitch. The anastomosis generally requires only eight to ten sutures.

Once the anastomosis is complete, a chest tube or drain is inserted through the lower cannula site and the tip is positioned under visualization near the anastomosis. The other ports are then removed and the sites are closed with absorbable sutures (Fig. 48-6).

POSTOPERATIVE CARE

The postoperative care is the same as for the open operation. The infants are left intubated postoperatively but are quickly weaned over the next 12 to 24 hours. If there is significant tension on the anastomosis, the infant can be paralyzed and intubated for a longer period to try to avoid disruption of the anastomosis. In general, we do not feed the infant through the nasogastric tube. Antibiotics are continued for 48 hours. On postoperative day 5, a water-soluble contrast study is obtained while

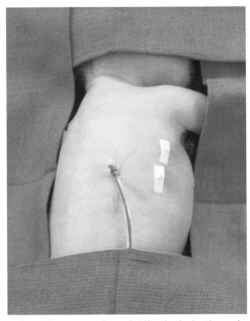

Figure 48-6. Placement of a soft Silastic drain through one of the incisions. The other two incisions have been closed with Steri-Strips.

withdrawing the tube (Fig. 48-7). If no leak is seen, oral feedings are started and the chest tube or drain is removed. If a leak is present, the patient is not fed and antibiotics are resumed. The contrast study is repeated in 3 to 5 days. The patient is discharged after tolerating full feedings for 48 hours. The majority are placed on an acid-reducing agent for 2 to 3 months because of the high incidence of gastroesophageal reflux.

PEARLS

1. Insufflation should start at 4 mm Hg. However, if the lung does not adequately collapse, the pressure can be increased to 7 or 8 mm Hg. Once the lung is

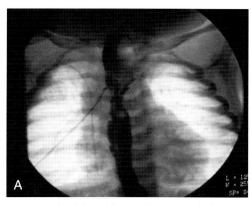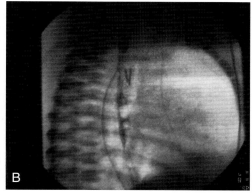

Figure 48-7.   Posteroanterior (**A**) and lateral (**B**) views of the postoperative esophagram show an intact anastomosis with minimal narrowing at the anastomosis. This infant did not require postoperative esophageal dilations and recovered uneventfully.

collapsed, it will stay collapsed until the anesthesiologist actively tries to inflate it with increased positive pressure.

2. After division of the fistula, gently dilate the distal esophageal orifice with a Maryland dissector. This makes it easier to see the mucosa and obtain full-thickness esophageal tissue when performing the esophageal anastomosis.

3. If the gap between the two ends seems too long, rather than trying to bring the two ends together with the first stitch, a slip knot can be placed and the esophageal ends only approximated. A second stitch is then placed and the tension is shared between the two sutures as the two esophageal ends are brought together.

4. The greater magnification afforded by the telescope may show some evidence of perforation or tear at the site where the suture passes through the esophageal wall. These are often not clinically relevant. If there is concern about a potential leak at the anastomosis, a pleural patch can easily be created to cover the anastomosis. Fibrin glue may also be used to help seal the anastomosis.

PITFALLS

1. Not placing the patient far enough prone or the telescope port posterior enough will result in inadequate exposure of the posterior mediastinum. This will necessitate a fourth port to retract the lung.

2. Avoid removing the first stitch even if the two ends cannot be brought together. It is better to leave a gap that can subsequently be closed than to create a rent in the esophagus that must be repaired.

3. Obtaining expeditious closure of the fistula is as important as in the open procedure. Do not waste time looking around. Go right for the azygos vein as the fistula is underneath it.

4. The area of dissection is a small place to suture. If you have not been suturing routinely during laparoscopic operations, this is not the place to start.

RESULTS

Thirty-four of 35 procedures have been successfully completed thoracoscopically. The average operative time was 95 minutes (range, 55 to 120 minutes). All but three patients were extubated by postoperative day 2. Our first patient required reintubation 4 hours after extubation for increasing respiratory distress. He was extubated on day 3. The fifth patient had an extremely long gap (four vertebral bodies), with significant tension on the anastomosis. He was kept sedated and intubated for 4 days. Esophageal contrast studies were obtained on day 5 in 34 patients, and the anastomosis was patent with no evidence of a leak in 33 of the 34. Our first patient had clinical evidence of a leak (saliva in the chest tube) on day 4. The drainage stopped 24 hours later. He was studied on day 8 with no evidence of a leak. One patient with a long-gap isolated esophageal atresia (without fistula) had a small leak that sealed on a repeat study on day 9. The one conversion was performed in a patient with an unrecognized distal congenital esophageal stenosis. The esophageal anastomosis was successfully completed thoracoscopically. However, because the nasogastric tube could not be passed into the stomach, the case was converted to ensure there was not a false passage. Eight patients have required esophageal dilations and all are now on full oral feedings.

SELECTED REFERENCES

1. Rothenberg SS: Thoracoscopic repair of a tracheoesophageal fistula in a neonate. Pediatr Endosurg Innov Tech 4:150-156, 2000

2. Rothenberg SS: Thoracoscopic repair of tracheoesophageal fistula and esophageal atresia in newborns. J Pediatr Surg 37:869-872, 2002

3. Van der Zee DC, Bax NM: Thoracoscopic repair of esophageal atresia with distal fistula. Surg Endosc 17:1065-1067, 2003

4. Rothenberg SS: Thoracoscopic repair of esophageal atresia and tracheo-esophageal fistula. Semin Pediatr Surg 14:2-7, 2005

5. Holcomb GW 3rd, Rothenberg SS, Bax KM, et al: Thoracoscopic repair of esophageal atresia and tracheoesophageal fistula: A multi-institutional analysis. Ann Surg 242:422-428, 2005

49
Thoracoscopic Repair of Esophageal Atresia without Tracheoesophageal Fistula

Marcelo Martinez-Ferro

Neonates without tracheoesophageal fistula (TEF) represent 5% to 7% of all patients with esophageal atresia (EA). Depending on the author, these lesions are classified as type A or type I esophageal atresia. In most of these patients, the esophageal segments are too far apart to allow primary anastomosis. Thus, the term *long-gap* is also used to describe EA without fistula.

The first report of a thoracoscopic repair of a type A esophageal atresia was described by Lobe and associates in 1999. One year later, Rothenberg reported the first thoracoscopic repair of type C esophageal atresia. We published our initial experience with thoracoscopic repair of esophageal atresia without a TEF in 2002.

INDICATIONS FOR WORKUP AND OPERATION

Management of patients with isolated EA is centered on placement of an early feeding gastrostomy followed by a variable waiting period with continuous upper pouch suction and periodic assessment of the distance between the upper and lower esophageal pouches. This assessment can be done either by radiologic or by combined endoscopic and radiologic examinations. During the waiting period, the pouches eventually get close enough to permit a primary esophageal anastomosis. This waiting period can last from 3 to 6 months. Before repair is considered, the real distance between the gaps should be less than one vertebra to allow a low-tension anastomosis.

OPERATIVE TECHNIQUE

Before making an incision, both atretic esophageal ends must be adequately recognized for easy identification during surgery. Thus, while the patient is still in the supine position, the surgeon can introduce a radiopaque semirigid bougie through the gastrostomy up through the distal pouch under fluoroscopy. The bougie is then secured to the infant with tape, and the end of the bougie is positioned to allow its manipulation (through the sterile drapes) by the surgeon during the operation. A softer bougie is inserted through the mouth into the upper esophageal pouch. This bougie should be secured so as to be separate from the endotracheal tube, and it will be manipulated by the anesthesiologist (Fig. 49-1).

The infant is positioned in a three-quarter left prone decubitus position, with a mild upward rotation of the right side. The surgeon and his assistant stand at the left side of the table facing the monitor, which is located at the right side. The anesthesiologist stands at the head and the scrub nurse at the foot of the operating table (Fig. 49-2).

Three cannulas are positioned as seen in Figure 49-3. The first cannula (5 mm) is inserted in the 6th intercostal space at the midaxillary line and is the site for the insertion of a short (18-cm), 4-mm, 30-degree telescope. We use a wide-angle telescope because it provides better vision in such a small working space. This port is also used for initiating the CO_2 insufflation. A pressure of 5 mm Hg provides excellent lung retraction and is well

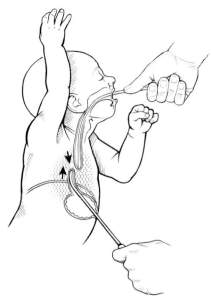

Figure 49-1. Semirigid radiopaque bougies are placed in each esophageal end to easily locate the two esophageal segments during thoracoscopic repair of esophageal atresia without fistula.

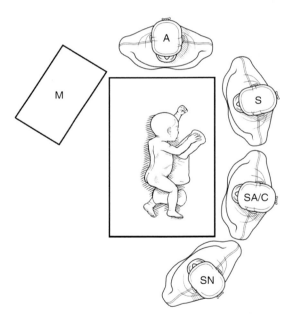

Figure 49-2. Operating room setup for thoracoscopic correction of isolated esophageal atresia. The surgeon (S) and surgical assistant/camera holder (SA/C) stand at the infant's front. The monitor (M) is over the infant's right shoulder. SN, scrub nurse; A, anesthesiologist.

tolerated by most, if not all, infants. A second port is placed in the axillary region at the 3rd intercostal space. We recommend using a 6-mm cannula with a 3-mm rubber reducer. If possible, we prefer this port to have an oblique thread outside the cannula that anchors the cannula securely in the thoracic wall. This cannula must have a silicone leaflet valve or a similar device that will

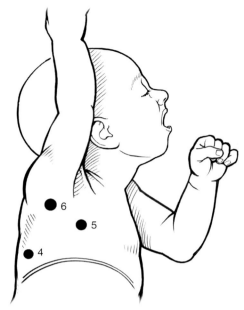

Figure 49-3. The infant is placed in a three-quarter left prone position. Three ports are inserted as shown in the figure. The first one is 5 mm and located in the 6th intercostal space. This port is for the telescope and camera. The other two ports are the working ports.

permit the introduction of a curved needle. This port is used for introducing the 3-mm needle holder and a C1 needle. The third and last port (4 mm) is placed at the 9th or 10th intercostal space in the posterior axillary line and is used for the introduction of grasping forceps. All the cannulas are fixed using the Shah-Neto technique, which involves a rubber sleeve around the cannula and a silk suture that is secured to the rubber sleeve and then tied around the insufflation stopcock. This stabilization of the cannula avoids dislodgment from the thoracic cavity and reduces the risk of CO_2 subcutaneous emphysema.

As a first step, the azygos vein is identified and divided with monopolar cautery or the 5-mm Ligasure (Covidien, Mansfield, MA) if available. The distal esophageal pouch is easily visualized by gently manipulating the bougie placed through the gastrostomy. The distal esophagus is dissected from the surrounding tissues by means of the monopolar hook, Maryland grasper, and scissors, all connected to cautery (Fig. 49-4A). Although there is controversy about dissection of the distal pouch, we strongly advocate extensive dissection down to the diaphragm (Fig. 49-4B). The upper esophageal pouch is then mobilized as cephalad as possible. Special care must be taken when dissecting between the anterior wall of the upper pouch and the posterior wall of the trachea. Extensive dissection cephalad into the neck is necessary to achieve enough esophageal length to perform a tension-free anastomosis. A rolling movement of the grasping forceps ("spaghetti maneuver") is

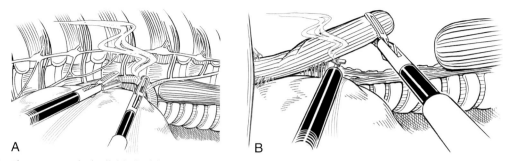

Figure 49-4. A, The azygos vein is divided with cautery or the Ligasure. **B,** The distal atretic esophagus is located and completely dissected from the surrounding tissues, down to the diaphragm, using the hook cautery.

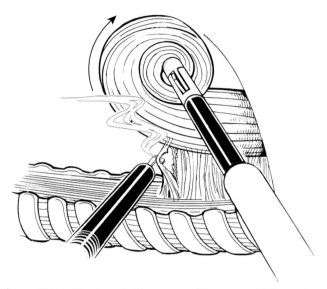

Figure 49-5.   The "spaghetti maneuver" is very useful for easier dissection of the upper pouch off the posterior tracheal wall.

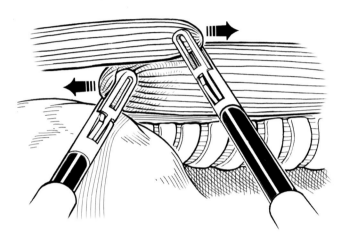

Figure 49-6.   When the esophageal ends overlap slightly, the anastomosis can be performed.

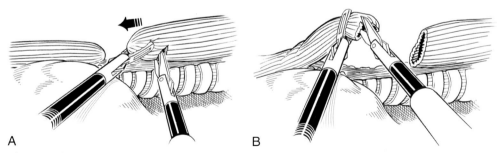

Figure 49-7. A, After complete mobilization of the upper pouch, its tip is transected transversely. **B,** The blind end of the distal pouch is transected as well.

of great help at this stage, thus providing an excellent view of the esophagus and the trachea (Fig. 49-5).

After thorough dissection of both pouches, the feasibility of an anastomosis is assessed by grasping both ends of the esophagus and sliding them together to feel the tension needed (Fig. 49-6). Then, the proximal end is transected transversely with scissors (Fig. 49-7A), followed by opening the distal esophagus (Fig. 49-7B).

The esophageal anastomosis is accomplished using 6 to 8 interrupted sutures of 5-0 PDS (Ethicon, Inc., Somerville, NJ) with a C1 needle. The first stitch

of the anastomosis is placed in the midline of the posterior wall (Fig. 49-8A). All knots are tied extracorporeally using a Roeder knot-tying technique, and the knot is secured with the needle holder (Fig. 49-8B).

Because the anastomosis is usually under significant tension, we have developed a way of avoiding all the force being applied to one single suture, thus preventing tissue tearing. The "twin-traction" suture (Fig. 49-9) is achieved by placing two simultaneous sutures in the posterior wall. Then, a Roeder knot is tied on each thread, and sequential tightening of the Roeder knot

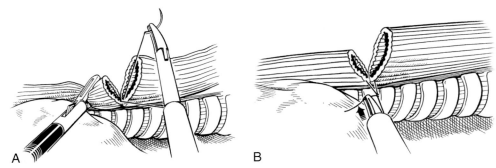

Figure 49-8. **A,** The first anastomotic stitch is placed in the midportion of the posterior esophageal wall in both the cephalic and caudal esophageal segments. **B,** The Roeder knot has been tied extracorporeally and is being slid down with the needle holder.

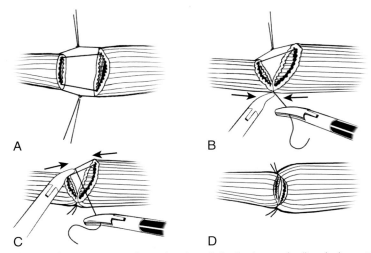

Figure 49-9. For the initial, high-tension sutures, we have developed the "twin-traction" technique. Two Roeder knots are sequentially tightened. The force is distributed on both sutures, thus preventing tissue tearing. **A,** Twin Roeder knots in place. **B,** Tension is applied to one knot, bringing the ends together. **C,** The second knot is brought down, distributing tension between both sutures. **D,** Esophageal ends are approximated. For **B** and **C,** The *arrows* illustrate knot being tightened.

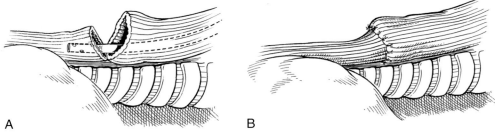

Figure 49-10. **A,** After completion of the posterior wall anastomosis, a transanastomotic feeding tube is advanced into the stomach. **B,** The completed anastomosis.

provides gentle traction with equal distribution of tension to both sutures.

After completion of the posterior wall of the anastomosis, a transanastomotic silastic tube is advanced to the stomach (Fig. 49-10A). Once the anastomosis is completed (Fig. 49-10B), a 12-French chest tube is inserted through the lowest port site.

POSTOPERATIVE CARE

All patients with a high-tension esophageal anastomosis remain fully relaxed, with airway intubation and mechanical ventilatory support for at least 48 hours. This management plan allows better pain management, prevention of cervical extension, and profuse swallowing during the early recovery period.

The transanastomotic silastic tube is used for several reasons. First, it serves as a tutor for the recently performed anastomosis. Second, it can be used to decompress the stomach in concert with the gastrostomy tube. Finally, if a leak or any other complication occurs, it can be advanced through the pylorus and provides an excellent delivery of food to the jejunum, avoiding gastroesophageal reflux (GER).

Because all patients with type A esophageal atresia already have a gastrostomy, it is mandatory to keep it functional until it is no longer needed. We recommend leaving the gastrostomy open and connected to drainage for the first 48 to 72 hours, or until feeding through the transanastomotic tube is initiated.

Early feeding is started on the third postoperative day through the transanastomotic feeding tube. On the fifth postoperative day, a barium swallow is performed (Fig. 49-11). If no leak is observed, oral feedings are started and the chest tube is removed.

PEARLS

1. For the right port (axillary position), use a 5-mm cannula with leaflet valve, as all sutures and needles will be exteriorized through this port. This type of valve is also ideal for sliding the extracorporeally tied Roeder knot into position.
2. Because of chronic irritation secondary to long-term pouch aspiration with the Replogle tube, most of these patients present with edema and periesophagitis. Dissection is dangerous and bleeding may be profuse. Hydrodissection of the tissues using high-pressure irrigation can be very useful.
3. To know if both ends are ready for anastomosis, grab the inferior pouch with the right-hand grasper and the upper pouch with the left-hand grasper. Pull them toward each other. Anastomosis can be performed if both ends overlap at least 1 or 2 mm.
4. Dissection of the upper pouch can be extended cephalad into the neck without risk.
5. For the posterior wall portion of the esophageal anastomosis, all the knots are tied extracorporeally.

6. Make sure that the mucosa is included in all the anastomotic stitches.

PITFALLS

1. Avoid tracheal perforation by staying on the esophageal side during dissection between the esophagus and trachea.
2. Avoid anastomotic stenosis by cutting the upper pouch transversally and resecting its distal tip.
3. Watch for vascular anomalies (e.g., vascular rings, double aortic arch), and convert if the anatomy is not fully understood.
4. Avoid using an excessive amount of stitches. Usually six to eight sutures are enough.
5. Be aware of the presence of the thoracic duct and avoid injuring it.

RESULTS

Four patients with esophageal atresia without fistula have been treated since March 2001, when we performed our first thoracoscopic repair of an EA with TEF. Correction was accomplished in all four cases and no conversions were needed. The results are shown in Table 49-1. No operative complications were encountered in any patient. CO_2 insufflation of the pleural cavity was well tolerated and allowed an excellent operative field in all cases. The mean operative time was 123 minutes (range, 90 to 180 minutes). No early or late postoperative complications were observed in this small series of patients. Three patients subsequently developed GER that required laparoscopic Nissen fundoplication without

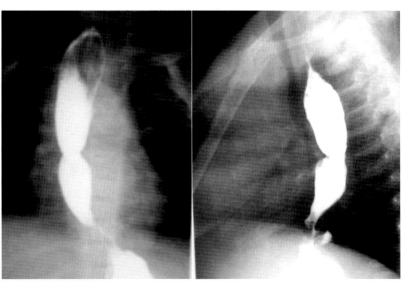

Figure 49-11.   A routine barium swallow is performed on the 7th postoperative day. The radiograph shows a patent anastomosis without leak.

Table 49-1 Four Patients Who Underwent Primary Thoracoscopic Repair of Isolated Esophageal Atresia without Fistula

| Patient | Age at Operation (mo) | Operative Time (min) | Conversion | Complications | | Follow-up |
				Intraoperative	Postoperative	
1	4	180	No	No	No	Laparoscopic Nissen
2	4	90	No	No	No	—
3	4	100	No	No	No	Laparoscopic Nissen
4	3	120	No	No	No	Laparoscopic Nissen

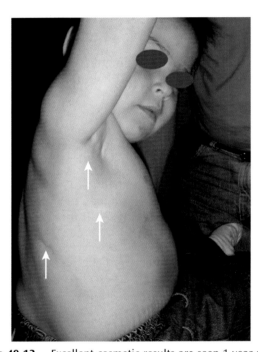

Figure 49-12. Excellent cosmetic results are seen 1 year after the operation in this child. The three incisions are marked with *arrows*.

complication. All patients had excellent cosmetic results (Fig. 49-12). At follow-up, these patients remain without symptoms. One patient exhibits symptoms related to mild tracheomalacia that does not require surgical treatment.

SELECTED REFERENCES

1. Shah R, Neto PN: An Innovative technique for reusable laparoscopic cannula stabilization and fixation. Pediatr Endosurg Innov Tech 1:59-61, 1997
2. Lobe TE, Rothenberg SS, Waldschmidt J, et al: Thoracoscopic repair of esophageal atresia in an infant: A surgical first. Pediatr Endosurg Innov Tech 3:141-148, 1999
3. Rothenberg S: Thoracoscopic repair of a tracheoesophageal fistula in a newborn infant. Pediatr Endosurg Innov Tech 4:289-294, 2000
4. Farkash U, Lazar L, Erez I, et al: The distal pouch in esophageal atresia: To dissect or not to dissect, that is the question. Eur J Pediatr Surg 12:19-23, 2002
5. Martinez-Ferro M, Elmo G, Bignon H: Thoracoscopic repair of esophageal atresia with fistula: Initial experience. Pediatr Endosurg Innov Tech 6:229-237, 2002

50
Thoracoscopic Aortopexy

Klaas (N) M. A. Bax

Aortopexy is considered to be necessary in patients with life-threatening tracheal obstruction secondary to severe tracheomalacia. The tracheomalacia may be primary or secondary. The secondary form is often seen in combination with esophageal atresia and with vascular rings. It has also been described in combination with congenital heart disease. Symptoms vary from mild and not requiring therapy, to severe and not allowing extubation or producing life-threatening events. Randomized controlled trials regarding the different treatment modalities do not exist. Continuous positive airway pressure ventilation is certainly not a therapy for the long term. Bronchial stenting has not gained popularity in view of its high failure rate and more severe morbidity and mortality. Aortopexy is a relatively simple procedure causing immediate relief of symptoms in about two thirds of cases. There is little doubt that this is the treatment of choice in severely symptomatic cases. Moreover, the thoracoscopic technique is much less traumatic than other approaches, such as left thoracotomy or a low cervical–upper sternotomy approach.

INDICATIONS FOR WORKUP AND OPERATION

Aortopexy is indicated in cases of life-threatening apnea on the basis of tracheomalacia. Once this diagnosis is made, not much time should be lost before the procedure is performed.

The diagnosis of tracheomalacia is made on clinical grounds supplemented by bronchoscopic signs of tracheomalacia. In children with esophageal atresia and distal fistula, clinical tracheomalacia can be documented in almost 100% of the patients. Tracheomalacia is also seen in aortic arch anomalies. A lateral chest radiograph shows the narrowed trachea in the thoracic aperture. Bronchoscopy should be carried out under general anesthesia but with the infant spontaneously breathing.

OPERATIVE TECHNIQUE

The patient is placed supine on the operating table. The midsternal line is marked on the skin (Fig. 50-1A). The left chest is elevated by 15 degrees, and the operating table is tilted in reverse Trendelenburg (Fig. 50-1B). The surgeon stands to the left of the patient with the camera person on the surgeon's left and the scrub nurse at the caudal end of the short operating table (Fig. 50-2). The most important monitor is positioned in front of the surgeon, at the right side of the patient. The equipment tower is placed behind the surgeon, and all cables enter the operating table along the surgeon's right side and the left edge of the table. The seven cables are bundled together (camera, light, CO_2, external monopolar electrocautery, internal electrocautery, suction, irrigation).

Three sleeved reusable ports are used (Fig. 50-2). The first 6-mm cannula with blunt trocar is inserted in an open technique in the midaxillary line at the level of the nipple. The cannula is fixed to the thoracic wall with a 2-0 Vicryl (Ethicon, Inc., Somerville, NJ) suture. The intrapleural position of the tip of the cannula is checked thoracoscopically before CO_2 insufflation. Pressure is set at 8 mm Hg and a flow of 1 L/min. If desaturation occurs, the chest should be desufflated and ventilatory settings adjusted. A higher ventilatory rate with higher oxygen concentration usually alleviates the problem. The surgeon needs to be patient. After 5 to 10 minutes,

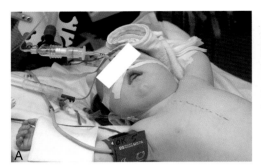
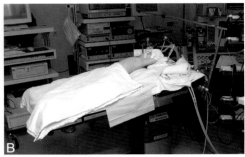

Figure 50-1.   **A,** The infant is placed supine on the operating table and the midsternal line is marked on the skin. **B,** A roll is placed under the left side of the abdomen to slightly elevate the left chest and the operating table is tilted in reverse Trendelenburg.

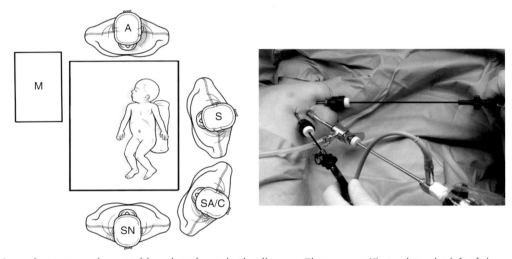

Figure 50-2.   Operating personnel are positioned as shown in the diagram. The surgeon (S) stands to the left of the patient with the assistant/camera holder (SA/C) at the surgeon's left. The scrub nurse (SN) is at the caudal end of the short operating table. A monitor (M) is positioned to the right of the patient, keeping the aorta in line between the surgeon and the monitor. A, anesthesiologist. The photograph shows port placement. Reusable, sleeved ports are used. A 6-mm cannula with blunt trocar is inserted in the midaxillary line at the level of the nipple. Two 3.8-mm cannulas are then inserted under endoscopic visualization, one cephalad to the initial port and one caudal and slightly anterior to the initial cannula. The working angles between these ports should be about 60 degrees. All cannulas are secured to the thoracic wall to prevent dislodgment.

the left lung will be completely collapsed and will not reexpand, even without CO_2 insufflation. Next, two 3.8-mm cannulas are inserted bluntly under endoscopic control after small skin incisions have been made, one more cephalad in the midaxillary line and one more caudal and anterior. The working angle between the ports should be about 60 degrees. These cannulas are also secured to the chest wall to prevent dislodgment.

The anatomy visualized is spectacular. A triangle is seen, with the anterior boundary being the internal mammary vessels and the posterior boundary being the phrenic nerve (Fig. 50-3A). The base of the triangle is formed by the pericardium. Care is taken not to injure the phrenic nerve. The surface of the triangle is formed by the mediastinal pleura overlying the left lobe of the thymus. The mediastinal pleura is opened in the middle

(see Fig. 50-3B). Next, the thymus is mobilized posteriorly until the ascending aorta with its pericardial reflection and the innominate artery are clearly seen (Fig. 50-4). The aortic arch itself is also seen but is not dissected free. The thymus can now be mobilized anteriorly and pushed into the right hemithorax. Alternatively, the lobe of the left thymus can be dissected free and amputated. At the end of the operation, the lobe can be removed piecemeal through one of the incisions.

The most difficult part of the operation is placement of the three 3-0 Ethibond (Ethicon, Somerville, NJ) sutures through the sternum, followed by securing a piece of the pericardial reflection or aortic adventitia, and then exteriorization of the sutures. To place these sutures, a small stab incision is made in the skin and soft tissue overlying the midsternum at the level of the ascending aorta. A 3-0 Ethibond suture on a V-5 needle

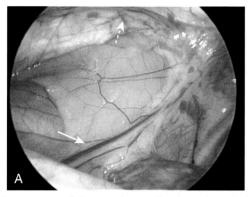 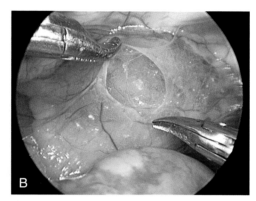

Figure 50-3. The anatomy of the anterior mediastinum is well visualized, especially in an infant. **A,** A triangle is formed anteriorly by the internal mammary vessels (*dotted arrow*) and posteriorly by the phrenic nerve (*solid arrow*). The base of the triangle is formed by the pericardium. **B,** The mediastinal pleura between the internal mammary vessels anteriorly and the phrenic nerve posteriorly has been opened.

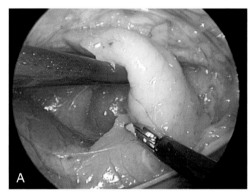 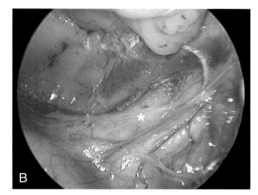

Figure 50-4. **A,** The thymus is mobilized to allow visualization of the ascending aorta. **B,** The ascending aorta (*asterisk*) is seen following removal of the thymus. Note the innominate vein coursing anterior to the aorta.

is then driven through this stab incision and through the sternum. It is secured in the mediastinum by a 3-mm needle holder. Using the 3-mm endoscopic needle holder, the pericardial reflection on the aorta is secured, and the needle is then driven up through the sternum a few millimeters from the other part of the suture. The needle is cut and the two ends of the Ethibond suture that course through the sternum and the pericardial reflection on the ascending aorta are secured extracorporeally with a hemostat. Two more sutures are placed in a similar fashion: one secures the adventitia of the innominate artery and the other grasps the adventitia of the ascending aorta (Fig. 50-5A). The sutures are then tied extracorporeally under bronchoscopic visualization, thereby elevating the aorta toward the sternum (Fig. 50-5B). The knots are anterior to the sternum and are secured in the soft tissue under the stab incisions. The stab incisions are then closed with 5-0 plain suture or Steri-Strips (3M Co., St. Paul, MN). The ports are then removed under visualization as well. The left lobe of the thymus is grasped with the instrument in the cannula in the upper axilla, and it is removed in segments.

CO_2 is aspirated by applying suction to the insufflation stopcock. Reexpansion of the lung is verified thoracoscopically, and the cannula and telescope are removed. The skin is closed with Steri-Strips. When the operation is successful, the effect is almost immediately evident. A chest drain is not routinely used, but a postoperative chest radiograph is obtained.

POSTOPERATIVE CARE

The child is kept in the intensive care unit overnight. Feeding is started the next morning and the child is discharged when feeling well.

PEARLS

1. The pericardial reflection onto the ascending aorta should be identified as well as the rest of the ascending aorta and innominate artery.
2. The three nonabsorbable sutures should be inserted just cephalad to the ascending aorta and innominate

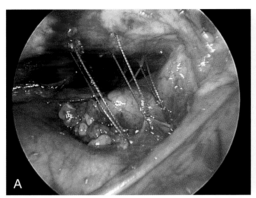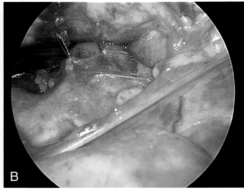

Figure 50-5. **A,** Sutures, 3-0 Ethibond, have been placed through the sternum into the tissues near the ascending aorta. Posteriorly, the sutures grasp the pericardial reflection on the ascending aorta, the adventitia of the innominate artery, and the adventitia of the ascending aorta. **B,** The aortic arch is elevated toward the sternum when these sutures are tied extracorporeally.

artery. One suture should secure the pericardial reflection on the ascending aorta, one the adventitia of the ascending aorta, and one the adventitia of the innominate artery.

3. The thymus is in the way but can be pushed to the right after thorough anterior and posterior mobilization. Alternatively, the left thymic lobe can be removed.

PITFALLS

1. The phrenic nerve runs along the anterior mediastinal pleura but is posterior to the area of dissection. Care should be taken not to damage this nerve.
2. The sutures should grasp adventitia only and should not include the vessel wall itself.

RESULTS

So far, six children, all with tracheomalacia in combination with esophageal atresia, have had a thoracoscopic aortopexy for life-threatening events. Four of the six children had an immediate and dramatic improvement in symptoms. Two children have responded less well and both have required a second aortopexy. Even after the second intervention, which was not very difficult, their symptoms have persisted. The success rate of aortopexy in the literature is quoted to be about 70%.

SELECTED REFERENCES

1. Applebaum H, Wooley MM: Pericardial flap aortopexy for tracheomalacia. J Pediatr Surg 25:30-32, 1990
2. DeCou JM, Parsons DS, Gauderer MWL: Thoracoscopic aortopexy for severe tracheomalacia. Pediatr Endosurg Innov Tech 5:205-208, 2001
3. Schier F, Korn S, Michel E: Aortopexy in esophageal atresia: Long-term experience of a parent support group. J Pediatr Surg 36:1502-1503, 2001
4. Vazquez-Jimenez JF, Sachweh JS, Liakopoulos OJ, et al: Aortopexy in severe tracheal instability: Short-term and long-term outcome in 29 infants and children. Ann Thorac Surg 72:1898-1901, 2001
5. Abdel-Rahman U, Ahrens P, Fieguth HG, et al: Surgical treatment of tracheomalacia by bronchoscopic monitored aortopexy in infants and children. Ann Thorac Surg 74:315-319, 2002
6. Kim YM, Yoo SJ, Kim WH, et al: Bronchial compression by posteriorly displaced ascending aorta in patients with congenital heart disease. Ann Thorac Surg 73:881-886, 2002
7. Schaarschmidt K, Kolberg-Schwerdt A, Pietsch L, et al: Thoracoscopic aortopericardiosternopexy for severe tracheomalacia in toddlers. J Pediatr Surg 37:1476-1478, 2002
8. Weber TR, Keller MS, Fiore A: Aortic suspension (aortopexy) for severe tracheomalacia in infants and children. Am J Surg 184:573-577, 2002
9. Masters I, Chang A, Masters IB: Interventions for primary (intrinsic) tracheomalacia in children. Cochrane Database Syst Rev 19;CD005304, 2005
10. Valerie EP, Durrant AC, Forte V, et al: A decade of using intraluminal tracheal/bronchial stents in the management of tracheomalacia and/or bronchomalacia: Is it better than aortopexy? J Pediatr Surg 40:904-907, 2005

51
Thoracoscopic Thymectomy

Thom E. Lobe

The traditional approach to thymectomy for a thymic mass or for myasthenia gravis has been through a median sternotomy or through a collar incision, or some combination of the two approaches. For patients with myasthenia, the sternotomy approach has been advocated because of the embryology of the thymus. Proponents of sternotomy assert that this approach maximizes the chance of finding all the potential thymic fragments that remain after migration from the neck. The advent of thoracoscopy has added another potential approach for surgery of mediastinal structures. The visualization provided by the telescope and the refinement in the operative technique allow adult and pediatric surgeons to adopt this approach to surgery of the thymus and other structures in the anterior mediastinum. The benefits of this approach include decreased postoperative pain and shorter hospitalizations.

INDICATIONS FOR WORKUP AND OPERATION

The indications for thymectomy include adenoma or other masses and failure of medical management for myasthenia gravis. When a mass is detected, either by palpation or in the course of evaluation for another problem, it is usually discrete. Ultrasound, computed tomography, and magnetic resonance imaging may all be useful in the detection and evaluation of a thymic mass. Metastases to the thymus are extremely rare.

Patients with myasthenia are usually initially treated with Mestinon (pyridostigmine bromide, ICN Pharmaceuticals, Costa Mesa, CA). In severe cases, plasmapheresis is useful in an effort to remove the autoantibodies against the acetylcholine receptor that results in profound muscle weakness. Thymectomy has been shown to eliminate or minimize symptoms when they persist despite maximal medical therapy. No specific diagnostic studies are required before performing a straightforward thoracoscopic thymectomy. In our experience, additional studies do not seem to add anything to the planning of the procedure. When patients are on steroids, appropriate precautions should be taken to support any potential perioperative endogenous steroid insufficiency.

OPERATIVE TECHNIQUE

ANESTHESIA AND PATIENT POSITION

Although many surgeons are satisfied with using CO_2 insufflation to collapse the lung on the ipsilateral side, we prefer to use a bronchial blocker for better maintenance of lung collapse and for better airway control. For all patients, standard monitoring includes a blood pressure cuff, a pulse oximeter, and conventional electrocardiographic leads. Many surgeons routinely use compression stockings to prevent embolic phenomena caused by venous stasis. There are no data, however, that show any advantage for such prophylaxis in children younger than 12 years. One intravenous line should be sufficient and we do not routinely have blood available for this procedure. These operations generally take less than 2 hours to complete so the use of an indwelling urinary catheter is not generally required.

Patients are induced using conventional methods and then either positioned for the operation if a bronchial blocker is not used, or a bronchial blocker is introduced after endotracheal intubation. For older or larger patients, a double-lumen endotracheal tube can be used. For smaller or younger patients, a 5 or 6 French Fogarty catheter is inserted into the trachea under direct vision immediately preceding the introduction of an endotracheal tube of the appropriate size for the patient. We then advance a flexible bronchoscope through the lumen of the endotracheal tube and position the Fogarty balloon just at the origin of the left mainstem bronchus. The Fogarty catheter and endotracheal tube are then secured with tape. We inflate the Fogarty balloon while watching with the flexible endoscope to make sure that the balloon occludes the bronchial orifice and has not advanced into the lumen of the bronchus. The position is rechecked (using the flexible endoscope if necessary) after the patient is positioned for the procedure. The goal is to block the left mainstem bronchus and prevent ventilation of the left lung while maintaining good ventilation of the right lung.

The patient is placed on a beanbag of the appropriate size to maintain the proper position on the operating table. We generally place a rolled towel or other object of similar size just under the left lateral chest, posterior to the posterior axillary line, to slightly elevate that side of the chest. In addition, the patient is positioned at the left edge of the operating table. The left arm can be flexed over the head to eliminate any stretch of the brachial plexus (Fig. 51-1). The goal of positioning is to slightly elevate the left side of the chest so that when the instruments are parallel to the floor, they are oriented somewhat anteriorly toward the thymus.

After being positioned, the patient is prepped and draped using the surgeon's sterile technique of choice. We do not routinely administer preoperative antibiotics for prophylaxis.

PORTS AND TELESCOPES

The surgeon and assistant are positioned side by side along the patient's left chest. The monitor is situated over the patient's right shoulder (Fig. 51-2A). We begin by inserting a 10-mm cannula in the fourth intercostal space at the level of the anterior axillary line on the left chest wall. We introduce this port in the same way we would introduce a thoracostomy tube, without insufflating CO_2 through a Veress needle first.

As soon as this port is inserted, we insufflate with CO_2 to 10 mm Hg, which collapses the lung and allows it to fall posteriorly. When a bronchial blocker has been placed, we inflate the balloon at this time to prevent the

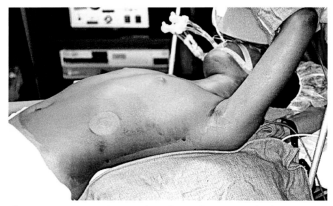

Figure 51-1. A patient undergoing a thoracoscopic thymectomy is positioned near the left edge of the table with a roll under the left lateral chest to elevate it slightly. The arm is positioned out of the way so as not to stretch the brachial plexus. Note the double-lumen endotracheal tube taped securely in position.

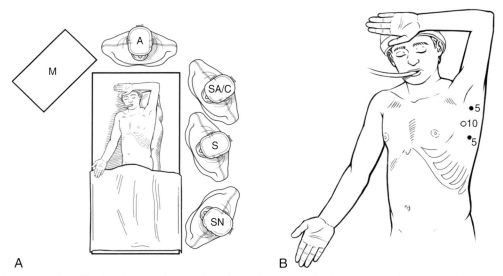

Figure 51-2. **A,** Personnel positioning for a patient undergoing a thoracoscopic thymectomy. The surgeon (S) and surgical assistant/camera holder (SA/C) are situated side by side along the patient's left chest. A, anesthesiologist; M, monitor; SN, scrub nurse. **B,** The location of the cannulas. A 10-mm cannula is inserted initially in the fourth intercostal space in the anterior axillary line (AAL). Next, two 5-mm ports are introduced. One is inserted in the 2nd or 3rd intercostal space just posterior to the AAL, and the other is positioned at the same level in the 5th or 6th interspace.

lung from expanding during the procedure. Two additional 5-mm cannulas are then inserted. One is placed in the 2nd or 3rd intercostal space just posterior to the anterior axillary line, and the other is introduced in the 5th or 6th intercostal space at the same level (Fig. 51-2B). A 5-mm, 0-degree telescope is inserted initially. If this fails to provide an adequate view, we switch to a 5-mm, 30-degree scope. The ports can be secured to the chest wall using whatever technique the surgeon feels comfortable with.

OPERATIVE STEPS

The first operative step is to incise the mediastinal pleura over the thymus and anterior to the phrenic nerve. We start this dissection with scissors and use blunt dissection to make the incision opening as large as necessary. We then identify the tail of the thymus and grasp it with an instrument placed through the left lateral port. Using primarily blunt dissection, the thymus is mobilized cephalad. Usually this is accomplished with minimal bleeding (Fig. 51-3). When the innominate vein is identified, we carefully search for the thymic vein. This is a short vein and care should be taken to ligate it securely to prevent hemorrhage that would obscure good visualization. The thymic vein can be divided with the Ligasure (Covidien, Mansfield, MA), or between endoscopic clips. Dissection is then performed to mobilize the right lobe of the gland. Cephalic to the gland are the thymic arteries that arise from the thyrocervical trunk. These arteries are then divided as far cephalad as possible, again with either the Ligasure or clips. With the thymus completely mobilized, we switch our telescope from its 10-mm port position to one of the 5-mm cannulas and introduce a retrieval bag through the 10-mm cannula.

The specimen is placed into the retrieval bag and extracted in its entirety through the 10-mm incision. A 10 French suction catheter is then introduced through one of the port sites to evacuate the CO_2 until the lung has fully expanded. The incisions are closed according to the surgeon's preference. As the anesthesiologist applies positive pressure to emulate a Valsalva maneuver, the suction catheter is removed.

Patients are then recovered in the usual location and fashion. There is usually no need for intensive care. A chest radiograph can be taken if there is the suspicion of a residual pneumothorax. If one is identified, either the patient can be observed or a thoracostomy tube or drain can be placed.

Because of their underlying disease, we keep patients with myasthenia overnight to make sure that they are fully awake and can ventilate adequately. Patients without myasthenia can be discharged the day of surgery. Analgesics are administered as needed for a day or two after the surgery. Results in patients with myasthenia may take several months to determine. Patients with a thymic mass are treated according to their pathology.

PEARLS AND PITFALLS

This is a straightforward operation with few potential complications. Care should be taken to identify the anatomy clearly so as not to divide important nerves, especially the phrenic nerve. The division of the thymic vein is the step associated with the most potential danger. Occasionally, a small residual pneumothorax is present after evacuating all the gas. This usually resolves spontaneously.

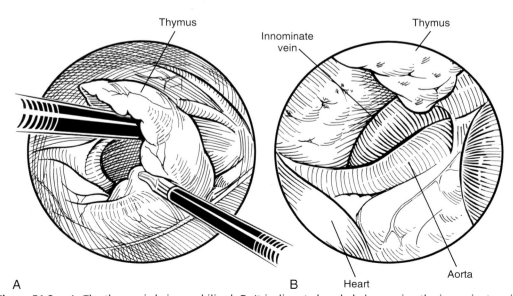

Figure 51-3. **A,** The thymus is being mobilized. **B,** It is dissected cephalad, exposing the innominate vein.

SELECTED REFERENCES

1. Kogut KA, Bufo AJ, Rothenberg SS, et al: Thoracoscopic thymectomy for myasthenia gravis in children. J Pediatr Surg 35:1576-1577, 2000
2. Kolski H, Vajsar J, Kim PC: Thoracoscopic thymectomy in juvenile myasthenia gravis. J Pediatr Surg 35:768-770, 2000
3. Kolski HK, Kim PC, Vajsar J: Video-assisted thoracoscopic thymectomy in juvenile myasthenia gravis. J Child Neurol 16:569-573, 2001
4. Skelly CL, Jackson CC, Wu Y, et al: Thoracoscopic thymectomy in children with myasthenia gravis. Am Surg 69:1087-1089, 2003
5. Seguier-Lipszyc E, Bonnard A, Evrard P, et al: Left thoracoscopic thymectomy in children. Surg Endosc 19:140-142, 2005

52
The Minimally Invasive Pectus Excavatum Repair (Nuss Procedure)

Donald Nuss and Robert E. Kelly, Jr.

Pectus excavatum is a depression of the anterior chest wall. It may be present at birth or may develop during childhood or early adolescence. The depression usually gets deeper as the child grows. During puberty, the deformity may worsen precipitously in as little as 6 months. Patients with a mild or moderate excavatum are generally asymptomatic and are treated with an exercise and posture program. They are seen annually to reinforce the value of the exercise program and to check for progression of the disease.

Patients with a severe pectus excavatum (approximately one third of the total) suffer from cardiac and pulmonary compression and frequently present with dyspnea on exertion, chest pain, decreased endurance, exercise intolerance, and frequent respiratory tract infections. Patients who are clinically diagnosed as having a severe deformity undergo a workup to confirm objectively the need for surgical correction.

INDICATIONS FOR WORKUP AND OPERATION

Evaluation of clinical severity includes a computed tomography (CT) scan of the chest, pulmonary function tests (PFTs), and cardiology evaluation (Fig. 52-1). The CT scan permits a three-dimensional evaluation of the anterior chest wall and vividly demonstrates cardiac compression and displacement. CT scanning permits objective assessment of the severity of the depression by comparing the ratio of the transverse internal thoracic diameter to the anteroposterior diameter at the deepest part of the depression (Haller index). Haller and associates have proposed that an index of greater than 3.25 constitutes a severe depression.

PFTs are obtained to evaluate for restrictive airway disease. Exercise pulmonary function studies may show a limitation of oxygen uptake (VO_{2max}) and a decreased ability to perform cardiopulmonary work.

A cardiology evaluation is sought on all patients. The electrocardiogram (ECG) and echocardiogram (ECHO) may reveal conduction pathway abnormalities, mitral valve prolapse, right ventricular wall abnormalities, or other effects of cardiac compression. Moreover, these tests help determine whether the patient is a reasonable candidate for a corrective operation.

Operative correction is indicated by the presence of two or more of the following criteria:

- A CT index greater than 3.25, with cardiac or pulmonary compression
- Pulmonary function studies that indicate restrictive airway disease
- A cardiology evaluation including ECG and echocardiogram showing that the compression is causing murmurs, mitral valve prolapse, cardiac displacement, conduction abnormalities, or other adverse functional effects
- Documentation of progression of the deformity with associated physical symptoms
- Failed previous repair

The operation is best performed between 6 and 25 years of age, and ideally at 12 to 14 years. At that age, the chest is still very malleable, allowing rapid recovery and maturation of the musculoskeletal system while the support bar minimizes the risk of recurrence. However, the Nuss procedure has been successfully applied to patients as young as 2 and as old as 50 years. At the present time, it is recommended that the support bar(s) remain in place for 2 to 4 years. Patients whose bars are removed before puberty have an increased risk of recurrence. Older patients sometimes require two and occasionally three bars.

All patients treated with an operation are also treated with an aerobic exercise, deep breathing, and a posture program starting at their first consultation. They are encouraged to continue with the exercise program until 1 year after bar removal. Before surgery, evaluate for metal allergy. If patients are allergic to metallic objects (usually a nickel or copper allergy), then a titanium bar should be used.

OPERATIVE TECHNIQUE

After induction of anesthesia, insertion of a thoracic epidural catheter and bladder catheter, and administration of intravenous cefazolin, the patient is positioned supine with both arms abducted at the shoulder and secured on arm boards. Photographs are taken of the chest before correction.

The surgeon is positioned on the patient's right, and the surgical assistant is on the patient's left. The deepest point of the pectus excavatum at the lower end of the sternum is marked. This mark sets the horizontal plane for bar insertion. At least one support bar should be under the bony sternum. If the bar is not under the sternum, there will not be correction of the deformity. It may be necessary to add a second bar superiorly or inferiorly, especially if the deepest point of the depression corresponds not to the inferior end of the sternum but to the xiphisternum or adjacent inferior costal cartilages. The intercostal spaces that are in the same horizontal plane as the deepest point of the pectus excavatum are marked with an X, slightly medial to the top of the pectus ridge. The Xs are the points where the bar will enter and exit from the mediastinum (Fig. 52-2A). The proposed incision sites are marked with a horizontal line from the anterior to the midaxillary lines. The chest is measured from the right midaxillary line to the left midaxillary line, and a Lorenz Pectus Bar (Walter Lorenz Surgical, Inc., Jacksonville, FL) is selected on the basis of this measurement *minus 1 inch (2 cm)* (Fig. 52-2B).

Following preparation and sterile draping, the bar is bent into a smooth convex shape leaving a 2- to 4-cm flat section in the middle to support the sternum. (If desired, the manufacturer will bend the bar at the factory

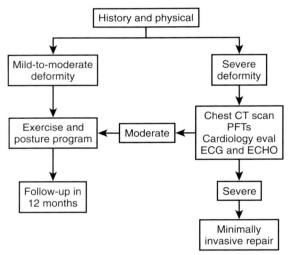

Figure 52-1. Algorithm showing evaluation of patients with pectus excavatum at Children's Hospital of the King's Daughters, in Norfolk, Virginia.

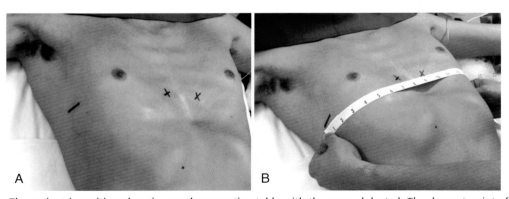

Figure 52-2. A, The patient is positioned supine on the operating table with the arms abducted. The deepest point of the depression at the lower end of the sternum is noted. The bar entry and exit sites into and out of the mediastinum are marked with an X, and the incisions in the midaxillary lines are marked with a horizontal line. **B,** The chest is measured from the right midaxillary line to the left midaxillary line.

on the basis of the patient's chest CT scan with CAD/CAM technology for an additional fee.) The bar should fit loosely on each side and not compress the chest wall muscles.

A 5-mm, 0- or 30-degree thoracoscope is inserted into the right lower chest through a clear plastic cannula one or two interspaces inferior to the proposed lateral thoracic skin incision. CO_2 is insufflated to a pressure of 6 mm Hg, which causes the right lung to collapse and improves visualization dramatically. The lungs, mediastinum, and anterior chest wall are carefully inspected for unrelated abnormalities. The scope is used to correlate the internal anatomy with the external markings. Pressure is applied over the proposed entry and exit sites of the bar (marked by the X) to ensure that they line up well with the deepest point of the pectus excavatum. Positioning of the bar at this site will allow good lifting pressure on the undersurface of the sternum by the bar.

Once the intercostal spaces selected for bar entry and exit are noted to line up well with the deepest point of the pectus excavatum, the scope is withdrawn, and bilateral lateral thoracic skin incisions are made (Fig. 52-3). Dissection is carried down to the pre-muscular fascia. Flaps are raised superiorly, inferiorly, and posteriorly, creating a deep subcutaneous pocket for the bar and the stabilizers. A deep subcutaneous tunnel is created from the anterior aspect of the incision to the point marked X that has been selected for entry of the bar into the mediastinum (Fig. 52-4).

It is important that the site selected for entry into the mediastinum be medial to the vertically (axially) directed ridge of the right chest wall created by the central depression. If the chest is entered lateral to that ridge, the bar has only the intercostal muscles to oppose the strong posterior force on the bar, and they will tear

under the load. Instead, this load must be borne by the ribs as they curve in toward the sternum.

The thoracoscope is reinserted into the chest. Under direct vision, a pointed clamp is used to create a small thoracostomy in the (right) intercostal space at the point marked with an X. The clamp is withdrawn and a Lorenz introducer of appropriate size for the patient is inserted into the subcutaneous tunnel (Fig. 52-5). It is pushed through the thoracostomy opening at the point marked X, turned over, and slowly advanced toward the mediastinum with the tip facing anteriorly (Fig. 52-6A). The ECG monitor is adjusted so that the heartbeat is clearly audible to hear arrhythmias. Very gently, under

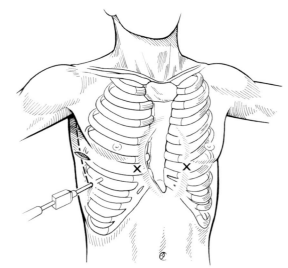

Figure 52-3.   After preparation and draping, bilateral axillary incisions are made. The thoracoscope has been introduced into the right chest a couple of interspaces below the right axillary incision.

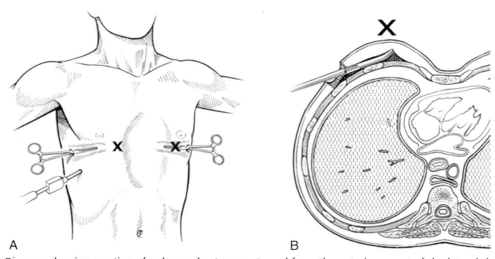

Figure 52-4.   **A,** Diagram showing creation of a deep subcutaneous tunnel from the anterior aspect of the lateral thoracic incisions to the X at the top of the pectus ridge on each side. **B,** The coronal diagram depicts the clamp in the subcutaneous tunnel just medial to the X. The clamp will be turned 180 degrees to penetrate the chest wall just medial to the X.

thoracoscopic visualization, the pleura and pericardium are dissected off the undersurface of the sternum. This should be performed under direct vision through the thoracoscope. Rotating a 30-degree thoracoscope passed medial to the pectus ridge may provide better visualization than a 0-degree scope. Occasionally, it is not possible to see the dissection with the thoracoscope. In this circumstance, a short subxiphoid incision may permit a finger to pass between the sternum and pericardium to guide the dissector, or a clamp may be attached to the xiphisternum and pulled anteriorly. Alternatively, a suction device may be applied to the anterior chest wall to elevate the sternum.

Once the avascular plane between the pericardium and sternum is entered, the bar introducer is advanced across the mediastinum. The introducer is pushed

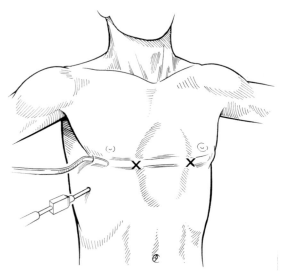

Figure 52-5.   After creation of the subcutaneous tunnel, the introducer is inserted through the tunnel and is advanced into the chest cavity just medial to the site marked by the X. The introducer will be passed from the patient's right to the left under thoracoscopic visualization.

through the left intercostal space marked with an X medial to the top of the left pectus ridge. The introducer is then advanced out of the left lateral incision until only the handle is protruding on the right side. This will elevate the sternum out of its depressed or sunken position (Fig. 52-6B).

The sternum is further elevated out of its depressed position by lifting the introducer in an anterior direction (toward the ceiling of the operating room) (Fig. 52-6B). The surgeon lifts the introducer on the right side and the assistant lifts the introducer on the left side. Simultaneously, pressure is applied to the lower costal margin below the introducer. This creates anterior bowing of the sternum. The introducer is lifted numerous times until the sternal depression has been completely corrected. Loosening up the chest wall in this manner prevents excessive torque on the pectus bar when turning it over (see later).

An umbilical tape is tied by the assistant to the end of the introducer, and the introducer is withdrawn from the subcutaneous tunnels and chest cavity (Fig. 52-7). The previously selected Lorenz pectus support bar is checked to make sure that it fits snugly on each side of the chest and that it is the correct length. It is then attached to the umbilical tape. Under thoracoscopic guidance, it is very gently guided through the right chest wall, across the mediastinum, and out on the left side (Fig. 52-8). The bar is inserted with the convexity facing posteriorly. Once it is in position with an equal amount of the bar protruding on each side, it is turned over either in a clockwise or a counterclockwise direction using the bar rotational device (or bar flipper).

After being turned over, pressure effects often cause the bar to straighten out, therefore requiring further molding to fit well against the chest wall. If further manipulation of the bar is needed, the bar is rotated again, and, using the bar benders, it is bent to fit loosely on each side of the chest without protruding under the skin. A stabilizer is attached to the bar. This can be placed on either side, but it is usually situated on the

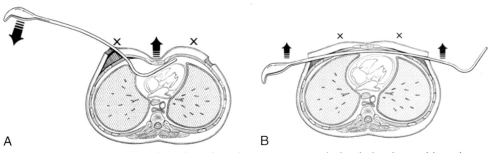

A   B

Figure 52-6.   **A,** After insertion of the bar introducer into the subcutaneous tunnel, the tip is advanced into the mediastinum just medial to the X and then is gradually advanced under the sternum. The tip of the introducer is kept under constant surveillance with the thoracoscope. **B,** The introducer has been passed out the patient's left midaxillary incision. The introducer is then lifted in an anterior direction by the surgeon and the assistant while they apply pressure over the lower costal margin. The introducer is lifted numerous times until the sternal depression has been completely corrected. Loosening up the chest wall in this manner prevents excessive torque on the anterior chest wall when the pectus bar is turned over.

left side because it is more difficult to place pericostal sutures on the left side given the presence of the heart (Fig. 52-9). It is essential to secure the stabilizer to the bar using #3 orthopedic wire/suture, which is placed in a figure-eight configuration. Otherwise, the stabilizer may slide right off the end of the bar.

If the stabilizer was placed on the patient's left side, several polydioxanone (PDS, Ethicon, Inc., Somerville, NJ) pericostal sutures are used to secure the bar to the underlying ribs on the right side. This is accomplished using the Endo-Close (Covidien, Mansfield, MA) device

under thoracoscopic visualization. In addition, several 0-Vicryl (Ethicon, Inc, Somerville, NJ) sutures are placed to secure the fascia of the lateral chest wall to the holes in the bar and stabilizer (Fig. 52-9). A needle, curved more than a semicircle, such as a UR-6 needle, greatly facilitates this suturing in a small working space.

The incisions are closed in layers with absorbable sutures to provide maximal soft tissue coverage over the bar and stabilizer, and the skin is approximated with subcuticular sutures. Once the incisions are closed, the thoracoscope is reinserted into the chest, and a thorough inspection is accomplished to ensure that there is no bleeding from the mediastinum, bar entry and exit sites, and the pericostal suture sites. The telescope is then withdrawn, the CO_2 insufflation tubing is cut, and the proximal end is placed in a basin of water to create a water seal. Positive end-expiratory pressure of 5 to 6 cm H_2O is administered through the endotracheal tube, the operating table is placed in Trendelenburg position, and the anesthesiologist re-inflates the lungs until no more air bubbles are escaping into the water. The lungs are held in full inflation when the port is withdrawn and the incision is closed. A chest radiograph is obtained on the operating table.

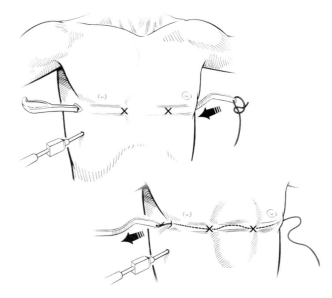

Figure 52-7. Umbilical tape is secured to the introducer, which has been exteriorized through the patient's left midaxillary incision. The introducer is then withdrawn, bringing the umbilical tape through the subcutaneous and substernal tunnel.

PEARLS AND PITFALLS

1. All patients are started on antibiotics at the beginning of surgery, they are continued until the patients are afebrile and show no signs of respiratory tract infection. Povidone-iodine solution is used for skin preparation and is also applied to the incisions before closure to minimize the risk of bar infection. This protocol has resulted in a bar infection rate of only 0.7% in more than 800 cases.

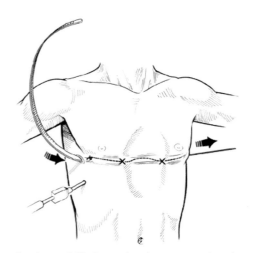

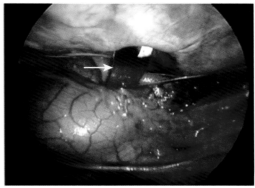

Figure 52-8.   Left, The umbilical tape has been secured to the pectus bar and is being advanced from the patient's right side through the subcutaneous and substernal tunnels and out through the left midaxillary incision. **Right,** The bar (*arrow*) is seen with the thoracoscope in the right chest and has been passed anterior to the heart. The tip of the umbilical tape is shown in this photograph as well.

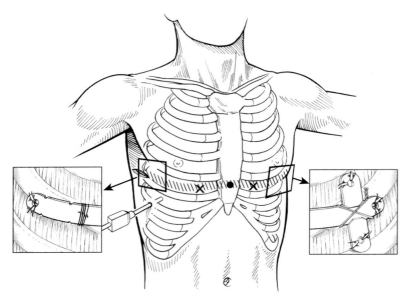

Figure 52-9.   After passing the bar, it is rotated so that its convexity faces anteriorly. The bar is stabilized to prevent displacement. Sutures (0-PDS) are placed around the bar and underlying ribs on the patient's right side. A stabilizer is wired to the bar on the left side. Both the bar and the stabilizer are sutured to the chest wall and fascia.

2. Evacuating the pneumothorax under a water seal system allows for complete evacuation of the pneumothorax. If there is an air leak, it becomes obvious because the pneumothorax does not evacuate completely, and a chest tube is then inserted at the time of surgery.

3. Bar fixation is absolutely essential at the time of surgery to prevent bar displacement. The bar and stabilizer need to be wired together—otherwise, the stabilizer will dislocate from the bar. Applying sutures around the bar and underlying rib on the right side, under thoracoscopic vision, minimizes the likelihood of bar displacement. The thoracoscope can be passed across the mediastinum to facilitate placement of sutures around the bar and underlying ribs on the left side as well.

4. Agitation during emergence from general anesthesia can result in bar displacement and should be avoided. The administration of morphine and midazolam in the operating room immediately before turning off the anesthesia is helpful for keeping the patient sedated while in the recovery room and emerging from the anesthesia.

5. Adequate pain control usually requires use of several drug classes. For example, epidural analgesia (fentanyl or bupivacaine), narcotics such as morphine, nonsteroidal anti-inflammatory drugs, sedatives such as diazepam, and muscle relaxants such as Robaxin may be used in varying combinations to allow the patients to participate with respiratory therapy and ambulation on the day after surgery.

6. Constipation is a predictable side effect of the narcotics and must be vigorously treated with daily laxatives starting on the morning after surgery.

Gastrointestinal hemorrhage might result from the nonsteroidal anti-inflammatory medication and necessitates histamine receptor blocking agents such as ranitidine.

7. Patients are discharged home with instructions to perform breath-holding exercises every morning and evening and to refrain from sporting activities for 6 weeks. After 6 to 8 weeks, the patients are encouraged to continue with their breath-holding exercises and to participate in aerobic sports. Patients are encouraged to participate in swimming, soccer, basketball, and other noncontact aerobic sports. Football is not allowed while the bar is in place.

SELECTED REFERENCES

1. Haller JA Jr., Kramer SS, Lietman SA: Use of CT scans in selection of patients for pectus excavatum surgery: A preliminary report. J Pediatr Surg 22:904-908, 1987
2. Nuss D, Kelly RE, Croitoru DP, et al: A 10-year review of a minimally invasive technique for the correction of pectus excavatum. J Pediatr Surg 33:545-552, 1998
3. Hebra A, Swoveland B, Egbert M, et al: Outcome analysis of minimally invasive repair of pectus excavatum: Review of 251 cases. J Pediatr Surg 35:252-258, 2000
4. Miller KA, Woods RK, Sharp RJ, et al: Minimally invasive repair of pectus excavatum: A single institution's experience. Surgery 130:652-659, 2001
5. Park HJ, Lee SY, Lee CS, et al: The Nuss procedure for pectus excavatum: Evolution of techniques and early results on 322 patients. Ann Thorac Surg 77:289-295, 2004
6. St. Peter SD, Weesner KA, Sharp RJ, et al: Is epidural anesthesia truly the best pain management strategy after minimally invasive pectus excavatum repair? J Pediatr Surg 43:79-82, 2008

Index

Page numbers followed by an *f* or *t* indicate figures and tables.